*No amount of word-making will ever make a
single soul to know these mountains.*

— *John Muir*

Your mountain is waiting.
So . . . get on your way!

— *Dr. Seuss*

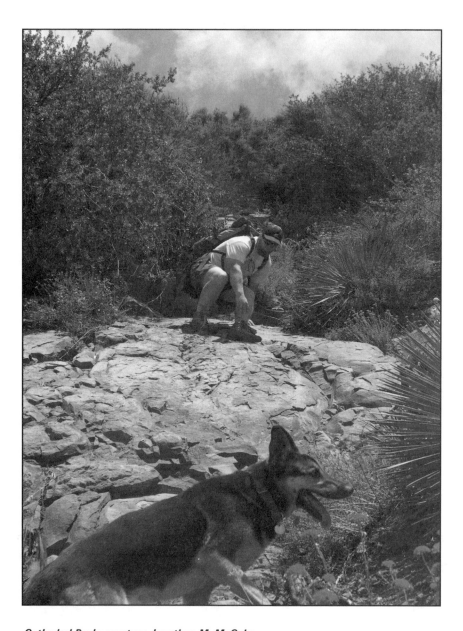

Cathedral Peak; courtesy Jonathan M. McCabe

SANTA BARBARA & VENTURA

A complete guide to the trails of the southern Los Padres National Forest

CRAIG R. CAREY

 WILDERNESS PRESS ... *on the trail since 1967*

Travel
_917.94_
CAR 2012

Hiking & Backpacking Santa Barbara & Ventura

1st EDITION, 1st printing

Copyright © 2012 by Craig R. Carey

Front and back cover photos: front cover upper right, courtesy Jonathan M. McCabe; all other cover
  photos by Craig R. Carey
Interior photos by Craig R. Carey unless otherwise noted
Maps: Craig R. Carey
Cover design: Scott McGrew
Book design: adapted by Annie Long
Book editors: Holly Cross and Amber Henderson

Library of Congress Cataloging-in-Publication Data
Carey, Craig R.
 Hiking & backpacking Santa Barbara and Ventura : a complete guide to the trails of
the southern Los Padres National Forest / Craig R. Carey.
    p. cm.
 Includes index.
 ISBN 978-0-89997-635-8
 ISBN 0-89997-635-2
 1. Hiking—California—Los Padres National Forest—Guidebooks.
 2. Backpacking—California—Los Padres National Forest—Guidebooks.
 3. Los Padres National Forest (Calif.)—Guidebooks. I. Title.
 GV199.42.C22L675 2012
 796.5209794—dc23
                          2012013018 <tel:2012013018>

Manufactured in the United States of America

Published by: **Wilderness Press**
                  Keen Communications
                  P.O. Box 43673
                  Birmingham, AL 35243
                  (800) 443-7227; FAX (205) 326-1012
                  info@wildernesspress.com
                  www.wildernesspress.com

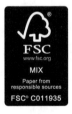 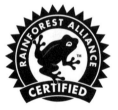

Visit our website for a complete listing of our books and for ordering information.

Distributed by Publishers Group West

SAFETY NOTICE: Although Wilderness Press and the author have made every attempt to ensure that the
information in this book is accurate at press time, they are not responsible for any loss, damage, injury, or
inconvenience that may occur to anyone while using this book. You are responsible for your own safety and
health while in the wilderness. The fact that a trail is described in this book does not mean that it will be
safe for you. Be aware that trail conditions can change from day to day. Always check local conditions and
know your own limitations.

ACKNOWLEDGMENTS

■ ■ ■ ■ ■ ■ ■ ■ ■ ■ ■ ■ ■

As with any project, many deserve credit, thanks, and/or a cold beer once the dust settles.

First are my folks—college sweethearts in the Bruins Mountaineering club—who one summer strapped a little Kelty frame pack to my 6-year-old shoulders, led me across a stretch of the Eldorado National Forest, and planted the seed. Billy Monster and Doug—who didn't have to haul their little brother along on all those multiweek treks or mountain bike trips but still did—in many ways laid the groundwork for this project with their enthusiasm, encouragement, and vetting.

Thanks to BeasT, JP-san, Maestro, Bo, DAW-G, Herr Wessen, Sas, M Aurelius, and most of all RSO Jonny for years of support, camaraderie, and an unflagging willingness to venture down those paths less traveled (even the ones we wish we hadn't, and there were a few); Clan Cook, always with a well-timed *craic* when it was needed most; Mr. Carney, who didn't need to take attendance (because we all wanted to be there); Messrs. G., G., S., Allen, and Dr. J., for the patience to lead a rowdy troop of Scouts and for somehow knowing when to let those rowdy Scouts lead; Roslyn Bullas for taking a chance on a new guy and guiding this project in its nascent stages; and Holly Cross for picking it up and seeing it through to the tome you now hold.

John Boggs (ret.), Kerry Kellogg (ret.), Heidi Anderson, Robert Cermak (ret.), Steve Galbraith, Warren Gibbs, and Rick Howell of the US Forest Service for intel and insight; Rick Bisaccia, Ojai Valley Land Conservancy preserve manager; Kevin Hyde at the USFS Rocky Mountain Research Station Forestry Sciences Lab; Russell Stevens and Evelyn Cuevas of the Ventura County Library (Saticoy Branch), for tending to a ridiculous amount of interlibrary logistics; Lara Otis at the University of Maryland Architecture Library, Christopher Winters at the University of Chicago Library, and Cynthia Moriconi of the University of California—Santa Cruz Library's Maps Unit for cartographic assistance above and beyond the call of duty; and Dave and the staff at the Full of Beans in Ojai and Ale and Tony at the Reyes Creek Bar & Grill for sustenance after a hard slog.

To gain the perspective necessary to draft this guide, I stood on the shoulders of giants (and their works/research). Among those giants are the late Dennis R. Gagnon, David L. Magney, Ray Ford, as well as a handful of others who directly contributed to various aspects of research—Bryan Conant and Mickey McTigue—and Robert A. Burtness, who was kind enough to lend me a great deal of material from his personal archives over the course of this project. Thanks also to Eldon M. Walker, PhD, LPE, SVP, for insight, commentary, and inspiration.

Thanks also go to the pack—for always taking point and remaining ever-vigilant—and to Li'l G and Jack, who allow me to view the wilderness and its gifts through fresh eyes and remind me to not see it as a project but rather as a refuge and a place full of wonder.

Lastly, thanks to K, who in the 2 years it took to write this book (and the 16 years previous) has always been my biggest supporter and source of encouragement, my work's toughest critic, and my rock.

This book is for Mom. And the butterflies.

C O N T E N T S

PART I SANTA BARBARA AND WESTERN MT. PINOS RANGER DISTRICTS

PART II EASTERN MT. PINOS AND OJAI RANGER DISTRICTS

CHAPTER one

Introduction to the Southern Los Padres

■ ■ ■ ■ ■ ■ ■ ■ ■ ■ ■ ■ ■

NAMED FOR THE SPANISH PADRES who established a network of missions along California's southern and central coasts, the Los Padres National Forest is the second-largest national forest in the state, encompassing approximately 1,950,000 acres.

In 1903, the General Land Office in California established the Santa Barbara Forest Reserve through the consolidation of the 1,644,594-acre Pine Mountain and Zaka Lake Forest Reserve and the much smaller 145,280-acre Santa Ynez Forest Reserve. After transfer to the stewardship of the US Forest Service (USFS) in 1905, the Santa Barbara Forest Reserve was proclaimed a national forest in 1907.

Forest Reserve boundary post, set in 1905

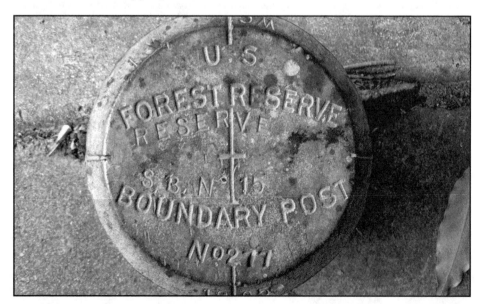

Subsequent absorption of the San Luis National Forest in 1910 and Monterey National Forest in 1919 made for a large stretch of land running more than 200 miles along the California coast. Renamed the Los Padres National Forest in 1936, these lands have been added to and reduced here and there over the years but have remained a welcome refuge for generations of area outdoors enthusiasts.

Nearly half of the Los Padres is now federally designated wilderness and stretches from Big Sur's rugged coast to Lake Piru near the edge of Los Angeles County. The southern section of the Los Padres—the focus of this guide, and comprising the Mt. Pinos, Ojai, and Santa Barbara Ranger Districts—features five such wildernesses (including part of the San Rafael, the first primitive area designated as wilderness after the 1964 Wilderness Act) in a diverse swath of forest, ranging from only a few hundred feet above sea level to nearly 9,000 feet in elevation. The forest contains countless natural and archaeological resources, numerous endangered species (among them the magnificent California condor), as well as the last major undammed river in Southern California, the Sespe.

But the Los Padres is also the only national forest with sizable natural gas and petroleum reserves, and drilling occurs on some 15,000 acres of the forest. This juxtaposition of preservation interests, land management, and industry has become one of many points of contention between conservationists, the U.S. Department of Agriculture (USDA), and those who've secured rights to extract such resources. Further, numerous access issues and their associated drama afflict various corners of the forest, leaving some historically accessible sites in a legal limbo and often restricting availability to the public.

Much of the Los Padres is dominated by chaparral, that fire-susceptible, non-deciduous blanket of shrub defined by the coastal areas' Mediterranean climate, the hillsides of which seem to erupt into wildfire every few years. Other landscapes are represented as well, of course: riparian sycamore- and alder-dotted ravines abound, lush pine forests dominate the higher elevations, the largest piñon forest in Southern California spreads out over the Cuyama badlands and the San Emigdio Mesa, and the Sespe drainage is home to some of the most impressive slot canyons and sandstone geology in the state.

Geography & Geology

MOST OF THE SOUTHERN LOS PADRES stretches across the western section of the Transverse Ranges, a section of the Coast Ranges considered unique due to its east-west orientation. Starting at Point Conception on the coast, the range—which includes the Santa Ynez, San Rafael, and Sierra Madre Ranges through Santa Barbara County and the Topatopa Mountains, Pine Mountain, and the Mt. Pinos area in Ventura County—extends into Los Angeles County, terminating among the high peaks of the San Bernardino and San Gabriel Mountains.

In very simplified geologic terms, the orientation and form of the range is the result of faulting along the San Andreas, with the Transverse caught between the forces of the Pacific and the North American Plates.

The mountains and all that come with them result in varied terrains ranging from a few hundred feet in elevation (the Santa Barbara frontcountry) to nearly 9,000 feet above sea level (the Mt. Pinos area, or San Emigdio Mountains), with terrain crossing sedimentary stone (e.g., the Santa Ynez Mountains) to granitic and metamorphic rock (e.g., the San Emigdio Mountains). And while there is no active volcanism in this stretch of Southern California, there are numerous hot springs through the forest (most of which are detailed herein).

Climate (And When to Go)

MOST OF THE SOUTHERN DISTRICTS fall within the Mediterranean climate and are characterized by cool, wet winters and hot, dry summers. Precipitation falls primarily between November and April, with annual totals averaging anywhere from 8 to 38 inches in the southern districts. In winter, high-elevation areas such as Pine Mountain, Mt. Pinos, Big Pine, Madulce Peak, and the Mission Pine Ridge are not practical for backpacking, as they remain under heavy snow until the spring. Further, the backcountry can be brutally hot in the summer, with most water sources bone-dry until the autumn rains. Plan accordingly, and call the local ranger station for conditions and updates.

Plant & Animal Communities
Flora
Plant Communities of the Southern Los Padres (with credit and thanks to the Los Padres National Forest Supervisor's Office)

The Los Padres is often touted as one of the most botanically diverse US national forests. The USDA identifies eight communities in this area, detailed on the next pages.

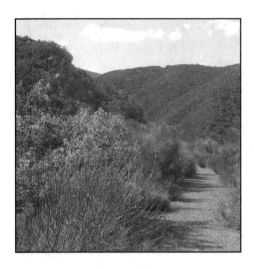

Chaparral

No plant community quite defines the Los Padres as does chaparral. Covering nearly two-thirds of this book's scope, this drought-adapted collection of plants dominates the frontcountry and is the ground cover visible to the majority of passersby driving through the forest along the highways or viewing the USFS lands from afar. Chaparral includes numerous varieties of manzanita, chamise, scrub oak, mountain mahogany, sugar bush, monkeyflower, toyon (also known as California holly), laurel sumac, buckwheat, and the true sages. Plants of this community feature moisture-conserving leaves and a large root system. Several of the plants also produce large amounts of terpenes and oils: this makes many of them aromatic but also extremely fire-prone.

Conifer Forests

Conifer forests occur in all districts of the Los Padres at high elevations—typically on cooler and wet north-facing slopes and canyon bottoms. This community consists of pure and mixed stands of Jeffrey pines, ponderosa pines, sugar pines, knobcone pines, Coulter pines, white firs, incense cedar, and bigcone Douglas-firs.

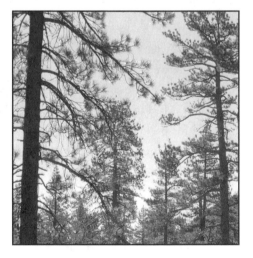

Camper's Note: While the sugar pine is known to produce the longest cones of any conifer, it's the cones of the Coulter (and the tree itself) of which you should be mindful when camping, especially in fire-scarred areas. Studies indicate Coulter pines demonstrate less drought tolerance than other conifers in Southern California, and when further weakened by air pollution, many Coulters have succumbed to bark beetle infestations. These compounded factors result in compromised trees quite susceptible to toppling in high winds, and their massively heavy and spiked cones can rain down on unsuspecting campers with little warning. They hurt, and tent walls are no match (trust us on this one).

Bigcone Douglas-firs, while related to the northern Douglas-firs, occur only in Southern California in a thin stretch ranging from San Diego to Santa Barbara. They are typically found in steep and fairly inaccessible north-facing drainages.

Grassland

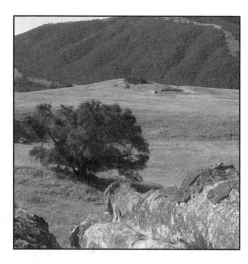

Native California grasses have been drastically supplanted by farmland and European annual grasses over the past few centuries. Botanists concede it has proven difficult to pinpoint when the peak of the invasion occurred, even noting foreign grasses mixed into the adobe bricks made during the Mission era. Remaining native species include needlegrass, melic grass, and wild rye. These can be found in some areas throughout the forest, along with annual species of wild oats, barley, and brome, which dominate the forest grassland.

Oak Woodland

Visitors to the forest will observe woodlands composed of pure and mixed stands of blue oaks (*Quercus douglasii*), black oaks (*Quercus kelloggii*), valley oaks, coast live

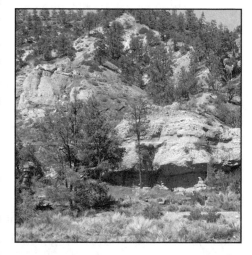

oaks, interior live oaks, and canyon live oaks. Oak acorns were once a major food source for Native Americans, and today numerous wild animals, including deer, squirrels, bears, and birds, consume acorns and rely upon the woodlands for shelter.

Piñon-Juniper Woodland

Piñon-juniper woodland occurs primarily in the Mt. Pinos Ranger District, and the district is in fact home to the largest piñon community in Southern

California. It thrives in the hostile badlands here, weathering snow and the brutally cold winters as well as the hottest summer temperatures in the forest. Piñon pines (specifically, single-leaf piñon, or *Pinus monophylla*) occupy the cooler north-facing slopes, and their seeds were once a staple for the Native American communities that occupied the region. Junipers tend to dominate the south-facing slopes. Other plants found in this woodland include Great Basin sagebrush, rabbitbrush, and scrub oak. Often depicted as a barren land, this community actually provides abundant food and shelter for many animal species: from the rare blunt-nosed leopard lizard to bighorn sheep. It also provides habitat for many rare plant species.

Riparian Woodland

Riparian woodland is one of the most productive and diverse plant communities in the forest. Dense stretches of willows, alders, cottonwoods, and sycamores are typically the few survivors of wildfires . . . saved by the very watercourses on which they depend.

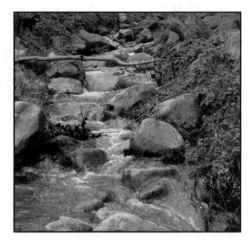

Serpentine Plants

Serpentine soils occur in scattered locations in the Santa Barbara Ranger District (as well as in the Monterey and Santa Lucia Districts to the north). Serpentine soils possess a high magnesium content and a low calcium content, a rare chemical composition most plant life finds intolerable. Of those plants that have adapted, several grow exclusively on these soils. Of the six botanical areas in all the Los Padres, three were established specifically to protect this unique plant community.

For those interested in learning more about the plant life of the southern Los Padres, the University of California Press's *Introduction to the Plant Life of Southern California (Coast to Foothills)* is an excellent place to start. The guide is part of the California Natural History Guide series, which also includes volumes detailing desert and mountain wildflowers, native trees, and other topics of interest and relevance to the forest.

Subalpine Fell-Fields

This community occurs at elevations above 8,000 feet in the Mt. Pinos Ranger District. Fell-fields are characterized by undulating flats and scree slopes covered with highly porous soil, rock, and/or gravel. These terrain features are shaped by cold winter winds and snow, both of which limit the majority of plant life to small, ground-hugging perennials. In summer, small flowers bloom in abundance and attract prolific pollinators. Limber pines can also be found in this community. The Mt. Pinos Ranger District offers a "Plants of the Mt. Pinos Summit" leaflet detailing ferns, conifers, and flowering plants above the 8,500-foot contour atop Mt. Pinos. The leaflet can also be downloaded in PDF format from the Internet.

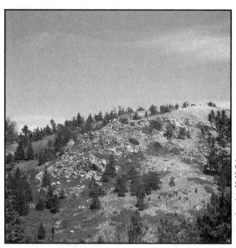

courtesy Jonathan M. McCabe

Lions, (no) Tigers, and Bears . . . Oh My!

THERE ARE SOME LARGE ANIMALS in the forest, some larger (or more dangerous) than you. In the southern Los Padres, these include black bears and mountain lions (also known as pumas or cougars).

The last California grizzly was killed in 1922, but the black bears of the Los Padres are still a presence and should be a consideration when planning trips into the wilderness. Black bears are nowhere near the nuisance as the conditioned bears of Yosemite and other national parks nor as dangerous as the grizzlies in the higher latitudes of North America. The American black bear is a nonconfrontational, almost shy opportunist—if he (or she) can secure an easy meal from your nonsecured cache of food, it will so long as there's no danger involved. Bear canisters may be overkill, but at a minimum food and other "smellables" should be hung overnight or when otherwise unattended, and all the usual rules apply—eat those sardines around the campfire rather than in your sleeping bag. Bears will seek to avoid you, so don't give them a reason to visit (e.g., don't leave that freeze-dried blueberry surprise unattended next to the fire overnight).

If you encounter a bear, more often than not the bear will retreat—they have little interest in humans and their racket. Make yourself heard and back away slowly. Don't run (you can't outrun a bear) and don't climb a tree (he can climb it better than you). Don't make threatening gestures or display threatening behavior.

Scat, prints, and claw-raked trees are common sights in the Los Padres backcountry. But given that hunting and dogs (both of which bears typically view as negatives) are allowed in our national forests, sightings are uncommon and instances of bears stealing food are rare. Attacks or other negative accounts are almost unheard of. Let's keep it that way.

Mountain lions are predators, most often seen at dusk and dawn. Sightings are uncommon and attacks incredibly rare. If you encounter a cougar, stand still, control any dogs, and pick up your children. Present yourself as large as you can. Do not run. If attacked, fight back with everything you have.

Endangered Species

WHILE NOT KNOWN FOR ITS PRODIGIOUS big game wildlife, the southern Los Padres has a unique wildlife population and is ground zero for several preservation programs.

Among the fauna are steelhead trout, California condors, California red-legged frogs, arroyo toads, western pond turtles, and two-striped garter snakes. In terms of restricting access, the California condor of course takes the most precedent, having two sanctuaries within the forest dedicated to its preservation (see below). Over the past few decades, the arroyo toad has also been cited as the reason for several campground and road closures, including Lion Campground (now Piedra Blanca Trailhead) and Blue Point, Hardluck, and Juncal Campgrounds and the roads leading to them, to name but a few.

As disappointing as the loss of some great recreation spots may be, please respect the efforts of the USFS and other agencies working to preserve these endangered species.

Condors

THE CALIFORNIA CONDOR (*Gymnogyps californianus*) is a massive scavenger with a 9-foot wingspan, and one of the greatest symbols of modern conservation efforts in the western United States.

As recently as the 1800s, the condor ranged from what is now southern British Columbia to present-day Baja California, and it is thought to have roamed over much of North America during the Pleistocene era. But as early as the 1850s, the decline of the condor population was being noted, and over the next century that decline only accelerated. The population dwindled to 22 by 1982, and the U.S. Fish & Wildlife Service (USFWS) spearheaded the rather controversial step of capturing the remaining condors for captive breeding. The last wild condor was captured in 1987. Progress has been sometimes slow and there have been setbacks, but the intensive captive breeding efforts—bolstered by public education programs—have seen a steady increase in both the captive and wild condor population. As of 2011, the population hovers near 400 (approximately half of which live in the wild).

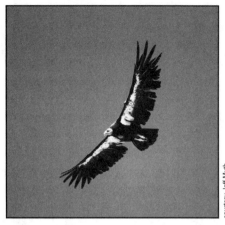

Numerous factors contributed to the condor's precipitous fall toward extinction, chief among them poisoning (lead, cyanide, and others), shortage of food, habitat loss, DDT, shootings, and nest disturbance. One particularly infamous death in recent years was that of condor 358 in July 2009, who died after getting tangled in some rope left by climbers or hikers in the Tar Creek area, a popular—but legally forbidden—Los Padres climbing spot within the Sespe Condor Sanctuary.

Abandoned webbing, rope, and straps can prove especially deadly to these giant birds, and it is imperative that users of such items *pack it out*. As condors are curious creatures, they are also attracted to shiny objects, including aluminum can pop-tops, litter, glass, and other small items of refuse which they sometimes ingest. These items cause horrific damage to the bird's digestive tract and can result in an agonizing death for the threatened bird. In this vein, volunteer groups have participated in several microtrash clean-up events, from Cuyama Peak to Tar Creek. Help these birds on their route to recovery by packing out all trash, and consider taking the extra step of carrying out more than your own.

Condors are distinguishable not only by their great size and bald, vulturelike heads, but also by the white or mottled lining on the underside of their massive wings. Further, if one is close enough, the condors' numbered wing tags are easily discernible.

Two sanctuaries in the forest—the 1,200-acre Sisquoc Condor Sanctuary in the San Rafael Wilderness (Santa Lucia Ranger District) and the massive 53,000-acre Sespe Condor Sanctuary (primarily in the Sespe Wilderness, Ojai Ranger District)—provide vast expanses of rugged terrain in which the condors can roost and live without interference from humans. Unauthorized human entry into either sanctuary is prohibited. Bitter Creek and Hopper Mountain National Wildlife Refuges adjacent to USFS lands (managed by the USFWS) provide additional grounds for the condor.

Nature-goers are reminded that all large dark birds are protected by law. If you witness anybody harassing or otherwise distressing or attempting to harm a condor, you are encouraged to contact any of the following agencies:

U.S. Fish & Wildlife Service: (805) 644-5185

Los Padres National Forest (Supervisor's Office): (805) 968-6640

California State Police: (213) 620-4700 (24-hour number)

Highly recommended is Noel Snyder and Helen Snyder's *Introduction to the California Condor* (University of California Press).

CANNABIS COUNTRY ▪ ▪ ▪ ▪ ▪ ▪ ▪ ▪ ▪ ▪ ▪ ▪

No matter your position or politics, the illegal marijuana harvest in the Los Padres backcountry presents a tenuous situation for both law enforcement and those who recreate in the national forest. It presents a genuine danger in some areas, one of which backpackers and cross-country trekkers especially need to be cognizant.

While Humboldt County and other more-traditional environs are well known for their cultivation of cannabis, the Ventura and Santa Barbara County backcountries have become a prime location for Mexican cartels looking to grow the product locally but with (relatively) low overhead and limited accountability if the product is discovered by law enforcement. Growing marijuana on secluded public property with all the necessary conditions fulfills those requirements . . . in the form of huge tracts of the southern Los Padres.

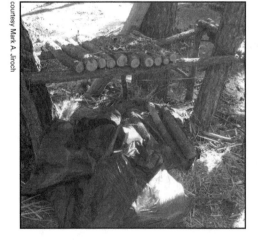

courtesy Mark A. Jiroch

Shrewd drug traffickers and those in their employ typically aren't so foolish as to establish their pot groves within easy access of the masses; therefore, such groves are not within immediate reach of the many trails the USFS has cut and maintains through the forest. These secret gardens are in seldom-traveled stretches of the wilderness, but where water is available or can be easily diverted. When off-trail, one of the first signs you are nearing a pot field is litter.

Growers often establish makeshift campsites at many of the grow sites; most of these sites and the guerrilla trails leading in and around them are often beset with trash and debris, irrigation pipe, camping equipment, and chemicals used to fertilize the plants (or empty containers therefrom).

The preparation of sites for cannabis growing causes significant damage to the environment (stream diversion, the cutting and removal of various trees and brush, as well as aggressive and disruptive landscape terracing), practices lamented by local forest officials and environmental concerns throughout the region.

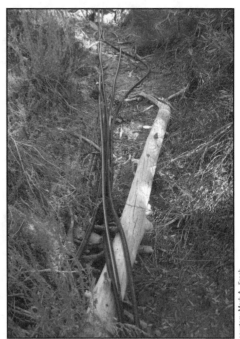

courtesy Mark A. Jiroch

Every year the USFS—in conjunction with the Drug Enforcement Administration and local authorities' air and narcotics units—identify, remove, and ultimately destroy thousands of pounds of marijuana sourced from the remote grow sites of the Los Padres. Law enforcement agencies urge hikers who inadvertently come across such sites to exercise caution. Leave the area immediately (and certainly don't help yourself to any samples, no matter how tempting!).

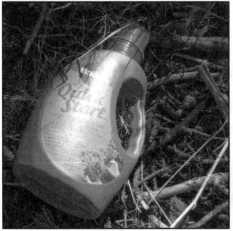

courtesy Mark A. Jiroch

When back in communications range, hikers are asked to notify the sheriff as to the location.

Ventura County Sheriff's Department
vcsd.org; (805) 654-9511

Santa Barbara County Sheriff's Department
sbsheriff.org; (805) 681-4150

LOOKOUT! ▨ ▨ ▨ ▨ ▨ ▨ ▨ ▨ ▨ ▨ ▨ ▨ ▨ ▨ ▨

Lookout Towers in the Forest

The primary purpose of a lookout tower is to provide the occupant (the actual lookout) a vantage point from which to spot fires and/or lightning strikes so that they may be reported in time to prevent widespread destruction. Though fire lookouts have been utilized since man has walked this earth, the modern concept of the fire lookout has been impressed upon the general American public by way of the US Forest Service (USFS) and its stoic lookout man.

The vast majority of lookouts in California (and thereby the Los Padres) consisted of the live-in 14-by-14-foot duBois design cabs conceived by New York–born forester Coert duBois in 1917 (one very notable exception being the La Cumbre Peak lookout; see *Route 18*). After the formation of the Civilian Conservation Corps (CCC), one of the CCC's tasks in addition to all the other work done in the forest (trails, roads, bridges, etc.) was the construction of fire lookout towers. From the CCC's inception into the second year of World War II, the Corps built approximately 250 towers in 10 years.

The lookouts were also used for aircraft spotting during the war by the Aircraft Warning Service (see the Thorn Point entry for one of the few remaining AWS cabins).

Over the last century, the number of lookouts in the southern Los Padres has diminished from several dozen to but a handful. Notable losses range from the Reyes Peak lookout burned in September 1932 during the infamous Matilija Fire to the Topatopa Peak lookout, consumed in the 2006 Day Fire. The Nordhoff Peak tower—visible from downtown Ojai—was lost in the 1948 Wheeler Springs Fire, rebuilt, and then dismantled in the 1970s. Only the metal frame remains today.

Numerous lookout towers were dismantled by the USFS to accommodate radio and radar facilities (Santa Ynez and McPherson Peaks) or removed due to general disrepair and/or vandalism (West Big Pine).

McPherson Peak Lookout, 1984

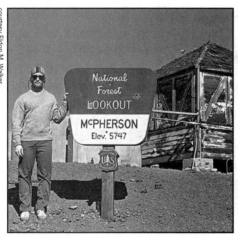

courtesy Eldon M. Walker

Last of their Kind

Following is a brief rundown of the remaining fire lookouts in the southern Los Padres National Forest.

CUYAMA PEAK (5,880')

The Cuyama Peak lookout was erected in 1934, but—like the few lookouts still standing in the southern Los Padres—fell into disuse in the 1960s. Utilized by the AWS during WWII, the site's cabin still (barely) stands, and is one of very few remaining in California. The modified L-4 cab typically remains open, and both it and the platform on which it stands still remain ideal vantage points for bird-watchers. Condors can on occasion be spied from here. While the tower is vehicle-accessible via Dry Canyon, the road is not advised for passenger cars.

FRAZIER MOUNTAIN (8,013')

Named for William T. Frazier, an 1850s miner in the area, this dilapidated tower is now dwarfed by neighboring communication towers. Built in 1934, the current lookout replaced an earlier structure from the 1910s.

The tower is accessible via Frazier Mountain Road, heading up the mountain from near the Chuchupate Ranger Station. The road, which turns to dirt after Chuchupate Campground, is typically open April–November and is passable via passenger car, but something with a bit more clearance is recommended.

LA CUMBRE PEAK (3,993')

A one-off design constructed in 1945, the current La Cumbre Peak lookout stands upon a 20-foot tower. Its staircase has been removed to prevent access. Its immediate surroundings are dominated by broadcast arrays, but the USFS does maintain a picnic area here, and there is a restroom. See *Route 18*.

Frazier Mountain Lookout

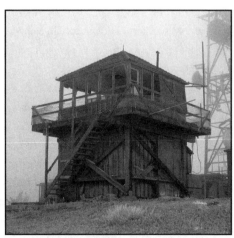

SLIDE MOUNTAIN (4,631')

An anomaly among the remaining towers, Slide Mountain lookout is the new kid on the block, built in 1969 in conjunction with the creation of the Pyramid Lake reservoir. It stands in a stretch of the Los Padres administered by the Angeles National Forest (Santa Clara/Mojave Rivers Ranger District), and the tower is maintained and occasionally staffed by volunteers of the Angeles National Forest Fire Lookout Association. See *Route 96*.

THORN POINT (6,935')

The Thorn Point lookout dates from 1933. The 14-by-14-foot L-4 cab on a 20-foot H-braced tower is in poor condition as of this writing, with some of its furniture and cabinetry intact, but certain elements (e.g., the telephone) long removed. During WWII it was staffed 24 hours a day, and a ground cabin was added for the off-duty observer during 12-hour shifts. Now within the Sespe Wilderness, the lookout has also been used as a condor monitoring station given its proximity to the Sespe Condor Sanctuary. See *Route 80.*

THE CLOSING DOWN OF SUMMER ■ ■ ■ ■ ■ ■ ■ ■ ■ ■ ■ ■

Even with flood, fire, and the inevitable human manipulation, the forest and its topography remain largely static. The same cannot be said for its numerous trails and camps. Over several decades some trails have been rerouted (or closed altogether) only to be again rerouted (or reopened), and numerous camps have come and gone over the years. Many sites formerly accessible by passenger car or 4WD are now limited to foot traffic.

Camps and trails are closed for numerous reasons. Some closings are in response to legislation or administrative changes intended to protect the various endangered species native to the forest; see "Endangered Species" on page 8 for the most recent changes in access. Others are for lack of use (or overuse) or a combination of factors. Sites such as Cow Springs (closed to vehicles in 1973 due to recurring vandalism and its proximity to the Sespe Condor Sanctuary) and Mine Camp (closed to vehicles in the 1970s) have had their access limited but are still very much in use and still retain some of the amenities they offered when accessible by vehicle.

Newer sites, such as the Valley View trail camp along the Pratt Trail (see *Route 56*), have been built in response to increased use (in Valley View's case, after the 1985 Wheeler Fire).

The largest contraction of forest services since WWII occurred at Los Padres in 1974, when numerous campsites (primarily trail camps) in the southern Los Padres were closed as a result of federal spending cuts prompted by the fiscal crisis of the time. Some are now nothing more than historical footnotes; others continue to be heavily used without USFS maintenance. The trip entries in this guide address relevant abandoned or historical sites in the trip descriptions.

Looking Forward
Condor Trail

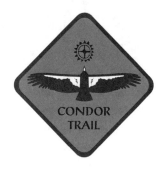

AN AMBITIOUS PROJECT conceived by local hikers, backpackers, and backcountry advocates, the Condor Trail is a projected 400-mile through-route traversing the Los Padres National Forest from Botchers Gap (Monterey Ranger District) in the north to Lake Piru (Ojai Ranger District) in the south, crossing through nearly every terrain the Los Padres has to offer. For more information, visit **condortrail.org.**

Into the Woods: Hazards

IN ADDITION TO BEARS AND MOUNTAIN LIONS (see page 7), there are a few other (admittedly smaller) hazards of which you should be aware.

Rattlesnakes

THESE SHY BUT VENOMOUS PIT VIPERS are on that flag for a reason: don't tread on them. Lethargic at night and in the cold, rattlesnakes can be found sunning themselves across stretches of trail in the morning and hunkered down in a coil under the shade of a bush or a tree during the heat of the day. Their buzz/rattle is unmistakable. Watch where you step (especially in grassy areas) and watch where you put your hands if bushwhacking, climbing, or otherwise scrambling off-trail. If struck, stay calm and seek medical attention immediately. Snakebite kits are overrated and typically do more damage than good.

Poison Oak—"Leaves of Three, Let them Be"

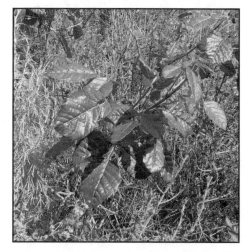

POISON OAK (*Toxicodendron diversilobum*) is easily identified by its shiny leaves in clusters of three and its small white berries. The leaves, which range from green to red depending on the season, contain the oil urushiol, which causes an allergic reaction with most humans. The severity of the reaction varies, but it typically entails an inflammation of the skin (with a maddening itch!) and blisters. During winter the shrub can lose its leaves, making avoiding it more difficult (the bare branches also carry the oil).

Another plant of concern is poodle-dog bush (*Turricula parryi*), a fire-follower that can cause contact dermatitis. The effect is similar to that of stinging nettle; however, the rash and duration of poodle-dog bush inflammation typically last much longer (often for at least a week). It can be identified by its rather skunky smell, an

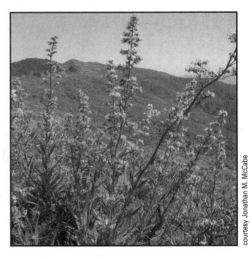

courtesy Jonathan M. McCabe

Poodle-dog bush (Turricula parryi)

appearance somewhat reminiscent of cannabis, and its telltale purple flowers.

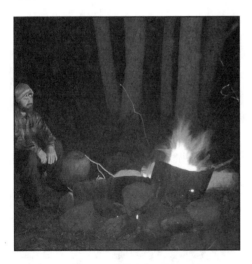

Permits
Fire Permits

EVER-SUSCEPTIBLE TO FIRE, the Los Padres National Forest is subject to fire restrictions every year, and regulations governing campfires change with weather and season. There are times in the summer when all fires are forbidden.

Even when fire restrictions are not in effect, visitors are required to carry a California Campfire Permit to use a stove or lantern outside any developed recreation area or campfire use site (i.e., established car campgrounds and day-use areas). This means any backcountry hikers and campers will need a permit (they're free). Fortunately, the USFS offers a downloadable, self-validating California Campfire Permit that can be retrieved from their website. The permit is valid until the end of the calendar year and may be used in any national forest in California. You may also apply for a permit in person at any USFS, CALFIRE, or BLM office during regular business hours.

Neither tracer ammunition nor fireworks are permitted in the forest at any time.

You are encouraged to contact your local USFS office for updates with regard to restrictions.

The Adventure Pass

IN 1997, THE NATIONAL FORESTS in Southern California (Los Padres, Angeles, Cleveland, and San Bernardino) instituted the Adventure Pass program, a pilot recreation fee program that required visitors to purchase a pass and display it on any vehicles parked alongside roads or at trailheads within the four forests, ostensibly to augment funding for trash collection, maintenance, improvements, and the like.

The subsequent uproar and backlash over the Adventure Pass fee program resulted in a better-defined and smaller area in which the pass would be required; now only high-impact recreation areas, 4WD routes requiring permits, and some campgrounds require the pass (in the case of many campgrounds, the pass is required in lieu of a camp fee).

Adventure Passes cost $5 for a day pass and $30 for an annual pass and are available at many outdoor retailers. Further, bear in mind that if you hold a federal Interagency Pass (or one of the equivalents, e.g., Senior, Lifetime Access, or Volunteer Passes), it will suffice in place of an Adventure Pass.

Trail Etiquette

COMMON COURTESY GOES A LONG WAY.

Sharing the trail with other hikers can be approached like driving in American traffic: stay to the right and pass on the left. If you're stopping to enjoy the view, do so in a way that does not impede traffic. Hikers heading uphill receive right-of-way. While there are vast sections of the southern Los Padres where you're not likely to see many other hikers, there are some stretches—especially the Santa Barbara and Montecito frontcountry and the Santa Ynez Recreation Area—where you'll often be sharing it with dozens of other users.

Love them, hate them, or be indifferent, but mountain bikers, equestrians, and dog owners have access to much of the Los Padres trail network. Everybody yields to horses, and mountain bikers are to yield to everybody. That puts hikers in the middle. Give right-of-way to horses. You *should* be granted right-of-way by mountain bikers, but for your own safety, don't assume it has been given until you're certain.

HIKING   WITH   DOGS ▪ ▪ ▪ ▪ ▪ ▪ ▪ ▪ ▪ ▪

Dogs are great hiking companions and often enjoy venturing into the wilderness as much as—or perhaps even more than—their biped cohorts. They are a good friend in any weather, find great joy in the simplest pleasures, have no compunctions following us through questionable terrain, and are more loyal to us than we deserve. Further, of all the federal lands, those managed by the USFS typically offer some of the greatest accessibility and provide opportunities for hiking with dogs second only to the BLM. It's a great place for dogs!

But it's the responsibility of the humans to not allow their dogs to be a nuisance to others or to be a detriment to the forest and its wild denizens. I hike with at least one dog nearly 90% of the time, but I am also consistently disappointed not by the conduct of other dogs I meet on the trail, but rather the conduct of their human companions.

Know the Rules

Every agency—from California State Parks to the National Park Service—has specific rules and conditions with regard to dogs. Know them and abide by them. Also bear in mind that simply because your dog is allowed within the

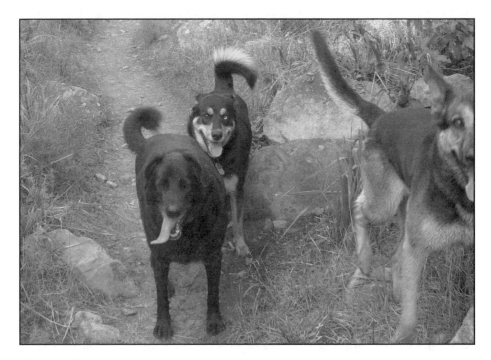

Semper volens

boundaries of a given area, that does not give him or her free roam (e.g., dogs are usually allowed within national parks but seldom on trails or even dirt roads, and almost never in creeks, lakes, and so on . . . and that's not much fun for an active pooch). Check with your local office to learn the specifics.

Control Your Dog

If your dog doesn't obey, don't bring him. Don't allow your dog to jump on others, chase other dogs, or act up. A dog that is not under voice control should be leashed or—better yet—left at home. Aggressive dogs (leashed or not) have no place in the forest.

Clean Up After Your Dog

Simply grabbing a poop bag at the trailhead and collecting your dog's waste isn't enough, especially if you collect it and then leave the plastic bag alongside the trail. Be considerate of others and the environment: *pack it out.* If odor is a concern, carry a few heavy-duty quart-size zip-top freezer bags with you to carry the pick-up bag. If that doesn't sit well with you, Rover shouldn't be on the trail.

That said, if your pooch is hearty enough to join you on a multiday trek through the wilderness and you're far removed from civilization, it is acceptable to treat the waste as you would treat your own. Dig a cathole (if Rover will pardon the expression) at least 8 inches deep and bury your dog's waste at least 200 feet from water and 50 feet from the trail or camps.

Finally, two key things to remember when you bring your canine companion into the forest: first, you and your dog(s) are ambassadors for others who would bring their dog to the wild; and second, do not expect everyone to love your dog as much as you do.

■   ■   ■   ■   ■   ■   ■   ■   ■   ■   ■   ■   ■   ■   ■

Leaving No Trace (Boiled-Down Edition)

THIS IS THE PART OF THE BOOK dealing with outdoors etiquette—specifically, your treatment of the actual outdoors. It's quite simple, so little word count will be spent here.

If you're holding this book, you presumably have some interest in the outdoors. Plain common sense tells us to not cut switchbacks, to clean up after our dogs, to not deface trees, to not scrawl on rocks, and to not leave litter. Don't justify an exception; just don't do it. You're not being cool going against the grain—nor being an independent thinker, nor a free spirit—you're part of the problem. Don't be lazy, and do the right thing.

If you can't abide these basic principles, stay home. For more information, visit **lnt.org.**

Maps and Navigation

FOR DECADES, THE BEST MAPS for backcountry navigation were the 15- and 7.5-minute topographic quadrangles published by the U.S. Geological Survey (USGS). Eventually the 15-minute quads were phased out and the 7.5-minute maps were the gold standard. But demand changes, technology improves (and the focus of various public agencies' efforts shifts), and suddenly those who swore by the "old reliables" find themselves with maps that have not been updated for some time. Before the recent USGS update, a number of private efforts have provided some very useful maps (see below).

After years without updates, the 1991 series of USGS quads were published, but they often included only the most popular or heavily traveled trails and excluded most trail camps, making them barely more useful than the Army Corps–derived quads of the 40s and 50s.

For 1993's USGS-USDA Forest Service Single-Edition Quadrangle maps update (wherein the two agencies embarked on a single-edition joint mapping program), the USFS provided many of the updates for lands within its jurisdiction. The majority of the Los Padres–area maps were released in 1995, and ironically enough, maps of this edition are notable for their chronic misplacement of campsites: for every trail camp corrected from previous editions (e.g., Shady Camp on the Devils Heart Peak quad), there seem to be two or three added that have been plotted incorrectly (e.g., Bear Creek and Oak Flat on the Topatopa Mountains quad).

Yet despite the chronic misplacements that almost make the 1995 Single-Editions a liability to users on the ground, what that series did provide—perhaps unknowingly—was very detailed insight into legacy and use trails the USFS had recorded or plotted over the years, because now not only did the 7.5-minute quads have nearly every campsite and designated trail, but the maps were crisscrossed by a veritable spiderweb of one-offs, routes that led nowhere, and spur trails into remote regions most hikers might otherwise never have considered. A handful of those historical or legacy routes have been addressed herein.

The launch in 2001 of the USGS's *National Map* and now the 2009–2011 rollout of the US Topo maps ("next-generation" 7.5-minute digital quads based on *The National Map*) finally bring the legacy maps of the USGS into the 21st century after what seems like a very long interval. These new maps, laid out to the same dimensions as the more traditional paper maps, are constructed with multiple layers of geographic data (e.g., topographic contours, hydrographic features, and USDA orthoimagery), which the user can toggle on/off at his or her discretion. Users can also select the reference systems (latitude/longitude, UTM, or MGRS) of their choice, and the maps include interactive capabilities with Google Maps, along with numerous other features. The maps are intended to be updated regularly based on changes to the data contained within *The National Map*.

Preliminary versions of the US Topo maps, referred to as Digital Maps–Beta, do not include contours and hydrographic features. The beta maps have been made available at the **usgs.gov** site and will be replaced by US Topo maps when they are fully revised.

There are also a handful of options to complement the USGS map resources.

The mainstay of Sespe-area hikers is the tried and trusted *Sespe Wilderness Trail Map* by Tom Harrison Maps (**tomharrisonmaps.com**). Last updated in 2012, the Harrison Map, as it is more often known, is printed on waterproof and tear-resistant plastic. Harrison's maps are well regarded throughout the state, and other editions cover dozens of other regions in California (most notably Sierra Nevada destinations and the Angeles National Forest). The large maps at several of the new wilderness trailheads throughout the Ojai district are custom maps rendered by Harrison specifically for the USFS.

Relative newcomers to the southern Los Padres map shelves are those designed and published by Bryan Conant (**bryanconant.com**). A local backpacker and cartographer, Conant has over the past decade produced two fine maps, one detailing the Matilija and Dick Smith Wildernesses (last updated in 2008) and another detailing the San Rafael Wilderness (last updated in 2009). These maps are a welcome addition to the local hiker's library, as they fill a much-lamented gap in local cartographic coverage. An added feature of Conant's maps is the inclusion of fire perimeters. Given the Santa Barbara backcountry's high incidence of major fires in the past decade, this additional layer of information is extremely useful in plotting and planning trips.

The BLM also produces a series of 1:100,000 cadastral survey maps that—while not necessarily practical for on-trail use—can prove useful in general planning and in gaining some perspective as to drive times for long shuttles and net elevation gains over the course of longer treks. They're known officially as the BLM Surface (or Mineral) Management Maps, and their small scale means that three of the quads—Santa Barbara, Cuyama, and Lancaster—cover nearly all the area of this guide's content, with a miniscule portion of the very southeastern portion spilling onto the Los Angeles quad.

Now, armed with all these navigational resources, one must bear in mind that maps (and GPS receivers, compasses, etc.) are of course only as good as the user's ability to use such tools and the ability to navigate when any (or all) prove incorrect, unreliable, go missing, or simply run out of batteries.

GPS Receivers

WITH THE TERMINATION of Selective Availability in 2000, the Global Positioning System's network of 24–32 satellites now enables civilian users to pinpoint their location within 20 meters. But as great as this has proven for wilderness navigation, 20 meters can still prove a massive margin of error when you're pushing through unrelenting brush 10 feet high, in the rain, at night, and with your headlamp failing. Overreliance on the electronic gadgets that technology has given us continues to be a problem for backcountry travelers, as well as those who are called in to perform the rescue when a given hiker ventures beyond his or her scope of competence and/or capability. Do not rely overly on these devices and stay within your ability levels.

HISTORIC SITES IN THE FOREST ■ ■ ■ ■ ■ ■ ■ ■ ■ ■

The lands that now fall within the boundaries of the southern Los Padres were once the home of numerous indigenous Americans, chiefly the various bands of the Chumash. With very few exceptions, this guide neither discusses nor divulges the locations of any Chumash sites, be they middens, mortars, or rock art (petroglyphs/pictographs).

The very basic tenets of the Leave No Trace principles should govern how you treat any Native American site you encounter—whether in the Los Padres or elsewhere, and whether by accident or intentionally. Don't take anything, don't touch anything, don't disturb anything, and certainly don't deface or alter anything. To drive home the point a bit further, know that the American Antiquities Act of 1906 protects any and all artifacts, with the exception of shards or arrowheads washed out along a trail. Leave them be. If areas are cordoned off, respect those boundaries—you needn't be the exception to any rule, and your wilderness experience won't be lessened because attempts at preservation aren't in line with your desire to visit a specific site.

Contact the forest archaeologist or your local ranger station if you believe you've discovered a "new" site, and do not disturb or remove any items.

■ ■ ■ ■ ■ ■ ■ ■ ■ ■ ■ ■ ■ ■ **GETTING IN TOUCH**

Santa Barbara Ranger District
3505 Paradise Rd.
Santa Barbara, CA 93105
(805) 967-3481

Ojai Ranger District
1190 East Ojai Ave.
Ojai, CA 93023
(805) 646-4348

Mt. Pinos Ranger District
34580 Lockwood Valley Rd.
Frazier Park, CA 93225
(661) 245-3731

■ ■

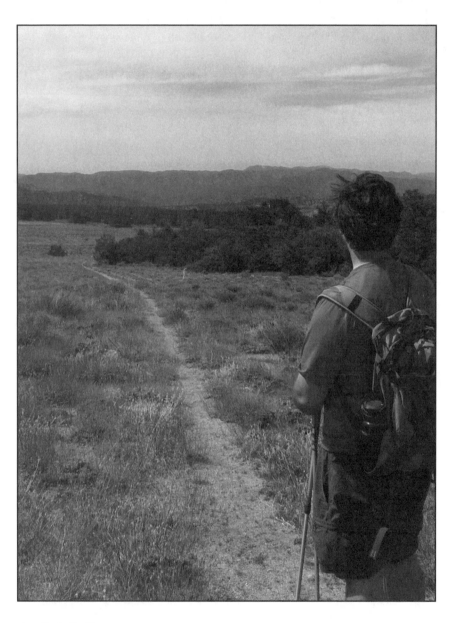

San Emigdio Mesa

CHAPTER two

About This Guide

IN THIS BOOK, trips in the southern Los Padres National Forest are described in two parts:

Part I details the Santa Barbara Ranger District and the western Mt. Pinos Ranger District (including the Santa Barbara frontcountry, the Upper and Lower Santa Ynez Recreation Areas, the Little Pine Mountain area, Carpinteria, Lake Casitas, the western Santa Ynez Mountains, the southern stretch of San Rafael Wilderness, and the Dick Smith Wilderness).

Part II details the eastern Mt. Pinos and Ojai Ranger Districts (including the Ojai frontcountry; the Sespe, Matilija, and Chumash Wildernesses; Pine Mountain; Lockwood Valley and Mt. Pinos; and Rose and Cuyama Valleys).

Each part is divided into chapters detailing routes numbered from west to east and accompanied by detailed maps. Each trip entry also includes a detailed route summary and instructions, along with waypoints and side trips as relevant. The routes detail trails ranging from easy, family-friendly day hikes of less than 1 mile to strenuous, multiday backpacking treks of 20 miles or more, and everything in between.

This guide doesn't cover *every* trail within the subject three ranger districts, but it does cover a vast majority of them. Rather than confine the reader to a prescribed itinerary, nearly all the entries are descriptions of the trail from point A to point B, allowing the reader the freedom to choose his or her target mileage and/or destination. Use the entries—paired with the accompanying maps—to devise your own trip as you see fit (e.g., rather than simply following the upper Cold Spring Trail to Forbush Flat and back, you can devise a route combining Routes 24, 11, 10, and 20 for a challenging near-circuit along which you'll witness numerous geologic features and plant communities).

Forest-Speak

A SHORT GLOSSARY OF RELEVANT TERMS

CAMPSITE: For the purpose of this book, campsites are defined as trail sites with few or no amenities. There is no car access. Water, when available, must be purified.

CAMPGROUND: These are camping areas to which one can drive. Some campgrounds are detailed in this guide only in that they may serve as a trailhead or provide a base from which to launch backcountry explorations.

SYSTEM TRAILS: Routes officially maintained and recognized by the US Forest Service (USFS), usually with a trail designation (see "Forest Road- and Trail-Naming Conventions" on page 28). These are the opposite of non-system trails.

NON-SYSTEM TRAILS: Unofficial use or "guerrilla" trails not maintained by the USFS but kept in use (and possibly even maintained) by historical traffic. The Cathedral Peak trail (*Route 19*) in the Santa Barbara Ranger District is one example.

Anatomy of a Trail Entry
Summary

EACH TRAIL ENTRY BEGINS with a summary index. These indexes include:

ROUTE NUMBER: As determined (roughly) by its west-to-east order within its group.

ROUTE TITLE: The common route name and—if applicable—its USFS trail designation (see page 28 for a brief summary of trail-naming conventions).

LENGTH AND TYPE: The route length and whether it's presented as a loop, out-and-back, one-way trip, and so on.

DIFFICULTY: The physical exertion demanded by the trip: easy, moderate, strenuous, or challenging.

TRAIL CONDITION: The trail's general condition at time of writing. *Well-maintained* trails are those regularly traveled with a clear route and regular maintenance or which follow service roads and the like. *Clear* trails are well defined with some possible obstacles (fallen trees in the off-season, etc.) but without any major impediments. *Passable* trails are those that receive little use and may require some navigation and those that do not receive regular maintenance. *Difficult* trails are those that have been abandoned by the USFS and/or are no longer in use, are cross-country routes, or are those that follow a stream or river and may require Class 3 scrambling, rock-hopping, and/or swimming. Navigation skills are a must.

MAP(S): The USGS 7.5-minute (1:24,000) topographic map(s) covering the route. In many cases, relevant USFS or other (e.g., Harrison or Conant) maps will also be noted here.

CAMP(S): Backcountry campsites along the described route. Sidebars detailing such camps accompany the trip descriptions as appropriate.

HIGHLIGHTS: Natural features, views, or other items of interest worth noting during the course of the trip.

TO REACH THE TRAILHEAD: Detailed directions (including UTM 10 or 11 way-points) to reach the trailhead from the nearest major town, highway, or other landmark. Details regarding facilities, water accessibility, and fees as applicable.

TRIP SUMMARY: A brief overview of the route.

Maps

EACH TRIP IS DEPICTED on a map (typically shared with the nearest trips in the area). Latitude/longitude (degree-minute-second) and UTM 10 or 11 coordinates (NAD83/WGS84) are included along the axes for all maps. The map is provided at the beginning of its representative group of trips; see also the List of Maps on page 398.

See the legend below for details about the map symbols.

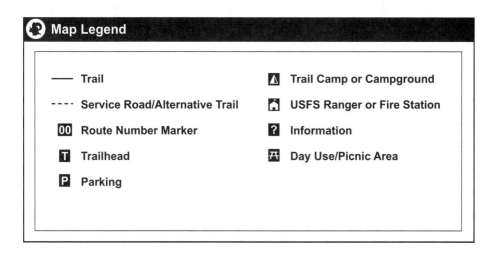

Map Legend

——	Trail	⚠	Trail Camp or Campground
----	Service Road/Alternative Trail	🏠	USFS Ranger or Fire Station
00	Route Number Marker	?	Information
T	Trailhead	⌗	Day Use/Picnic Area
P	Parking		

Trip Description

EACH TRIP ENTRY details the route and trail, including trail conditions, navigational considerations, travel hazards, seasonal considerations, geology, flora, fauna, and historical notes (including relevant fire history and any "legacy" comments). The route description also includes spur trails, trail camps, junctions, major river convergences or forks, and other considerations. The key points of the description are noted in **boldface** and are accompanied by a parenthetical notation usually including mileage from your starting point, elevation, and UTM coordinates, e.g., **Raspberry Spring Camp (0.4 mile, 6,640', 288021E 3835588N)**.

Because many routes are interconnected or overlap with another, notes will often guide the reader to reference other trip entries for the continuation of a given route or optional spur or side trip. Conversely, directions from a previous entry may provide the first portion of the relevant directions, in which case the reader will be directed to that entry first, e.g, "see *Route 31* for the first 9.1 miles of this route [to Mission Pine Spring]."

Sidebars detailing side trips, toponymy, and historical anecdotes are distributed throughout the text.

FOREST ROAD– AND TRAIL-NAMING CONVENTIONS ▦ ▦ ▦ ▦

Trails, in addition to their route name (e.g., Alder Creek Trail or West Camino Cielo Road), also receive a trail designation (e.g., 20W11 or 5N19). Though some might think twice as to how or why forest roads and trails receive their designations, there *is* a (relatively) simple method to the alphanumeric madness. The designations come from the **township** and **range** as defined by the Public Land Survey System (PLSS). The PLSS is the method by which public lands (those held by the United States for the benefit of the public) are divided and legally described. The PLSS is regulated by the Bureau of Land Management (BLM) and covers most of the western (postcolonial) US, though most of these lands have since transferred to private ownership.

Under the PLSS, most land is divided into 6-mile-square **townships**, and the townships are in turn divided into 36 1-mile-square (640-acre) **sections**. The PLSS is a series of separate surveys, each with an initial point; the townships are surveyed in the four cardinal directions from that point. The north-south line running through the initial point is the **principal meridian** (of which there are 37 in the PLSS). The two meridians relevant to the southern Los Padres are the

Mt. Diablo and the San Bernardino. A perpendicular east-west **base line** (parallel of latitude) also runs through the initial point.

Each township is identified with a township and range designation. Township designations indicate position north or south of the base line and Range designations indicate position east or west of the meridian.

In the case of trails, the first half of the designation is derived from the Range of the route's origin or terminus; 20W11 indicates the trail is in Range 20 West, and is one of at least 11 trails to originally begin or end within the range.

Roads are similarly named, but receive their designations from the Township of its origin or terminus.

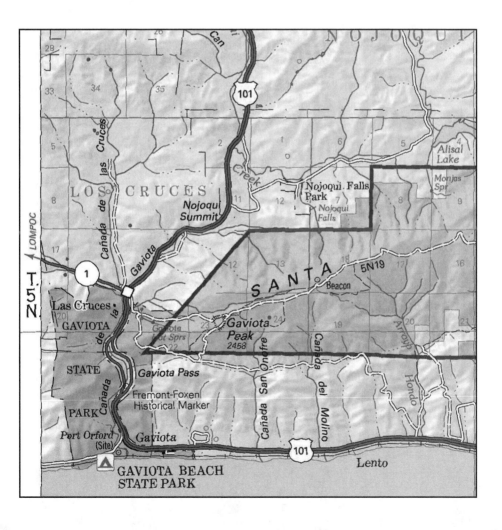

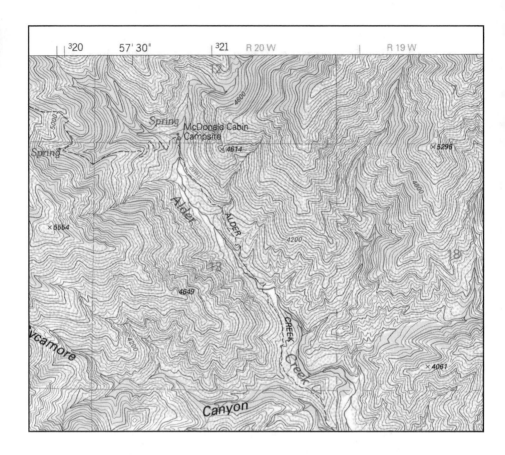

You may notice in some cases that a trail or road does not enter the township or range for which it received its designation; in most cases this is due to the route having been shortened (e.g., converted to trail use after a wilderness designation) or a section of the original route having been abandoned or rerouted over the past century.

PART ONE

■ ■ ■ ■ ■ ■ ■ ■ ■ ■ ■ ■ ■

Santa Barbara and Western Mt. Pinos Ranger Districts

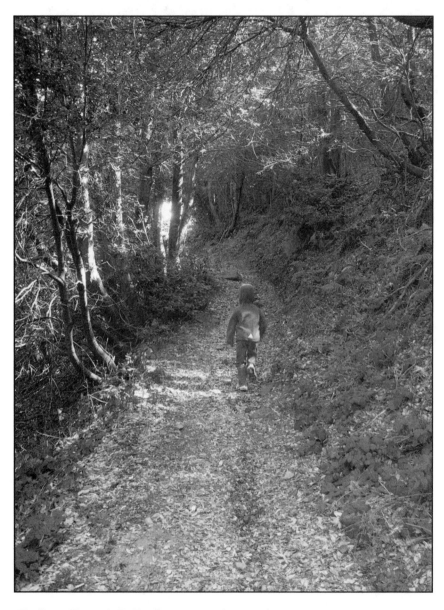

The Upper Tequepis Trail, prime banana-slug territory!

CHAPTER three

Western Santa Ynez Mountains

This chapter details routes in the western Santa Ynez Mountains portion of the forest.

REPRESENTING THE WESTERNMOST EDGE of the southern Los Padres, the western Santa Ynez Mountains are a rugged and largely undeveloped stretch of forest. Hemmed by the Gaviota Pass (US 101) on the west and San Marcos Pass (CA 154) on the east, the area (like the rest of the range) consists almost exclusively of Miocene-era sedimentary geology, and the resultant boulder and rock formations are extremely popular with sport climbers.

See the individual entries for trailhead specifics.

Route 1

GAVIOTA PEAK via Gaviota Hot Springs

LENGTH AND TYPE:	6.1-mile out-and-back
RATING:	Moderate
TRAIL CONDITION:	Clear
MAP(S):	USGS *Solvang*
CAMP(S):	—
HIGHLIGHTS:	Hot springs; expansive ocean views from Gaviota Peak

TO REACH THE TRAILHEAD(S): From Santa Barbara, follow US 101 north along the coast approximately 34 miles to the split for CA 1 (Exit 98A; Vandenberg AFB/Solvang). Turn right (east) at the stop sign, and immediately right again onto the frontage road. Proceed 0.3 mile south along this frontage road to the small Gaviota State Park **parking area** (**350', 754678E 3821616N**). The route begins in the southeast corner of the parking area. As of this writing, California State Parks system charges $2 for parking; make your payment using the envelopes provided. There are no facilities here.

TRIP SUMMARY: From the Gaviota State Park trailhead, this hike follows a very clear route by way of the old Gaviota Peak Fire Road (with a side trip to Gaviota Hot Springs) into the national forest to Gaviota Peak (2,458').

Trip Description

Note: UTM coordinates in this entry are Zone 10.

This hike begins on California State Park property; dogs are allowed on this trail but are to be leashed at all times until reaching the forest boundary.

From the **parking area** (**350', 754678E 3821616N**) head east along the service road. The track here is composed largely of road base. You'll note various nonnative plants (in addition to the ubiquitous fennel) alongside your route, among them Peruvian pepper and eucalyptus trees. Massive sycamores, live oaks, and the occasional valley oak—many skirted with poison oak—line your early progress along the southern bank of Hot Springs Creek to the first **fork** (**0.3 mile, 460', 755001E 3821560N**).

Continue left (east) here until you cross the culvert over Hot Springs Creek and reach the Hot Springs **spur trail** on your right (**0.6 mile, 600', 755265E 3821425N**). Follow this trail, which at times can be overgrown with various grasses, blackberries, and poison oak. Continue along the shady and moist creekside through a small grassy flat ringed by oaks until you reach **Gaviota Hot Springs** (**0.7 mile, 700', 755391E 3821410N**). This pleasant spot—shaded by

MAP 1 Gaviota Peak 35

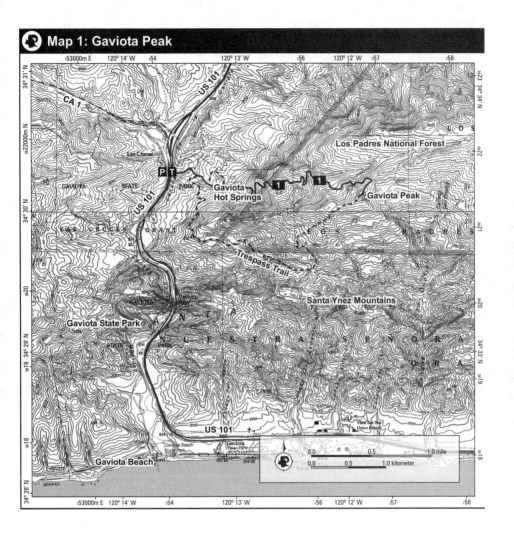

Map 1: Gaviota Peak

a nonnative palm and ensconced by rough New Deal–era masonry—consists of one soaking tub and a larger natural-bottom pool.

From the hot springs, continue up-canyon along the short connector trail (stay left at the fork) until you reconnect with the **fire road** (**0.8 mile, 760', 755439E 3821487N**). The climb is steady from here; hike around an old road gate and begin the first series of switchbacks while the road leads you up the northwestern flanks of Gaviota Peak. Because you'll be hiking along north faces for much of your ascent, opportunities for shade are plentiful. The area has not burned since the 1955 Refugio Fire, and the hillside growth here is thick—but for the road, it would prove an impenetrable barrier of ceanothus, chamise, and flat leaf summer holly for most of this side of the peak. Five-fingered ferns abound in many north-facing

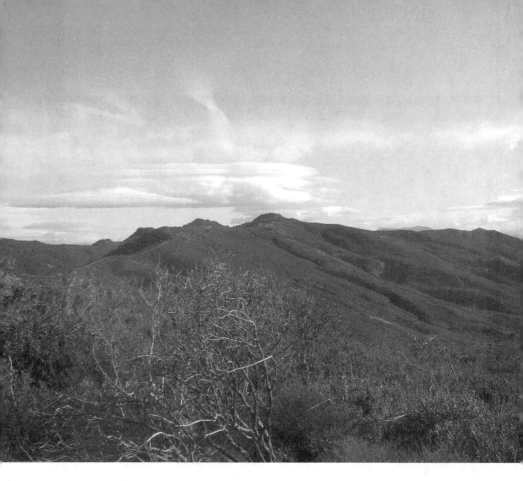

Eastward views from the Gaviota Peak Trail

nooks, and the road alternately consists of rough rock surface where more exposed and firm, and then compacted soil in the sheltered stretches.

In addition to increasingly spacious views of CA 1 and the Gaviota Pass below, you'll begin to gain a good view of Las Cánovas Creek's geology to your north (left) just as you are coming into the national forest. Continue until you reach the **ridgeline (2.8 miles, 2,300', 757368E 3821568N)**, where views of the ocean and miles of the Santa Ynez range spread out before you.

The wind here can be quite fierce; Gaviota Pass is known for its wind, but it feels especially forceful standing atop this ridgeline. Follow the trail to your right (south) and up the rutted track to **Gaviota Peak (3 miles, 2,458', 757368E 3821568N)**. There is a metal canister here with a trail register; views southward from the summit extend from Isla Vista and Santa Barbara in the east to Point Conception in the west, as well as Anacapa, Santa Cruz, Santa Rosa, and the San Miguel Islands. To the northeast, Big Pine Mountain and an array of Los Padres ridgelines fade into the distance.

Once you've soaked up your fill of the view (or wind), return the way you came.

Route 2

BROADCAST PEAK via Tequepis Trail (29W06)

LENGTH AND TYPE:	8.2-mile out-and-back to trail's end at Camino Cielo; 11-mile out-and-back to Broadcast Peak
RATING:	Moderate to strenuous
TRAIL CONDITION:	Clear
MAP(S):	USGS *Lake Cachuma*
CAMP(S):	—
HIGHLIGHTS:	Panoramic views of Lake Cachuma, the Santa Ynez Valley and mountain range, Santa Barbara, and the Pacific

TO REACH THE TRAILHEAD(S): From Santa Barbara, follow CA 154 (San Marcos Pass Road) toward Lake Cachuma. At the junction with **Forest Route 6N04 (780', 229216E 3829077N)**, turn left (south) and continue along the leftmost of the two forks. Numerous NO TRES-PASSING and PRIVATE PROPERTY signs dot the route, but the road proper is public access. Follow this rough asphalt-and-dirt road 1.2 miles to a small **parking area (1,180', 228686E 3827393N)** outside the gates of Circle V Ranch Camp, operated by the Society of St. Vincent de Paul. There are no facilities at this trailhead. (Though some brazen hikers do use the camp's restrooms, please be considerate and simply hike through.) Dogs should absolutely remain on-leash through this portion of the hike.

TRIP SUMMARY: From the Circle V Camp, the Tequepis Trail steadily ascends Broadcast Peak's northern flank through high chaparral and deciduous hardwoods. An elevation gain of nearly 3,000 feet is made pleasant by a great deal of shade and cool canyons. The trail tops out at Camino Cielo Road just east of Broadcast Peak.

Trip Description

From the Circle V **parking area (1,180', 228686E 3827393N)**, pass through the pedestrian access to the immediate left of the camp's entrance gates (not the road off to the right, which is private and leads to camp housing). Follow the gravel-and-dirt road past the facility's swimming pool and recently constructed cabins and bear left at the signage in the middle of camp indicating the trail's direction. Follow the road out of camp, crossing the creek bed (note the small pipe paralleling your route here), and proceed along the canyon by way of an old roadway. Stay right/straight at the first split in this road.

The road is heavily eroded in spots, and big-leaf maples, sycamores, and huge live oaks track your progress as you climb fairly easily to a **flat (0.8 mile, 1,680', 228650E 3826086N)** that makes a fine spot for your first water break. There is a rusting steel sign here indicating an old

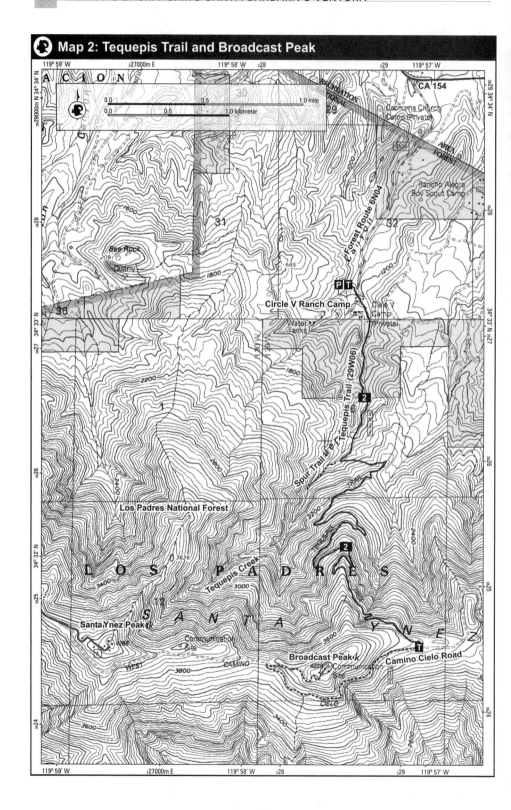

Map 2: Tequepis Trail and Broadcast Peak

oil lease. A little farther on, once you've moved beneath a canopy of live oaks, is a **fork** in the trail (**0.9 mile, 1,750', 233135E 3825876N**). The main trail leading up to Camino Cielo and to Broadcast Peak is on the left, but it's worth considering the short spur trail (outlined below).

■ ■ ■ ■ ■ ■ ■ ■ **TEQUEPIS CREEK SPUR TRAIL**

From the Tequepis Creek fork, this short trail follows a shaded and (even on hot days) rather cool and dark route, tracing the progress of the old metal pipes used to bring water down-canyon. It's an easy 0.25 mile to **Tequepis Creek (1,850', 228255E 3825743N)**, a dark and narrow-walled ravine lined with tall bay trees straining for the limited sun. This quiet and pleasant spot is your last access to water along this route.

■ ■ ■ ■ ■ ■ ■ ■ ■ ■ ■ ■ ■ ■ ■ ■ ■ ■ ■ ■

From the fork, continue left (east). The trail noticeably narrows as you leave Tequepis Creek and begin to climb in earnest. Soon you'll come to a well-shaded flat from which the trail climbs alongside a fenced property line. The first Pacific madrones along the route begin to appear here. Emerging from the other side of the flat and starting a short set of switchbacks, you'll gain your first good views of Lake Cachuma to the north. Continuing along Broadcast Peak's flanks, your route leads like a rope laid across the ridgeline; climb steadily along the west side, cross over to the east, cross over again, and so on. Poison oak and blackberries intermittently populate the shady trailsides, along with the usual ceanothus and scrub oaks. This continues for numerous switchbacks, providing great views of Santa Ynez Peak, the Santa Ynez Valley, and Lake Cachuma when on the west side and views of your eventual destination when on the east. Soon enough you'll spot the cut of Camino Cielo Road eastward across the canyon.

The final stretch is a series of switchbacks lined with bays, various ferns, and rather uncommon (in this region) tan bark oaks. You're likely to see a banana slug or two along this cool and moist stretch before breaking into a rocky section and emerging from the chaparral to find yourself at the **firebreak (4 miles, 3,550', 229096E 3824588N)**. Views here are fantastic—to the east and south especially—and Broadcast Peak looms to your right (west).

Some older-generation guides and trail accounts allude to a thin spur trail leading along the firebreak to Broadcast Peak from the northeastern approach here (with the concession that the trail is oft-overgrown and the hard chaparral tough going). This remains the case; a thread of trail does lead westward along the firebreak to the first rock formation, but thereafter disappears altogether, with nary a hint of more than a few game trails tunneling beneath the unforgiving foliage. Even the adventurous would be best-suited to bushwhack

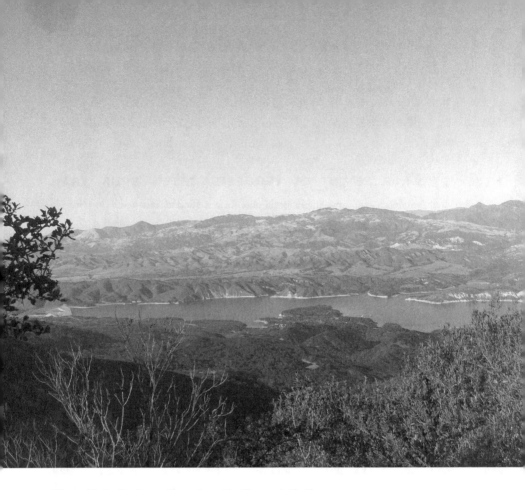

View of Lake Cachuma from along the Tequepis Trail

this portion when *descending* Broadcast Peak, for at least then you'd be able to see over the next bloodletting hedge of whitethorn ceanothus or impassive manzanita while navigating.

Tequepis Trail from here can be difficult to follow in this clearing; the condition of the firebreak (primarily how recently it was graded) can make navigating a bit of a guessing game for the first-time visitor, but the trail leads another hundred yards southeast to its formal upper trailhead with the dirt **Camino Cielo Road** (**4.1 miles, 3,500', 229167E 3824511N**).

If Broadcast Peak is your goal, continue right (west) another mile along Camino Cielo Road. Views en route to Broadcast Peak are wonderful; while Lake Cachuma has been obscured from view, the entire Pacific and many of the Channel Islands are laid out before you. A long stretch of the Central Coast is also visible far below this 270-degree vantage point. At the first fork, take the **service road** (**5.1 miles, 3,790', 227908E 3824450N**) right (east) to **Broadcast Peak** another 0.5 mile to the array of broadcasting towers and equipment (**5.5 miles, 4,025', 228397E 3824406N**). The actual peak of Broadcast Peak is behind the barbed-wire fence.

Santa Ynez Peak is another 1.5 miles from the junction along the Camino Cielo.

Route 3

LIZARD'S MOUTH

LENGTH AND TYPE:	0.25 mile + meander/loop
RATING:	Easy
TRAIL CONDITION:	Clear to passable (not officially maintained)
MAP(S):	USGS *San Marcos Pass* and *Goleta*
CAMP(S):	—
HIGHLIGHTS:	Climbing, scrambling, and bouldering opportunities; fantastic views

TO REACH THE TRAILHEAD(S): From the junction of US 101 and CA 154 in Santa Barbara, follow CA 154 (San Marcos Pass Road) northward approximately 7.1 miles to West Camino Cielo Road (the turnoff is also marked Kinevan Road). Turn left (west) here and continue along West Camino Cielo approximately 3.5 miles to a small **parking area (2,850', 237046E 3821510N)**. Additional parking can be had up and down the route on either side, as necessary. If you reach the Winchester Gun Club shooting range, you've missed the parking area by approximately 100 yards. There are no facilities here.

TRIP SUMMARY: One of the easiest routes in this guide, the Lizard's Mouth is a sandstone boulder field with numerous overhangs, crevices, and other spots for picnicking, exploring, or just lounging.

Trip Description

This destination is less a trip than a general meandering and exercise in exploration. Children will love the various boulders over which they can scramble and nooks in which one can hide; ambitious bouldering enthusiasts and sport climbers come to the Lizard's Mouth formation to practice their moves. Do be mindful of the occasional broken glass bottle, as this site is a well-known late-night party destination for area high school and college students.

From the **parking area (2,850', 237046E 3821510N)**, follow the boulder field to the southwest (the use trail just to the east here doesn't lead to the main formation as one might expect). From the road the formation seems a tad unimpressive, and you won't see the formations fully until you've gained a bit of altitude. After 100 yards or so, however, you'll spy the maze this sandstone outcrop provides as you drop down into the main collection of cobbles and massive boulders. The actual **Lizard's Mouth (2,760', 236684E 3821592N)** is approximately 0.25 mile to your southwest.

Views here are some of the best available with so little labor; to the south Santa Barbara, Goleta, and the Pacific are laid out before you, and to the west Broadcast and Santa

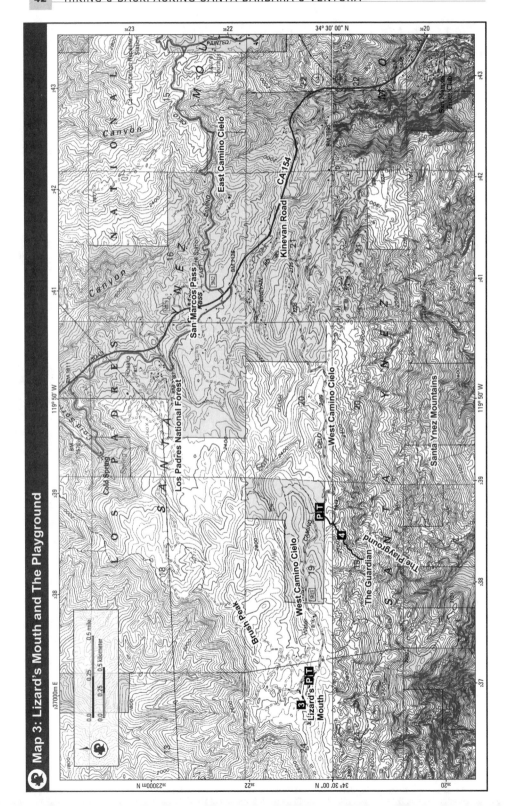

Map 3: Lizard's Mouth and The Playground

Ynez Peaks are easily distinguishable for their various transmission arrays. Damage from the 2008 Gap Fire is still evident, but as the area isn't heavily vegetated, the impact was relatively minimal.

In the spring, much of the interior area (where there is soil) is carpeted by fine green grass. The usual chaparral species (most notably manzanita) line the various paths, which snake throughout the labyrinth of sandstone boulders and crevices, with the occasional mature oak providing additional shade. After rains, numerous pools form atop many of the boulders.

Bolt hangers and other climbing hardware are sometimes left on the larger formations, so be mindful of those while scrambling about. Also be mindful of numerous drop-offs, especially if you have little hikers in your party.

Straight from the Lizard's Mouth; courtesy G. Carey

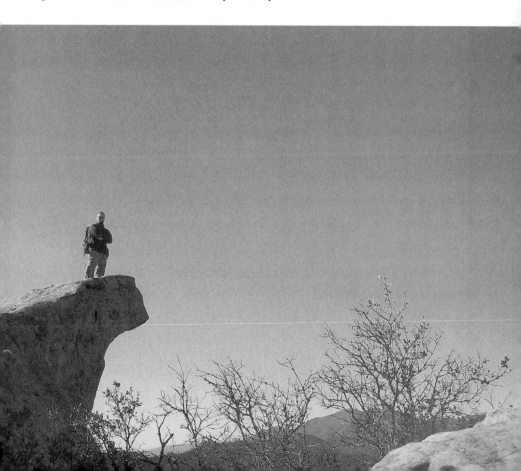

Route 4

THE PLAYGROUND

LENGTH AND TYPE:	0.5 mile to start of formation
RATING:	Easy and up
TRAIL CONDITION:	Clear to passable
MAP(S):	USGS *San Marcos Pass* (*Note:* Use trails not shown on map)
CAMP(S):	—
HIGHLIGHTS:	Possibly the best rock-hopping, scrambling, and bouldering in the Santa Barbara area; excellent seaward views

TO REACH THE TRAILHEAD(S): From the junction of US 101 and CA 154 in Santa Barbara, follow CA 154 (San Marcos Pass Road) northward approximately 7.1 miles to West Camino Cielo Road (the turnoff is also marked Kinevan Road). Turn left (west) here and continue along West Camino Cielo approximately 2.5 miles to a small **parking area (2,680', 238634E 3821391N)** on your left (south) just as you cross beneath a series of power lines. There are no facilities here.

TRIP SUMMARY: A short 0.5-mile approach leads to sublime rock formations. One could spend an entire day exploring and barely scratch the figurative surface of what the Playground holds.

Note: In addition to your usual provisions, if you intend to explore the Narrows, you may wish to bring a headlamp or flashlight, as well as a 20-foot length of rope (and know how to use it) for any hiker not comfortable with some of the free climbs/descents. The Narrows are also not recommended for the claustrophobic.

Trip Description

From the **parking area (2,680', 238634E 3821391N)**, follow the thin use trail leading southwest, along a small creek bed cut into exposed sandstone, staying west as it disappears into the brush to cross a **creek (0.1 mile, 2,600', 238514E 3821318N)**. From here you'll climb and then descend easily over both open terrain burned clear during the 2008 Gap Fire and more dense, canopied stretches (in the draws) to a **junction** just yards from the north face of the Guardian (**0.5 mile, 2,540', 238155E 3820986N**). This huge stone formation is the first as you approach the complex jumble of sandstone boulders, overhangs, tunnels, and caverns comprising the Playground. A dozen yards farther to your left (east) is a gap in this massive rock wall, through which you can access the rest of the rock field.

From this point, your excursion is largely of your own accord. Climbers tend to gravitate toward the dozens of set challenges throughout the area. The most popular destination for non-climbers is the **Narrows**, a thin gap extending for hundreds of yards into a small, nearly lightless antechamber beneath massive sandstone slabs. When looking from the northern vantage point, take a bearing on the cluster of trees visible along the eastern edge of the "spaceship"—local custom and sensitivities (compounded by numerous incidences of vandalism in recent years) preclude specific directions. They almost prompted the author to exclude this route altogether. Show respect.

Oak and bay trees tend to dominate the shadier stretches of the region, while farther south and along the exposed stretches, what little vegetation is left tends to be manzanita and the hardier chaparral species.

Looking out from the Guardian; courtesy John Cook

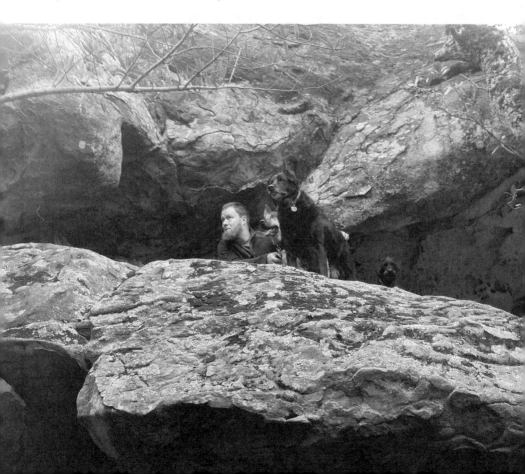

Santa Ynez Recreation Area

This chapter details the trails beginning (or ending) in the Santa Ynez Recreation Area.

THE SANTA YNEZ RECREATION AREA (sometimes abbreviated SYRA) is a stretch of forest popular with day-trippers and car-campers, as well as more seasoned outdoor adventurers. It is situated (appropriately enough) alongside the Santa Ynez River, which is often lauded as the longest stretch of publicly accessible river in Southern California.

Numerous sites dot the **Lower Santa Ynez Recreation Area** (accessed via Paradise Road)—including six day-use picnic sites (all with restrooms, tables, and barbecues), five car-accessible overnight campgrounds, and numerous trailheads to hiking trails and off-highway vehicle (OHV) routes. The Santa Barbara Ranger District office is also situated here, at 3505 Paradise Road (between Fremont and Paradise Campgrounds). *Note:* The 1995 *San Marcos Pass* quad and several online mapping sites show the ranger station on the south side of Paradise Road. The current station is north of the road.

The **Upper Santa Ynez Recreation Area**—accessed via Romero-Camuesa Road by way of East Camino Cielo—provides another four car campgrounds, the Big Caliente day-use area, and access to numerous hiking trails, OHV routes, and some hot springs for good measure. Because its access is more difficult, it receives far less traffic and the sites are much more rustic. Toilets are vault rather than flush, and all trash must be packed out when you depart. Reservations are not necessary to camp at Middle Santa Ynez, P-Bar Flats, Rock, or Mono Campgrounds.

Reaching the trailheads of either portion of the Santa Ynez is fairly straightforward, as there are only two points of entry (one for each section). All directions for points within the Lower SYRA begin at the intersection with Paradise Road at **CA 154 (1,200', 237727E 3825030N)**. All directions for points within the Upper SYRA begin at the **Romero**

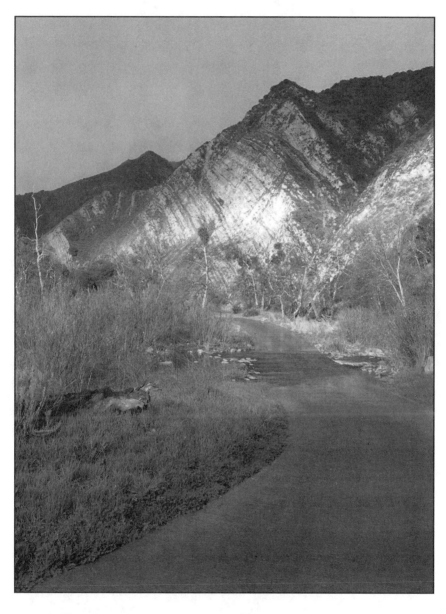

Paradise Road

Map 4: Lower Santa Ynez Recreation Area

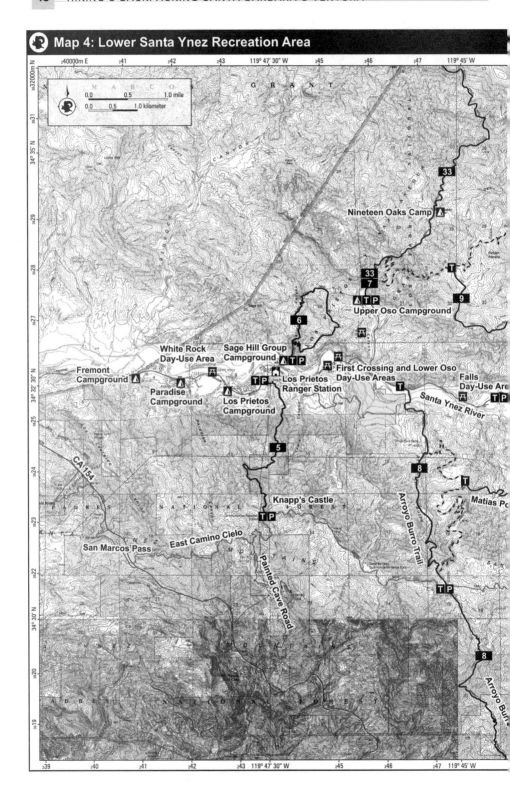

MAP 4 Lower Santa Ynez Recreation Area   49

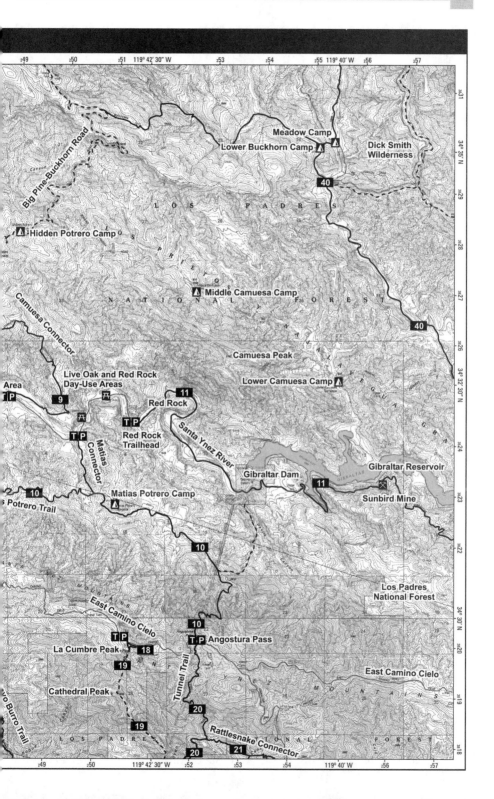

Big Pine-Buckhorn Road

Meadow Camp
Lower Buckhorn Camp

Dick Smith
Wilderness

40

L O S   P A D R E S

Hidden Potrero Camp

Camuesa Connector

Middle Camuesa Camp

N A T I O N A L   F O R E S T

40

Camuesa Peak

Live Oak and Red Rock
Day-Use Areas

Lower Camuesa Camp

Area
P
9

11
Red Rock

T P
Red Rock
Trailhead

Santa Ynez River

Gibraltar Reservoir

Matias Connector

T P

10
Potrero Trail

Matias Potrero Camp

Gibraltar Dam
11

Sunbird Mine

10

Los Padres
National Forest

East Camino Cielo

10

T P
La Cumbre Peak
18

T P Angostura Pass

19

East Camino Cielo

Tunnel Trail

Cathedral Peak

19

20

Burro Trail

Rattlesnake Connector

L O S   P A D R E S

20
21

N A L   F O R E S T

Saddle (**3,060', 261638E 3818018N**), where the paved East Camino Cielo turns to the graded dirt Romero-Camuesa Road (Forest Route 5N15).

A US Forest Service (USFS) Adventure Pass, federal Interagency Pass, or equivalent permit is required to park a vehicle anywhere within the Santa Ynez Recreation Area.

Lower Santa Ynez Recreation Area

Trailheads

Snyder Trailhead (1,050', 243543E 3825739N)

From CA 154, continue along Paradise Road 4.1 miles to a small parking area along a wire fence on the right (south) side of the road. There are no facilities here, but facilities are available at some of the nearby USFS campgrounds (e.g., Paradise or Los Prietos). This is the lower access for the Snyder Trail (see *Route 5*) and Wellhouse Falls.

Aliso Canyon/Sage Hill (980', 244231E 3826212N)

From CA 154, continue along Paradise Road 4.5 miles to the Los Prietos Ranger Station. Turn left (north) here and follow the road (and signage) 0.25 mile (passing the station), turning right and across the Santa Ynez River (this is often a wet crossing) to Sage Hill Group Campground. The trailhead is in the northeast corner of the grounds, past Loop 5 (Caballo) and in its own space. There are facilities (including flush toilets and potable water) here.

First Crossing (990', 244906E 3826210N)

From CA 154, continue along Paradise Road 5.5 miles to the signed parking lot for the First Crossing day-use area. Though not typically used as a trailhead, this day-use area is often the end of the road whenever the river level or road conditions beyond are determined to be impassable (usually after the winter storms). The space has ample parking, barbecues, restrooms, and potable water.

Lower Oso (990', 245376E 3826130N)

Just across the river from First Crossing (5.7 miles from CA 154), this campground-turned–day-use area is an option for those seeking to hike the Arroyo Burro route from the northernmost end (see *Route 8*). It features restrooms, water, and 23 day-use sites.

Upper Oso (1,200', 245736E 3827459N)

The Upper Oso Trailhead provides access to the Santa Cruz National Recreation Trail (see *Routes 7* and *33*); there is also a car-accessible campground here. From CA 154, continue along Paradise Road 5.7 miles to the split with Buckhorn Road. Follow Buckhorn Road another 1.3 miles to the Upper Oso parking area; the trailhead is on the north end of the pavement. There are restrooms and water here.

Arroyo Burro Turnout (1,075', 245619E 3826023N)

This parking area is notable for the large live oak situated beside the road and is 6 miles along Paradise Road, just past the split with Buckhorn Road. There is room enough for a few vehicles on the left (north) side of the road, but little more (parking is not allowed along the road for a few miles eastward due to frequent rockfall). There are no facilities here.

Falls Day-Use Area (1,080', 247573E 3825367N)

Falls, 7.3 miles along Paradise Road, is another day-use area that isn't overly close to any trails in the area. It is, however, a fine spot for enjoying the namesake falls on the south side of the Santa Ynez.

Camuesa Connector Trailhead (1,100', 249002E 3825014)

This easy-to-miss trailhead, 8.3 miles from CA 154, provides access to the Camuesa Connector trail (27W22; see *Route 9*). Parking is available along the shoulder farther up and down the road; there are no facilities here.

Matias Connector Trailhead (1,100', 249863E 3824597N)

This trailhead, 9 miles along Paradise Road, provides access to the Matias Connector (27W25; see *Route 10*). One or two vehicles can fit here, but be sure to not block the gate. Otherwise, parking is available along the shoulder farther up and down the road. There are no facilities here.

Live Oak Day-Use Area

This fairly new day-use area, 9.2 miles along Paradise Road, doesn't provide access to any local trails, but it's a really pleasant spot to enjoy a dip in the river.

Red Rock Day-Use Area

A former campground, this day-use area features 28 sites with tables and barbecues, vault toilets, and good access to the river.

Red Rock Trailhead (1,130', 251027E 3824763N)

This parking area, 10.4 miles along Paradise Road from CA 154, rather confusingly shares its name with the day-use area farther back along the road (site of a former car campground) and is named after the formations upstream. This trailhead provides foot, mountain bike, and equestrian access to the Gibraltar Reservoir area. There are toilets and trash receptacles here. From here one can access the Red Rock formation along the Santa Ynez as well as the Gibraltar Reservoir area (see *Route 11*).

Campgrounds of the Lower Santa Ynez

Popular to the point of being overcrowded on holiday weekends and during the summer months, the campgrounds of the Lower SYRA can make great bases if you're inclined to spend more than just a day or two in the area exploring the numerous trails.

As of this writing, Rocky Mountain Recreation Company manages all campgrounds and day-use areas in the Lower SYRA—including the Fremont, Los Prietos, Paradise, Upper Oso, and Sage Hill Group Campgrounds. All camps in this part of the SYRA have barbecues and/or fire pits, tables, garbage bins, flush or vault toilets, and RV space. Most have water. Reservations for the sites can be made at **recreation.gov** or by calling (877) 444-6777.

FREMONT (1,000', 241100E 3826094N)   2.5 miles from CA 154   **15 sites**

PARADISE (1,055', 241990E 3825966N)   3.1 miles from CA 154   **15 sites**

LOS PRIETOS (1,075', 242865E 3825769N)   3.7 miles from CA 154   **37 sites**

SAGE HILL GROUP (980', 243889E 3826213N)   4.7 miles from CA 154   **5 group sites**

UPPER OSO (1,200', 245736E 3827459N)   7 miles from CA 154   **23 sites**

Upper Santa Ynez Recreation
Trailheads
Blue Canyon Pass (2,125', 264961E 3819093N)

Upper Blue Canyon Trailhead, 3.8 miles from Romero Saddle, is located just west of Blue Canyon Pass and is easy to miss coming from the saddle. There are no facilities here.

Juncal (1,800', 266738E 3819092N)

This roadhead/trailhead, 5.6 miles from Romero Saddle, is near the site of the former Juncal Campground. The Juncal Road (closed to public vehicular traffic) heads east here up the Santa Ynez River drainage, providing access to the old Franklin Trail (see *Route 16*), as well as to the Upper Santa Ynez camp and the Murietta Divide. Parking can be tricky, as you must stay off the roadway. The best spot is often another third of a mile down the road to a small turnoff (**266375E 3819426N**). There are no facilities here.

Big Caliente Day-Use Area (1,875', 264644E 3824942N)

This small day-use area, 11.2 miles from Romero Saddle and along the Pendola/Agua Caliente Road (5N16), features one space with a table and vault toilet. Its main attractions are the hot springs, one just off the road and another set just up the trail. The Agua Caliente Trail (see *Route 13*), as well as La Carpa Potreros (for the hearty), can be accessed from this trailhead.

Little Caliente Spring (1,650', 259519E 3825184N)

Past Mono Campground and then along a short spur road (5N33), 14.4 miles from Romero Saddle, this unofficial trailhead (and former campground) has no facilities (but there is the nearby hot spring). Use this parking area for the closest access to the hot spring as well as one of two access points for *Route 12: Mono-Alamar Trail.*

Mono Creek Gate (1,520', 258686E 3824656N)

This gate, 13.7 miles from Romero Saddle, marks the farthest the public can currently drive an auto along the Romero-Camuesa (in decades past one could drive all the way into the Lower SYRA via this route). Just east of the road's crossing of Mono Creek, this small road-side parking area is the staging ground for trips into the lower Dick Smith Wilderness, lower Indian Creek (see *Route 40*), and the closed portions of the Romero-Camuesa Road.

Campgrounds of the Upper Santa Ynez

Use of these sites requires only a US Forest Service Adventure Pass, federal Interagency Pass, or equivalent permit; they are first come, first served with vault toilets but no water.

ROCK (1,920', 264756E 3824529N)   10.9 miles from Romero Saddle and along the Pendola/Agua Caliente Road (5N16); formerly known as Little Caliente   **1 site**

MIDDLE SANTA YNEZ (1,500', 263272E 3821648N)   8.7 miles from Romero Saddle **13 sites**

P-BAR FLATS (1,500', 262150E 3822269N)   9.7 miles from Romero Saddle   **4 sites**

MONO (1,450', 258814E 3823850N)   13.1 miles from Romero Saddle (camps are a few hundred yards' walk to the southwest)   **3 sites**

Map 5: Upper Santa Ynez Recreation Area

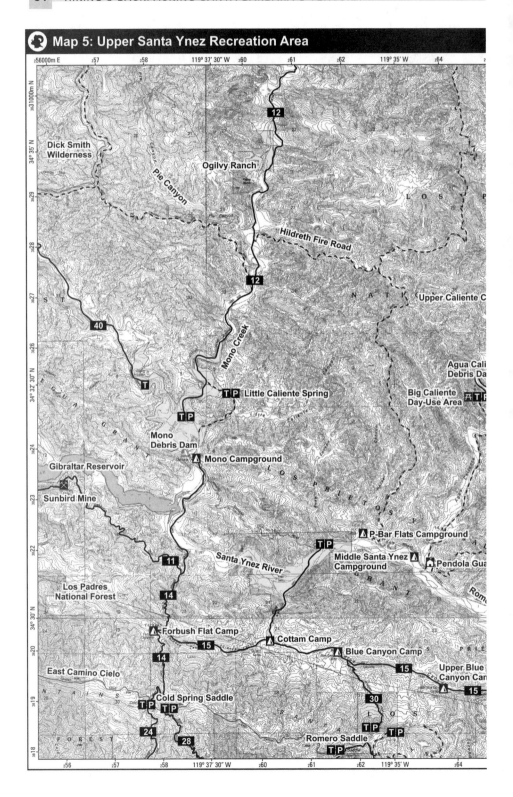

MAP 5 Upper Santa Ynez Recreation Area   55

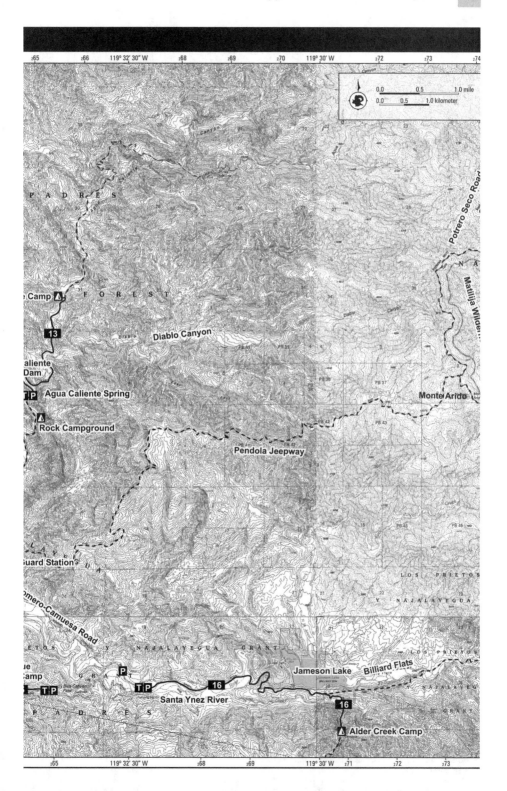

Route 5

SNYDER TRAIL and KNAPP'S CASTLE

LENGTH AND TYPE:	0.7-mile round-trip from Camino Cielo;
	6.2-mile round-trip from Paradise Road via Snyder Trail
RATING:	Easy from Camino Cielo; moderate from Paradise Road via Snyder Trail
TRAIL CONDITION:	Well maintained (service road) to clear
MAP(S):	USGS *San Marcos Pass*; Conant's *Matilija & Dick Smith Wilderness*
CAMP(S):	—
HIGHLIGHTS:	Ruins of the Knapp Mansion; panoramic views of the Santa Ynez River Valley; great hike for children from Camino Cielo

TO REACH THE TRAILHEAD(S): *Camino Cielo:* From the junction of US 101 and CA 154 in Santa Barbara, follow CA 154 (also San Marcos Pass Road) north 7.8 miles to East Camino Cielo Road (also Forest Road 5N12). Turn right (east) here and continue along East Camino Cielo 3 miles to a small **parking area (2,960', 243582E 3823200N)** on the left (north) side of the road. There is also space alongside the road in both directions. There are no facilities here.

    Paradise Road: From Paradise Road in the Santa Ynez Recreation Area (SYRA), use the Snyder Trailhead.

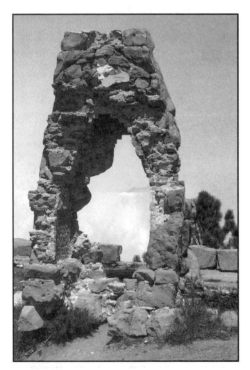

TRIP SUMMARY: This very easy walk from atop East Camino Cielo Road leads to the ruins of the once-magnificent Knapp mansion. A longer option is to approach from the SYRA to the north. Be mindful of mountain bikers when on the main fire road. The Knapp ruins are on private property, but the current owner allows hikers to visit (this may change without notice). The site is occasionally used as a filming location.

Trip Description

From Camino Cielo

From the parking area, follow the service road north past the gate, descending easily along the ceanothus- and scrub oak–lined route to the **junction (0.25 mile, 2,880',**

243584E 3823509N) of the main route and the spur leading to Knapp's Castle. The left option leads along the Snyder Trail, eventually dropping to the Santa Ynez valley floor and Paradise Road, some 3.5 miles distant.

Head right (up) here and past another gate, continuing easily up the grade another 0.1 mile to **Knapp's Castle (0.35 mile, 2,920', 243624E 3823691N)**. Enjoy wandering through what is left of the mansion's stone frame and foundations and soak in the fantastic views of the Santa Ynez River Valley. Live oaks and Coulter pines dot the perimeter of the grounds, and poppy displays are impressive in the spring.

■ ■ ■ ■ ■ ■ ■ ■ ■ ■ ■ ■ **A MAN AND HIS CASTLE**

George Owen Knapp, president of Union Carbide, arrived in Santa Barbara in 1912, part of a wave of East Coast transplants mesmerized by the region's beauty. By all accounts a very civic-minded philanthropist, Knapp contributed heavily to the construction and improvement of local schools, churches, and infrastructure, and he was instrumental in the construction of the Camino Cielo Road built along the spine of the Santa Ynez Mountains.

One of Knapp's most ambitious endeavors in his adopted hometown, however, was the construction of a massive five-bedroom mansion high atop the Santa Ynez ridge, built on a 160-acre tract of land he purchased in 1916. Knapp's property also held a separate home for the groundskeeper, as well as servants' quarters and a private observatory. The impressive building commanded even more impressive views of the Santa Ynez Valley and what is now the San Rafael Wilderness.

Knapp sold the property in 1940, and only a few months later the Paradise Canyon Fire roared across the land, destroying the engineer's long-time home. The observatory remained for almost another quarter century before the Coyote Fire in 1964 destroyed it as well. Today, all that is left of Knapp's visionary home are crumbling and skeletal stone remains.

■ ■ ■ ■ ■ ■ ■ ■ ■ ■ ■ ■ ■ ■ ■ ■ ■ ■ ■ ■

From Paradise Road

From the **trailhead** alongside Paradise Road (**1,050', 243543E 3825739N**), pass through the fence opening and follow the service road south. Your route here is well shaded by mature oaks and winds up to a **junction (0.4 mile, 1,200', 243844E 3825768N**) beside a pair of fenced-off water tanks and an outbuilding. Follow the trail on your right up some rocky stretches above the creek to where the road comes in again on your left (east). You'll note throughout this route that some of the less-considerate members of the fat-tire community have continually cut the trail and in some spots even fashioned berms alongside and off the trail. Follow the designated route, making a left just past a third water tower, and up a series of lush and well-shaded switchbacks. Take a moment to enjoy the **vista (0.9 mile, 1,540', 243987E 3825243N)** providing 270-degree views of the surrounding Santa Ynez River Valley and mountains to the north.

The switchbacks continue to and then along a grassy hillock, after which you pass beneath the ever-present **power lines (2.1 miles, 2,270', 243722E 3824311N)** and the singletrack turns back to road. Here the route gets steeper but is easily navigated; enjoy especially the thick groves of bay trees as you ascend to the **turnoff (3 miles, 2,880', 243584E 3823509N)** leading to your left (northeast) toward **Knapp's Castle (3.1 miles, 2,920', 243624E 3823691N)**.

Route 6

ALISO NATURE TRAIL (28W05)

LENGTH AND TYPE:	1.9-mile out-and-back along Aliso Canyon Interpretive Trail; 3.4-mile round-trip via Aliso Loop Trail
RATING:	Easy along the interpretive trail; easy to moderate along loop (climb)
TRAIL CONDITION:	Clear
MAP(S):	USGS *San Marcos Pass*; Conant's *Matilija & Dick Smith Wilderness* or *San Rafael Wilderness*
CAMP(S):	—
HIGHLIGHTS:	Self-guided interpretive nature trail; cool riparian trekking

TO REACH THE TRAILHEAD(S): See directions for the Aliso Canyon (Sage Hill) trailhead.

TRIP SUMMARY: Named for the aliso (alder) trees that shade portions of the trail, this pleasant route offers an easy out-and-back interpretive trail ideal for children or those looking for a very easy hike. There is also an option for a marginally more exerting loop trip up to and then along the ridge separating Aliso and Oso Canyons.

Trip Description

From the **trailhead (980', 244231E 3826212N)** at the mouth of Aliso Canyon, follow the trail easily beneath the shade of large sycamores.

The lower portion of the trail—about a mile long—is also the Aliso Canyon Interpretive Trail, for which you can obtain informational brochures at the nearby ranger station and sometimes at the trailhead (don't depend on them always being available at the trailhead, however—it's best to get them from the station if you want your own copy). The relevant portions of the brochure are mounted to posts along the way as well. The interpretive trail is maintained (and repaired, as needed) by volunteers of the Santa Barbara–based Los Padres Interpretive Association. Members of the association also provide guided tours along the Aliso and other trails on occasion.

The brochure's narrative follows the footsteps of Khus and Tani'alishaw, two young Chumash collecting milkweed and other natural supplies along the route. This is an excellent experience for young hikers and any visitors interested in the plant and natural resources along the route, especially those used in Chumash life.

Follow these markers—crossing the creek a number of times along a very easy grade—to the **junction (0.25 mile, 1,015', 244227E 3826611N)** with the Aliso Loop Trail (if you're doing the entire loop, this will be where you rejoin the lower trail along your return).

The route continues easily until Post 15, at which time the interpretive trail heads left (west) away from the watershed to climb above the creek before returning to and crossing Aliso Creek just before reaching **Post 21 (0.9 mile, 1,140', 244432E 3827361N)**. This is the final marker along the route. Just beyond is a large bench-shaped chunk of rock inlaid with quartz veins and a final post indicating the terminus of the interpretive section of the trail. From this terminus, you can either return to the main trail to retrace your steps back to the trailhead for a 1.9-mile out-and-back, or head north from the junction to complete the Aliso Loop Trail.

Note: As of this writing, this final marker instructs that "if you choose to take the Loop Trail, go back across the creek to the trail junction." This is not accurate—you're on the trail at this point and there's no backtracking necessary. One can only surmise the terminus of the

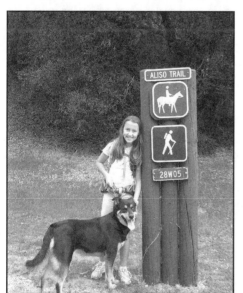

interpretive trail was somewhere across the creek when the brochures from which the little placards originate were initially printed in 1993 (this is confirmed by the US Forest Service's overview map of the route, which does show the final post being along a spur across Aliso Creek from the post's present position).

To continue along the Aliso Loop Trail, follow the singletrack as it makes its abrupt climb into the sharp rocks and yucca-lined route eastward, leaving the watershed. The first 0.25 mile of this section can be littered with small slides after rains, so do mind your footing. The trail here climbs steadily—you'll gain fine views of Sage Hill to your west and the sandstone bluffs to the north as you progress—before coming to a **meadow (1.4 miles, 1,550', 244815E 3827651N)**, which in the spring is filled with wildflowers (and in the fall and winter, often features star thistle along the trailside). Just beyond is the **junction (1.5 miles, 1,620', 244972E 3827638N)** with the Upper Oso Trail connector. You'll have a good view of the Santa Ynez River, lower Oso Canyon, and the Upper Oso Trailhead, as well as Little Pine Mountain and the approach of Santa Cruz Creek toward Alexander Peak and points north.

Head right (south) from this junction, climbing briefly through the low chaparral to a bald **knoll (1.6 miles, 1,710', 244943E 3827505N)**, from which your views are largely unobstructed. The trail southward from here feels like a service road (albeit rutted in areas), as it is wide and quite clear. Follow the trail south along the ridge dividing Aliso and Oso Canyons through a brief saddle and then up again briefly before dropping easily to the very edge of the **bluff (2.2 miles, 1,615', 244999E 3826707N)** overlooking the Santa Ynez River. Mind any children and/or pets here; the turn right (westward) is sharp and inattentive trail-goers could suffer a very long fall.

Follow the route easily along the bluff and then down toward Aliso Creek, following switchbacks full of fascinating marine geology back to the **junction (3.1 miles, 1,015', 244227E 3826611N)** with the lower trail. Retrace your steps along the interpretive trail back to the **trailhead (3.4 miles, 980', 244231E 3826212N)** and parking area.

"WELL, BACK IN MY DAY . . ." ■ ■ ■ ■ ■ ■ ■ ■ ■ ■

Hikers who have visited the Aliso Nature Trail in years past may remember the route a bit differently, and for a handful of reasons.

The original concept for the interpretive section of this trail was conceived and executed by students of the Santa Barbara Open Alternative School who studied the area in the spring of 1982. The signs—21 of them—were quite different from those that now populate the length of the trail, but they shared much of the same information with those that now chronicle the walk of Khus and Tani'alishaw.

■ ■

Route 7

UPPER OSO CANYON TO NINETEEN OAKS (27W09)

LENGTH AND TYPE:	3.6-mile out-and-back
RATING:	Easy
TRAIL CONDITION:	Clear
MAP(S):	USGS *San Marcos Pass*; Conant's *Matilija & Dick Smith Wilderness* or *San Rafael Wilderness*
CAMP(S):	Nineteen Oaks
HIGHLIGHTS:	Lush riparian hiking and varied geology; great for younger trekkers

Lower Oso Creek

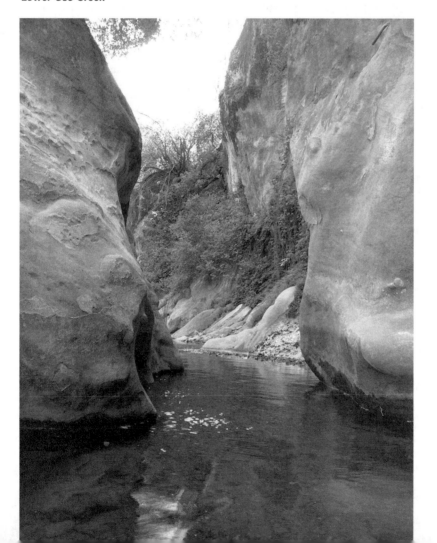

TO REACH THE TRAILHEAD(S): Use the Upper Oso Trailhead for this hike.

TRIP SUMMARY: This route follows the Buckhorn-Camuesa Fire Road and then the Santa Cruz National Recreation Trail (NRT) (27W09) an easy 2 miles to Nineteen Oaks Camp. The US Forest Service (USFS) publishes the 16-page "Geologic Trail Guide for the Upper Oso Canyon," which leads the reader on a self-guided tour through the Upper Oso drainage. These pamphlets are sometimes at the trailhead, as well as at the nearby ranger station (alternatively, they can be downloaded from the USFS website).

Note: This route is presented as a separate trip from the rest of the Santa Cruz NRT (*Route 33*) due to its accessibility and popularity.

Trip Description

From the **Upper Oso Trailhead (1,200', 245768E 3827395N)**, head north past the locked gate along Buckhorn-Camuesa Road (5N15). Note that the first 0.5 mile of your route is along this dirt service road, and as such, ATVs and mountain bikers also have access. Follow this road easily along the eastern bank of Oso Canyon, passing through a narrow gorge of towering sandstone. This stretch, while hot in the summer, does enjoy quite a bit of shade and features some nice sections where the creek can be accessed (though be mindful of poison oak).

Just as the service road begins its steep switchbacks up the northwestern flank of Camuesa Peak, you'll come to the **junction (0.7 mile, 1,350', 246261E 3828264N)** with the singletrack of the Santa Cruz NRT. Turn left (northeast) here and follow the singletrack along the creek. (While motorized vehicles are not allowed on this trail, mountain bikes are, so do mind the corners.) This stretch is well shaded, and in addition to big-leaf maples, oaks, and sycamores along the well-worn track, there are also numerous wildflower specimens and ferns. As described in the geology guide, serpentine rocks, Franciscan soils, and other examples of metamorphic geology present themselves as you follow the Oso drainage and cross the Little Pine fault.

Continue along this lush trail—crossing the **creek (1 mile, 1,400', 246713E 3828377N)** twice in rapid succession at one point—before reaching the **spur trail (1.8 miles, 1,600', 247197E 3829154N)** to Nineteen Oaks Camp.

CAMP :: NINETEEN OAKS

ELEVATION:	1,630'
MAP:	USGS *San Marcos Pass*
UTM:	247308E 3829100N

Set beside a small meadow just downstream from the confluence of two tributaries to Upper Oso Canyon, Nineteen Oaks is a frequently visited spot along the Santa Cruz

NRT. While the actual number of oaks is subject to debate, the site is true to its name in that it is shaded by a number of massive live oaks. Flowers—Indian paintbrush, yarrow, yellow lupines, and mariposa lilies, to name but a few—abound here in the spring and frame the monoliths standing sentinel over the edges of the meadow.

There are a few sites with stoves and fire pits distributed among the oaks; a few have picnic tables. Just upslope from camp you'll even find an old privy (it affords one very little privacy, be warned); the site also holds a spring-fed trough (water should be treated).

From camp, the trail continues north toward Little Pine Mountain, Happy Hollow, and the southern San Rafael Wilderness (see *Route 33*). Also see "Chapter 6: Santa Barbara Backcountry and Southern San Rafael Wilderness" for additional options.

Route 8

ARROYO BURRO (27W13)

LENGTH AND TYPE:	0.2-mile up-and-back from Arroyo Burro Turnout to East Camino Cielo; 11-mile up-and-back from Jesusita Trailhead to East Camino Cielo; 10.7-mile one-way for complete traverse
RATING:	Moderately strenuous (climb; steep at times)
TRAIL CONDITION:	Clear
MAP(S):	USGS *San Marcos Pass, Little Pine Mountain,* and *Santa Barbara* (route outdated; see sidebar on page 66); Conant's *Matilija & Dick Smith Wilderness*
CAMP(S):	—
HIGHLIGHTS:	Riparian trekking; great views from East Camino Cielo and numerous vantage points

TO REACH THE TRAILHEAD(S): *Jesusita Trailhead (Cater Plant):* From US 101 in Santa Barbara, take the Las Positas Road exit (Exit 100). If coming from the southeast, follow Calle Real for 0.33 mile before reaching Las Positas Road. Follow Las Positas Road (it becomes San Roque Road along the way) north 1.4 miles to the intersection with Foothill Road (CA 192). Cross Foothill Road and continue along San Roque Road another 0.5 mile (just past the Cater Water Treatment Plant) to a small **parking area (530', 249321E 3815921N)**. Parking is available on either side of the road; the trail begins at the north end of the left (eastern) parking area. There are no facilities here.

Arroyo Burro/Lower Oso Trailhead: See the Arroyo Burro Turnout for the Santa Ynez River (northern) trailhead.

TRIP SUMMARY: Arroyo Burro is really a tale of two trails: one lush that ascends the north-facing slopes of the Santa Ynez range to East Camino Cielo from the Santa Ynez River; the other a more exposed (and somewhat more challenging) ascent to East Camino Cielo from the outskirts of Santa Barbara. Both descriptions are presented as a climb from their respective trailheads to East Camino Cielo; if descending or doing the entire length, reverse the relevant description as necessary. Watch out for poison oak.

Note: The Jesusita Fire laid waste to the lower stretches of this route in 2009, and subsequent erosion has made sections of the trail of inconsistent quality and tread. Trail volunteers frequently repair and trim portions of the route, but be prepared for loose sections and various levels of regrowth in the years to come. Further, like many of the trails in the region, portions of this route (especially the northern half) are frequently traveled by mountain bikers, so do exercise caution (especially at blind corners).

Trip Description

Arroyo Burro Front (Jesusita Trailhead to East Camino Cielo)

From the **trailhead/parking area** (**530', 249321E 3815921N**), follow the trail (and old service road) northward and down under cover of coast live oaks and scrub. Follow the right fork at the first **junction** (**0.1 mile, 485', 249296E 3816039N**) to continue heading upstream. A number of spur trails—some tempting and well cut—provide alternatives, but stay low (left) to follow the course of San Roque Creek, through thistle- and fennel-lined trail, climbing very easily (and at times closely) along the stream's edge and passing by some avocado orchards on your right before coming to a very pleasant picnic area set beneath massive live oaks and with easy access to the creek. This spot is easily identified by the landmark wooden **table** (**0.4 mile, 620', 249397E 3816539N**).

From the table, continue through the well-shaded riparian cover of oaks and sycamores to the **junction** (**0.6 mile, 660', 249274E 3816623N**) of the Arroyo Burro and Jesusita Trails. Follow the left (north) fork (see *Route 17* for the route heading right) and drop immediately to a crossing of San Roque Creek and then up an old service road to the junction with **North Ontare Road** (**0.7 mile, 642', 249248E 3816598N**). This is a residential area, which the trail follows for a short while, so please respect the local residents—remain on the road and keep hold of any canine companions. Follow the road up to the west—switchbacking past an enigmatic stone bench—to where the trail departs the road just outside the gates of San Roque Ranch. This junction is usually signed, and there is a very obvious **fire hydrant** (**1.2 miles, 955', 248681E 3817172N**) here.

From the road, follow the trail in a long crescent along the headwaters of an eastern tributary to Barger Canyon, connecting with a **dirt road** (**1.5 miles, 980', 248514E 3817620N**)

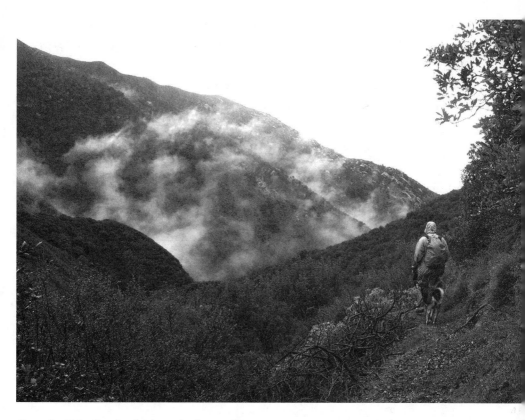

Dropping into the clouds along the Arroyo Burro

that runs along a low ridge. Access to this stretch was obtained through an easement with several of the local landowners, so respect their property and stay to the main road, passing avocado groves as you head northwest toward a pair of **water tanks (1.8 miles, 1,140', 248345E 3817875N)**. Again, this stretch is usually very well marked, with NO TRESPASSING signs at every "wrong" turn. Beyond the water tanks, continue climbing toward the end of the road, ducking under the final pylon of the power lines stretching across this portion of the land and heading up to the large sandstone formation known locally as **Autograph Rock (2.4 miles, 1,450', 248114E 3818598N)**, so named because vandals (well-meaning and not) have etched their messages in the soft sandstone here.

From these coarse sandstone clefts, continue climbing steadily through the thoroughly burned slopes with great views of San Roque Canyon; several of the darker red sandstone layers are composed of Sespe sandstone such as that found farther south in the Ojai district. Soon the trail levels off and leads eastward to a vista point with views of lower Barger Canyon. Continue down to the junction with a long-retired **service road (3.6 miles, 1,630',**

247563E 3819742N). There is often debris (large tree limbs, etc.) on the old road just below this junction as a reminder to hikers that they are progressing through private property and should only proceed up-canyon from this point.

The retired road here has been inundated with rockfall and debris from the slopes along its western edge since the Jesusita Fire; mind your footing as you progress to the first of three crossings of this, the easternmost fork of **San Antonio Creek** (**3.8 miles, 1,780', 247646E 3819862N**). This cool stretch is well shaded by alders, bays, and sycamores, and on warm days it can provide a welcome respite from the exposed climbing of the previous stretch. It may also prove an ideal lunch or rest spot before you embark on the climb toward East Camino Cielo.

After crossing San Antonio Creek for the third time and then passing an old concrete **spring box** (**4.2 miles, 1,980', 247911E 3820334N**), your route returns to singletrack and climbs steadily. This stretch was spared the ravages of the recent fire, and while no longer the shady riparian climes of the ravine below, it does provide slightly more cover (in the form of yucca, low oaks, and chaparral) than the earlier climb. Wildflower displays are often impressive in the spring; lupines and the less-common mariposa lilies especially thrive here (as do poison oak and a disproportionate number of ticks, so check your waistbands).

After a rather steep mile, you'll cross the headwaters of the creek and pass through the more exposed grass and talus of the canyon's upper reaches to reach the junction with **East Camino Cielo** (**5.5 miles, 3,050', 247246E 3821602N**).

THE "NEW" ARROYO BURRO ■ ■ ■ ■ ■ ■ ■ ■ ■ ■ ■

The Arroyo Burro route is one of the historical routes used by the Chumash to traverse the Santa Ynez range. Hunters, explorers, prospectors, and sundry others also used the route to access the Santa Ynez River area and what is now the San Rafael Wilderness. But in the early 1970s the corporate owner of the land (across which a significant portion of the front trail passed) fenced off the area to keep out trespassers. A few years later the County of Santa Barbara engaged the corporation in a drawn-out legal battle claiming the public had a right to the trail due to the historical precedent of use . . . but the county lost. Only in recent years—in conjunction with some land development along the contested stretch—has an easement been negotiated.

The 1995 *Santa Barbara* 7.5-minute quad shows the historical incarnation of the trail and should not be relied upon for trail-finding. Refer instead to Maps 4 and 6 on pages 48–49 and 94–95 or Conant's *Matilija & Dick Smith Wilderness* map.

■ ■

Arroyo Burro North (Lower Oso to East Camino Cielo)

From the **Arroyo Burro Turnout** (**1,075', 245619E 3826023N**), follow the road eastward to the old Arroyo Burro **service road** (**0.5 mile, 1,020', 246409E 3825661N**; also known as Forest Route 5N20), which departs from the sealed road and drops into the Santa Ynez (during or after any measurable rain, this can often entail getting one's feet wet). Just past the crossing you have the option to keep to the dirt road or take the trail that splits from the road on your left (east) to head up through the oak woodland for nearly a mile. Whichever route you choose, after 2 miles you'll again reach the **junction** (**1.7 miles, 1,340', 246925E 3824519N**) of the trail and road. Follow the road uphill (southward) here under the dappled shade of some rather impressively massive valley oaks. The private White Oaks Camp is on your right (west) here. Keep right at the junction just beyond, and again as the road splits between a short route to some water tanks or the singletrack (head for the singletrack).

Once on the trail proper, you'll steadily climb under cover of mature sycamores, bays, big-leaf maples, and oaks, crossing the creek after each series of switchbacks over the course of about 1.25 miles. After the third such creek **crossing** (**3.4 miles, 2,100', 246953E 3822723N**) you'll have gained a good view of your progress, the Santa Ynez River Valley, and the drainage to your west. Continue along the eastern edge of this drainage before another series of switchbacks leads you into the more exposed yucca- and chaparral-dotted terrain and to the junction with the upper stretch of the Arroyo Burro **service road** (**4.6 miles, 2,990', 247083E 3821926N**). Turn right (south) here and follow Arroyo Burro Road up and past the gate and then through the litter and detritus left by slack target shooters to **East Camino Cielo** (**4.8 miles, 3,050', 247258E 3821640N**).

Route 9

CAMUESA CONNECTOR TRAIL (27W09)

LENGTH AND TYPE:	8-mile out-and-back from Camuesa Connector trailhead; 10.2-mile loop via Buckhorn-Camuesa and Paradise Roads
RATING:	Moderate (climb)
TRAIL CONDITION:	Clear
MAP(S):	USGS *San Marcos Pass* and *Little Pine Mountain*; Conant's *Matilija & Dick Smith Wilderness* or *San Rafael Wilderness*
CAMP(S):	—
HIGHLIGHTS:	Excellent views of the Santa Ynez River Valley

TO REACH THE TRAILHEAD(S): Use the Camuesa Connector trailhead for this route.

TRIP SUMMARY: This route climbs along the southern flank of Camuesa Peak from the Santa Ynez River to Buckhorn-Camuesa Road. Hot and dry in the summer, this trail is better known as a mountain bike and/or equestrian route, but it can still make for a fine day trip on foot. Cyclists tend to make the trip in clockwise fashion (climbing the road and descending the singletrack). The route is described as an up-and-back from Paradise Road, but see Map 4 on pages 48–49 to consider other permutations.

Note: The 1995 *Little Pine Mountain* quad shows a different route; the trail as depicted on the map follows more of the firebreak than the actual trail described herein.

Trip Description

From the Camuesa Connector **trailhead (1,100', 249002E 3825014N)** on the north shoulder of Paradise Road, follow the singletrack to the banks of the Santa Ynez River and cross the riverbed. This crossing can entail wet feet or waist-deep wading in the winter and spring, or it can be a simple walk across bone-dry cobbles in the summer. Be prepared for both.

Across the river, signage directs you along the singletrack, which in the early stretch is a pleasant rolling affair through low chaparral and brush. While you are making a net elevation gain, there are numerous (usually dry) ravines and tributaries into which you'll drop and then out of which you'll climb, making much of this route something of a seesaw. A series of **serpentine formations (2.3 miles, 2,075', 248859E 3826758N)** marks a (relative) leveling off as the trail continues to lead upward on a slightly less taxing grade toward the **saddle (3.6 miles, 2,300', 248131E 3827107N)** that is your high point.

From the saddle, drop easily to the **junction (3.8 miles, 2,100', 247682E 3827484N)** with the firebreaks at the foot of the meadow. A quarter mile to the right (north) through the grasses here puts you at the junction with the **Buckhorn-Camuesa Road (4 miles, 2,210', 247489E 3827968N)**. Return the way you came.

Route 10

MATIAS TRAIL (27W19 and 27W25)

LENGTH AND TYPE:	2.2-mile out-and-back from Paradise Road to Matias Potrero Camp; 6.4 miles from Arroyo Burro Road to Gibraltar Road (Forest Route 5N25)
RATING:	Moderate
TRAIL CONDITION:	Well maintained and clear (partial former service road and shared-use singletrack, in recent years used for a popular local endurance run and maintained by volunteers)
MAP(S):	USGS *Little Pine Mountain* and *Santa Barbara*; Conant's *Matilija & Dick Smith Wilderness*
CAMP(S):	Matias Potrero
HIGHLIGHTS:	Excellent views of Santa Ynez River and surrounding ranges

TO REACH THE TRAILHEAD(S): *Arroyo Burro Road:* If starting from the western Paradise Road approach, see the directions for the Arroyo Burro Turnout. Follow the initial trail description for Arroyo Burro North in *Route 8*. At the junction just above White Oaks Camp where the service road splits, continue along the road (left fork) another 1.9 miles to the trail **junction (1,900', 247663E 3823787N)**. This adds 3.5 miles to your hike.

If starting from the eastern Paradise Road approach, use the **Matias Connector Trailhead** and refer to the sidebar on page 71.

If coming from East Camino Cielo near the **shooting range (3,050', 247258E 3821640N)**, hike northward down Arroyo Burro Road (Forest Route 5N20) 3.1 miles to the western trail **junction (1,900', 247663E 3823787N)**.

If coming from East Camino Cielo at **Angostura Pass (3,370', 252164E 3820489N)**, hike northward down Gibraltar Road 0.2 mile to the trail **junction (3,310', 252303E 3820930N)**.

TRIP SUMMARY: This moderately easy route leads from Arroyo Burro Road to the closed dirt stretch of upper Gibraltar Road, weaving in and out of drainages along the northern flanks of the Santa Ynez Mountains. The route seems uncommonly heavy with ticks.

Trip Description

If coming from East Camino Cielo (Angostura Pass), follow the closed dirt Gibraltar Road 0.2 mile north from the road's junction at East Camino Cielo to the **upper trailhead (3,010', 252301E 3820929N)**. *Note:* The 1995 *Little Pine Mountain* quad and most maps show the connector to be an additional 1.1 miles farther down the road from its actual location. This is an older (firebreak) route and no longer maintained (refer to Conant's *Matilija & Dick Smith Wilderness* or Map 4).

This route is described in two parts—the bulk being the main Matias Potrero, which traverses the northern flanks of the Santa Ynez Mountains from Arroyo Burro. This trail (27W19) is described from Arroyo Burro in the west to the eastern terminus at Forest Route 5N25. As neither end of the trail is accessible by passenger vehicle, the additional mileage should be accounted for when planning. You can also design a route utilizing the mile-long Matias Connector (27W25), which intersects the Matias Trail at about its halfway point, from Paradise Road (see sidebar on page 71).

From the Matias Trail junction at **Arroyo Burro Road (1,900', 247663E 3823787N)**, follow the trail eastward along a fairly well-worn trail. You're following a long-retired service road dating from the early half of the 20th century, originally graded for use by utilities trucks during the construction and early maintenance of the power lines that stretch across the river valley. Earlier guides have alluded to how the map and a quick mental calculation as to your mean elevation loss can be somewhat deceptive. Over the course of the next 2.5 miles—while neither losing nor gaining much elevation—you'll be dropping into one drainage, up the other side to gain the next ridge, and then back down into the next. This seesawing makes for a wonderful hike, but know that it's not as level as it may look.

Vistas of the various drainages—as well as the Santa Ynez River and mountains beyond—are nearly constantly in view as you make your way eastward. Ticks seem especially prevalent along this route, and nowhere does that hold true more than in the initial mile. The thirsty little arachnids will likely be found on your socks or lower extremities in little time, so be sure to check both you and any four-legged companions when taking breaks. There are three creek crossings along this route before you climb one final low ridge to reach the **Matias Junction (2.5 miles, 1,600', 250156E 3823427N)**, along a retired dirt road situated almost directly beneath the power lines.

From this junction, the route left (west) leads down to Paradise Road (see "Matias Connector (27W25)" opposite). The main Matias Trail continues to your right (east), climbing easily less than 0.25 mile to the junction with the **spur trail (2.7 miles, 1,700', 250334E 3823417N)** leading to Matias Potrero Camp.

CAMP :: MATIAS POTRERO

ELEVATION:	1,700'
MAP:	USGS *Little Pine Mountain*
UTM:	250525E 3823373N

This site, a fairly new one by this area's standards (meaning it's fewer than 80 or so years old), includes a small corral just east of the kitchen area. The site proper is set within a cluster of mature live oaks and contains a single fire pit with stove and (at this writing) an aging table.

From this junction, the trail leads you farther east, climbing steadily (but not steeply) and passing in and out of two more drainages. Pass through the handsome meadow that, were it not for the lack of water, one might think would have made a far better location for a camp than the site actually used. From the second of these crossings, you'll begin the steady climb to the southeast, hedged in for extended periods by chaparral and chamise, and soon arrive at the junction with **Devils Canyon Trail (4.7 miles, 2,450', 252248E 3822332N)**. It's not quite 2 miles of climbing through high chaparral and oak—with a smattering of big-leaf maples, bays, and madrones toward the very end—to reach **Gibraltar Road (6.4 miles, 3,310', 252303E 3820930N)**. It's another 0.25 mile to the gate at Angostura Pass and **East Camino Cielo (6.7 miles, 3,370', 252164E 3820489N)**.

■ ■ ■ ■ ■ ■ ■ ■ ■   **MATIAS CONNECTOR (27W25)**

From the Matias Connector **trailhead (1,100', 249863E 3824597N)** beside Paradise Road, walk around the gate and proceed southwest up the initially fairly steep and cobble-strewn road. Live oaks shade the lower stretches, and the banks are heavy with bigberry manzanita as you climb with less exertion toward the power lines to the south. After a steady mile of climbing, you'll reach the **Matias Junction (0.9 mile, 1,600', 250156E 3823427N)**, directly beneath those ubiquitous power lines. Refer to the main narrative for your options from here.

■ ■

Route 11

GIBRALTAR TRAIL (28W06)

LENGTH AND TYPE:	7-mile out-and-back to Gibraltar Dam from Red Rock Trailhead (via trail); 9.5-mile one-way from Red Rock Trailhead to junction with upper Cold Spring Trail
RATING:	Easy to moderate (distance)
TRAIL CONDITION:	Well maintained (service road), clear (heavily used singletrack), and passable (rock-hopping and some lightly used trail)
MAP(S):	USGS *Little Pine Mountain*, Conant's *Matilija & Dick Smith Wilderness*
CAMP(S):	—
HIGHLIGHTS:	Red Rock swimming area; Gibraltar Reservoir; abandoned Sunbird Mine; Santa Ynez River Valley

TO REACH THE TRAILHEAD(S): Use the Red Rock Trailhead to access this route.

TRIP SUMMARY: From Red Rock, this route follows the Santa Ynez River upstream to Gibraltar Reservoir, and then continues along retired roads of varying condition to the junction with the upper Cold Spring Trail.

Trip Description

From **Red Rock Trailhead (1,150', 251064E 3824758N)**, follow the trail eastward into the Santa Ynez riverbed. This stretch will be an exercise in some rock-hopping and numerous creek crossings, but the route is heavily traveled and therefore easy to follow. Alternatively, if you haven't any desire to get your feet wet or trek along the canyon floor, you can also follow Paradise Road (still Forest Road 5N18) to parallel the southern banks of the river (and save 0.5 mile of hiking), though the initial climb from the parking area and another just near the base of the dam are quite steep.

Follow the trail through the snaking riverbed, where the Santa Ynez cuts through a veritable laundry list of rock along the Little Pine Fault: limestone, serpentine, sandstone, and shale all compete for attention. This stretch can be especially crowded (and is perhaps best avoided) during holidays and summer weekends. At the next major right (south) bend in the river, you may notice the cut of an old route that switchbacks up the riverbank on your left (this route—marginally passable on foot—leads past an old mine along the northeast face of the knoll, and then down to a small man-made pond along the edge of the reservoir; it is not advised).

From Red Rock, continue following the trail upstream as your route crisscrosses the Santa Ynez River a handful of times over the course of 3 miles before a final impressive wading pool and a last **crossing** (**2.9 miles, 1,240', 253058E 3823347N**), which will reconnect you with the road near **North Portal** (**3 miles, 1,250', 253209E 3823357N**). The impressive pools at the base of the dam—like much of this area—are off-limits and property of the City of Santa Barbara. The North Portal is the starting point for the Santa Barbara Water Tunnel (also known as the Mission Tunnel) and travels 3.7 miles to the southwest to the appropriately named South Portal in Santa Barbara.

The oak-dotted flat on the left (north) side of the river directly across from here is where the Gibraltar Campground once stood. During the dam's and tunnel's construction, workers lived at the site, and the facility was opened as a campground in 1934. Tables, stoves, and a pit toilet were provided, even after the site was re-designated as a day-use-only area in 1974 in an attempt to curb the litter and wear to which the site was subjected. While the concrete footings of the main structure and even concrete steps of the toilet still stand, little else remains of the camp, and it faded out of use in the 1980s.

ROCKS OF GIBRALTAR ■ ■ ■ ■ ■ ■ ■ ■ ■ ■ ■ ■ ■

The Gibraltar Reservoir, known in its early decades as Santa Barbara Reservoir, was formed upon completion of the constant radius, concrete arch Gibraltar Dam. Begun in 1914 and completed in 1920, the dam is owned and maintained by the City of Santa Barbara and is second only to the massive Lake Cachuma project in volume provided to the city. The entire reservoir is closed to swimming, boating, and fishing. Numerous NO TRESPASSING signs abound to remind visitors of the fact.

According to the County of Santa Barbara Public Works Department, by 1945 sedimentation had reduced the reservoir's capacity by nearly half (from 14,500 acre-feet to approximately 7,800 acre-feet). This decrease in capacity led to the construction of a 23-foot extension in 1948, restoring the reservoir's capacity to roughly its original level. Since then, continued sedimentation reduces capacity by approximately 150 acre-feet per year.

The city did at one time utilize a dredge to clear sediment from the reservoir (the practice has since ceased). The 2007 Zaca Fire has further increased the rate of sedimentation and quite likely lowered the quality of water (which in turn will increase the treatment costs when the water reaches the Cater filtration plant).

Once on the road, follow it farther toward the reservoir. If you're looking for the lower trailhead for the **Devils Canyon Trail (1,280', 253223E 3823196N)**, it's an easy 0.25 mile south up the road. Climb eastward along the service road (views of the spillway here are excellent), passing the junction with the spur road leading to the dam outbuildings. Continue along the road past a private residence on your right (south) until you reach a **junction (4 miles, 1,600', 254236E 3823349N)** where the left (east) portion of road is gated.

This is the old road that traces the southern perimeter of the reservoir. Follow this retired service road with very little elevation gain—your initial drop down to and across **Gidney Creek (4.8 miles, 1,410', 254865E 3822940N)** is recovered with the climb back up on the other side. Once out of the Gidney drainage, it's a very pleasant and usually well-shaded trek beneath big-leaf maples, oaks, and sycamores to the intersection with the old road **spur (6.3 miles, 1,600', 256044E 3823455N)** leading to the abandoned quicksilver mine.

SUNBIRD MINE

The rusting, fenced-off ruins you see here are the long-abandoned facilities of the quicksilver mine formerly (most recently) operated by Sunbird Mines LTD.

A report filed by the California State Mining Bureau in 1918 described the property—the Milburn-McAvoy and Snow claims —as "somewhat inaccessible, being reached by trail over the Santa Ynez Mountains 13 miles from Santa Barbara, or by wagon road, 40 miles. It can also be reached via the Santa Barbara Water Tunnel, being two miles east of the north portal."

The mine was worked intermittently from the 1870s until 1992, by which time the remoteness of the operation and mercury prices rendered it patently unprofitable. Old engines, payload cars, rail, abandoned trucks, and the old mining buildings and smelter still stand

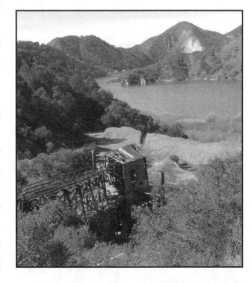

sentinel over this quiet corner of the Santa Ynez River Valley. The mine shafts are largely filled in with fallen timbers and dirt fill; a heavy-gauge steel barrier has been set at the entrance to deter those who may wish to explore the damp and dank cavern.

■   ■   ■   ■   ■   ■   ■   ■   ■   ■   ■   ■   ■   ■   ■   ■   ■   ■   ■

Continuing eastward past the mine turnoff, the old road slowly narrows (and the pink conglomerate across which you've been hiking eventually gives way to an increasingly faint graded road). At the end of the road, a lightly used singletrack leads rather easily southeast—the mature trees you enjoyed en route to the mine giving way to yucca, chamise, and manzanita—to the **junction** with the upper portion of the Cold Spring Canyon East trail (**9.5 miles, 1,650', 258391E 3821608N**; see *Route 24*).

Route 12

MONO-ALAMAR and ALAMAR HILL TRAILS (26W07, 26W16)

LENGTH AND TYPE:	23.4-mile out-and-back to Lower Alamar Camp; 13.8-mile one-way to Rollins Camp; 13.9-mile one-way to Dick Smith Wilderness and Alamar Trail
RATING:	Moderate
TRAIL CONDITION:	Passable (seldom maintained; receives little traffic)
MAP(S):	USGS *Little Pine Mountain, Hildreth Peak,* and *Madulce Peak;* Conant's *Matilija & Dick Smith Wilderness*
CAMP(S):	Lower Alamar and Rollins
HIGHLIGHTS:	Riparian trekking; access to Dick Smith Wilderness

TO REACH THE TRAILHEAD(S): Use the Mono Creek gate trailhead or Agua Caliente trailhead for this route; the trip is described from the Mono Creek gate.

TRIP SUMMARY: The Mono-Alamar Trail follows Mono Creek and then Alamar Creek upstream to the edge of the Dick Smith Wilderness.

Trip Description

From the **gate** (**1,520', 258686E 3824656N**) head west along the Romero-Camuesa Road (5N15) about 500 feet to the **junction** (**0.1 mile, 1,470', 258568E 3824735N**) with the Mono-Alamar Trail. Head north here along trail that can be a bit of a wander along the Mono Creek streambed. A mile of this will lead to the **junction** (**0.9 mile, 1,500', 259013E 3825424N**) with the abandoned stretch of 6N30 at another crossing. Continue following the track as it meanders time and again across Mono Creek. The route here is open and—while not typically maintained—still bears the grade of the old service road. Even when overgrown, this route can be navigated fairly well—the large trees and brush were cleared well enough in previous decades that the route still cuts a wide swath through the chaparral.

Follow the old road to a **junction (3 miles, 1,625', 259974E 3827280N)** with the steep spur trail and the main Mono-Alamar track; keep to the right (east) here. The track to the left leads to the Pie Canyon Fire Road, which at its western end connects with the Indian Creek Trail (see *Route 40*). Your route will also meet the **fire road (3.7 miles, 1,675', 260002E 3828044N)** but farther east near where the creek crosses the road and along an easier grade.

You'll merge with the **Hildreth Fire Road (3.9 miles, 1,680', 260063E 3828250N)** 0.25 mile farther. Head left (north) along this better-maintained (but at times, still brushy) road to the marked **turnoff (4.6 miles, 1,700', 260212E 3829174N)** just below Ogilvy Ranch. Drop into the creek and cross to begin the traverse of the east banks of Mono Creek.

■ ■ ■ ■ ■ ■ ■ ■ ■ ■ ■ ■ ■ ■ ■ ■ **OGILVY RANCH**

The Ogilvy Ranch—situated on the former Chumash village Sigvaya—has a colorful and at times bizarre history. Converted to Rancheria San Gervasio during the mission era and then abandoned, 160 acres of the site were homesteaded by the Hildreth brothers in 1894. It has passed hands several times since (retaining the Ogilvy moniker of its third owner) and still possesses numerous buildings. Once owned by an agricultural commune, and later some fringe religious interests, the site is known to have yielded numerous Chumash art sites, many of which were damaged during fire suppression efforts during the 1964 Coyote Fire.

In 1992, the US Forest Service (as part of its efforts to protect the habitat of the arroyo toad) closed the road leading up Mono Creek from the Romero-Camuesa Road. In reports, the U.S. Fish & Wildlife Service attributed the 18 crossings the road made along Mono Creek en route to the ranch as being "likely responsible for a depressed population of arroyo toads in Mono Creek." The subsequent closing of the road forced the owners at the time to use the Hildreth Fire Road, an exponentially longer and more difficult route to access the ranch. This and other factors ultimately led to the abandonment of the ranch. While still owned and occasionally visited by the owners, it is no longer regularly occupied.

That said, Ogilvy Ranch remains private property. Please respect the rights of the owners and stay on the bypass trail that skirts the eastern banks of Mono Creek while passing this unique corner of Los Padres history.

■ ■ ■ ■ ■ ■ ■ ■ ■ ■ ■ ■ ■ ■ ■ ■ ■ ■ ■ ■

The trail reconnects to the uppermost portion of the road north of the ranch, and then reduces to singletrack en route to the **departure from Mono Creek (9 miles, 2,200', 262251E 3833108N)**. While not an officially recognized camping area, there is often a serviceable guerrilla camp or two here along Mono Creek.

Here the trail climbs away from the creek, eschewing the old and rather challenging Mono Narrows route that lays ahead, instead continuing northward toward Alamar Hill. Now out of the riparian washes that were your route along Mono Creek, this stretch leads you through rocky oak-dappled scrub. Here, trail designations become a bit muddled, as what was once an extensive network of trails as late as the 1980s has been reduced to a collection of forgotten routes and official routes mangled by fire, regrowth, and general disrepair. Climb rather steeply for 2 miles—passing the old terminus to this route, which passes through the unique Caracole formation—and continue along an old dozer line to a cluster of oaks. Beneath these trees you'll find the **junction (10.9 miles, 2,850', 261645E 3835306N)** with the Alamar Hill Trail (see the "Alamar Hill" sidebar below for the trip description of the route climbing through Loma Pelona to the fire road and then descending to the Pens campsite on Indian Creek).

ALAMAR HILL ▨ ▨ ▨ ▨ ▨ ▨ ▨ ▨ ▨ ▨ ▨ ▨

The steep climb westward along Alamar Hill Trail is a small price to pay for the views commanded from Loma Pelona, a wide hilltop meadow. There are a number of metal posts rising above the grass to help guide you on your way, as the tread is often difficult to find. Climb from the junction through the grasses (minding your footing and watching for snakes) a steep mile to briefly join and then split again from an old doubletrack occasionally used by the private inholding here and then up to the **Don Victor–Loma Pelona Fire Road (1.6 miles from junction, 3,990', 259796E 3836087N)**. It's another mile down the west side to **Pens Camp** along Indian Creek **(2.7 miles from junction, 3,300', 258285E 3836285N)**.

Continue right (east) from this junction along the lowest portion of the Alamar Hill Trail, dropping along the grassy slopes and into the sycamore-, willow-, and alder-lined Alamar Creek watershed to **Lower Alamar Camp (11.7 miles, 2,890', 262697E 3835506N)**.

CAMP :: LOWER ALAMAR

ELEVATION:	2,890'
MAP:	USGS *Madulce Peak*
UTM:	262697E 3835506N

Formerly the site of a US Forest Service (USFS) administrative site, the iconic Alamar Tin Shack that once stood here was burned in 2007 (but not in the Zaca Fire). The 12-by-12-foot shack was used by the State Fish and Game field researchers in the early 20th century. The camp has received very little traffic and even less maintenance in recent years. Ruins of the corrugated tin building (siding, wood stoves, 50-gallon drums, etc.) are piled in the grassy meadow here; stoves hidden in the grass can be cleared out for a kitchen. Live oaks ring the meadow, and water can usually be had from Alamar Creek.

From Lower Alamar, the often-rough trail heads north along Alamar Creek to the **Don Victor–Loma Pelona Fire Road (13.4 miles, 3,070', 261977E 3836937N)**. Head right (east) 0.5 mile to reach **Rollins Camp (13.8 miles, 3,110', 262315E 3837083N)**. This stretch puts on a fairly impressive wildflower display in spring and early summer. Views along this road are excellent, revealing the grasses of Redondo Potrero and the folded geology of the Mono watershed up which you've just labored.

CAMP :: ROLLINS

ELEVATION:	3,110'
MAP:	USGS *Madulce Peak* (*Note:* Route not shown on most maps)
UTM:	262315E 3837083N

Though inexplicably dropped from recent USFS maps, Rollins is a pleasant site situated alongside the Don Victor–Loma Pelona Fire Road set within a ring of old live oaks (one of which still bears the old arc-welded steel camp sign). Named for the bulldozer operator who worked the jeepways in the areas, the site dates from the early 1980s.

Burned during the Zaca Fire, the site (as of this writing) features one rather charred (but functional) table and a newer additional table. Water can usually be retrieved from Alamar Creek.

Just the other side of the creek east along the road from Rollins is the start of the **Alamar Trail (13.9 miles, 3,125', 262351E 3837123N)**, which continues north to Alamar Saddle (see *Route 39*).

Route 13

AGUA CALIENTE TRAIL TO UPPER CALIENTE (25W06)

LENGTH AND TYPE:	0.6-mile one-way to Agua Caliente Debris Dam; 2.3-mile one-way to The Oasis; 5-mile out-and-back to Upper Caliente Camp
RATING:	Easy to moderate
TRAIL CONDITION:	Passable to Upper Caliente
MAP(S):	USGS *Hildreth Peak*; Conant's *Matilija & Dick Smith Wilderness*
CAMP(S):	Upper Caliente
HIGHLIGHTS:	Hot springs; debris dam; geology; the Oasis swimming hole

TO REACH THE TRAILHEAD(S): Use the Big Caliente Day-Use Area trailhead for this hike.

TRIP SUMMARY: This 5-mile round-trip travels up Agua Caliente Canyon past hot springs, a Depression-era debris dam, and a swimming hole to Upper Caliente campsite. This route can be brutally hot in the summer.

Trip Description

This area's hot springs were developed by George Knapp (of Knapp's Castle fame; see *Route 5*). The Big Caliente Hot Spring is just off the road. It is cemented, has a rail ladder and a picnic table set in the shade of palms and conifers, and is generally a nice place to relax (though the water is less refreshing in the summer). There is a small cinder-block building for use as a changing area as well. Agua Caliente is a more primitive set of tubs a few hundred yards up the old road, on the other side of the stream.

From **Big Caliente Day-Use Area (1,875', 264644E 3824942N)**, follow the trail heading upstream and pass all the hot spring tubs (save those for the return!). *Note:* The old trailhead sign alludes to La Carpa Potreros and Potrero Seco, destinations which in recent decades are rather difficult to achieve via this route; that portion of the trail is not described herein.

Follow the long-retired but well-trod service road through Agua Caliente Canyon, passing through chaparral, wildflowers, scrub, and fractured geology to cross the **creek (0.3 mile, 1,900', 264525E 3825344N)** at the first sharp bend. Continue eastward along the old road another 0.33 mile to the **use trail** leading down to the **Agua Caliente Debris Dam (0.6 mile, 2,000', 264895E 3825262N)**. Cottonwoods dominate the growth here.

■ ■ ■ ■ ■ ■ ■ ■ ■ ■ **DAM ALL THIS DEBRIS!**

The Agua Caliente Debris Dam, built by the Civilian Conservation Corps in 1936–1937 for the City of Santa Barbara to prevent sediment and debris from reaching the Gibraltar Reservoir, is a fascinating and nearly forgotten piece of watershed protection history. Rising 65 feet above the original creek bed, the single-arch concrete dam is 240 feet long and—like Mono Debris Dam to the west—is largely silted in after nearly a century of service.

■ ■ ■ ■ ■ ■ ■ ■ ■ ■ ■ ■ ■ ■ ■ ■ ■

Beyond the dam, the trail (now singletrack) leads through willows, cottonwoods, oaks, and grassy meadows along the snaking creek. You'll enter the Zaca burn zone just as you reach the **split (2.2 miles, 2,090', 265195E 3826530N)**, with one trail continuing toward camp and the other heading to the **Oasis (2.3 miles, 2,090', 265252E 3826789N)**. Take the left fork to reach the Oasis, once a magnificent swimming hole and one of the main attractions of this trail in years past. Unfortunately, the pool was heavily silted in after the Zaca Fire and as a result is presently far less impressive. When the creek has good flow, however, it still makes for a fine spot to wade, and the falls—which flow through a notch in the tilted sandstone strata—are refreshing. To reach Upper Caliente Camp or the upper stretches of the canyon, you can either backtrack to the junction or scramble back up to the trail on the east side of the creek. **Upper Caliente Camp (2.5 miles, 2,175', 265327E 3826946N)** is set 0.25 mile upstream.

CAMP :: UPPER CALIENTE

ELEVATION:	2,175'
MAP:	USGS *Hildreth Peak*
UTM:	265327E 3826946N

Already a fairly barren site when the Zaca Fire tore through in 2007, Upper Caliente offers the backcountry camper fairly little. There is a grate stove, and the two benches were replaced in early 2010.

Upper Caliente is effectively the end of this route; return the way you came at your leisure. From Upper Caliente, the old trail pushes through the wide expanse of grass to the north. The hearty may wish to pursue the old course, but it is not recommended lest you are prepared for a hard slog. The old USGS *Hildreth Peak* quad shows the route rather accurately—as do many GPS data sets—however, once onto USGS *Old Man Mountain* the trail is no longer shown. It's not impossible . . . just not overly recommended.

Route 14

FORBUSH-MONO (Upper Cold Spring East Trail [26W10])

LENGTH AND TYPE:	3.4-mile out-and-back to Forbush Flat; 5.3-mile one-way to Mono Campground
RATING:	Moderate
TRAIL CONDITION:	Clear to passable
MAP(S):	USGS *Santa Barbara* and *Little Pine Mountain*; Conant's *Matilija & Dick Smith Wilderness*
CAMP(S):	Forbush
HIGHLIGHTS:	Forbush orchard; fascinating geology; riparian trekking

TO REACH THE TRAILHEAD(S): *Cold Spring Saddle:* From the junction of US 101 and CA 154 in Santa Barbara, follow CA 154 (also San Marcos Pass Road) north 7.8 miles to East Camino Cielo Road (also Forest Road 5N12). Turn right (east) here and continue along East Camino Cielo 14.7 miles to the Cold Spring Saddle **parking area (3,400', 257657E 3818995N)**. The trail to access Forbush and Blue Canyons begins on the north side of the road. There are no facilities here.

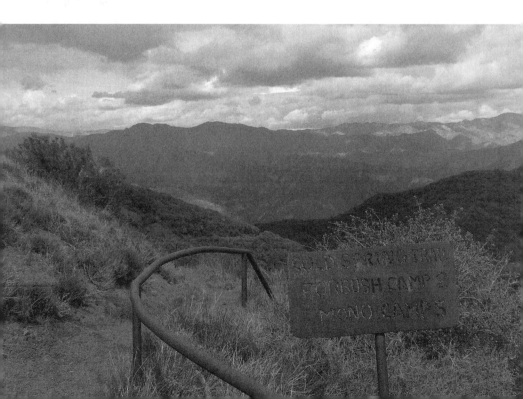

Alternately, from the junction of CA 192 and Mountain Drive in Santa Barbara, follow Mountain Drive north 0.2 mile to the junction with Gibraltar Road. Turn left (north) at this dogleg and continue along Gibraltar Road 7.3 miles (this is a slow and winding route) to its intersection with East Camino Cielo Road (also Forest Road 5N12). Turn right (east) here and continue along East Camino Cielo for 3.6 miles to the Cold Spring Saddle **parking area (3,400', 257657E 3818995N)**.

Mono Campground: Use the Mono Campground trailhead for the lower portion.

TRIP SUMMARY: From Cold Spring Saddle, the Forbush-Mono route follows a historical northward route along drainages to the Santa Ynez/Mono Creek confluence. Watch out for poison oak.

Trip Description

From the Cold Spring Saddle **parking area (3,400', 257657E 3818995N)**, cross East Camino Cielo to the trailhead directly across the western edge of the parking area. A rusted arc-welded sign posting rough mileages to Forbush Camp ("2 miles") and Mono Camp ("5 miles") guides you to the start. This trail is officially an extension of the 26W10 trail (see *Route 24: East Fork Cold Spring*) but is often simply referred to as the Forbush Trail or the Forbush-Mono Route.

Follow the trail southward down the fairly gentle descent. The trail here is usually clear and easygoing, with an easy series of switchbacks leading you along a low chaparral ridge and then looping back northward into the upper stretches of the drainage. Clusters of the fairly rare (and by some accounts, endangered) Humboldt's lily and brambles of blackberry usher you to the crossing at **Bulkley Spring (0.5 mile, 3,100', 257909E 3819194N)**, where an old concrete spring box and a small green wooden bench stand. (The spring is dedicated to Edward Addison Bulkley, a New York–born Harvard grad who died in Albuquerque in March 1916.)

This cool little spot is an ideal respite or first water break; for those coming from below it can prove a most welcome respite after their climb. This spot—which gladly sacrifices any views for nearly 360-degree shade—is also a sampler of numerous tree species. The usual bays, sycamores, and live oaks are omnipresent, but various species not often seen in such close proximity abound: Pacific madrones just to the north, numerous knobcone pines with a handful of the uncommon Bishop pines for good measure, as well as a cluster of poplars in the ravine immediately downstream from the spring.

From this cool retreat, continue along the east bank of this drainage—passing through a grove of pines and then crossing two tributaries in quick succession—along more of the classic hillside chaparral. After a mile of easy hiking during which you'll cross a few bands of geologic conglomerate, you'll then reach a **gap (1 mile, 2,900', 258002E 3819824N)** with expansive views not only of your destination but also of Forbush and Blue Canyons to your east (along with the ubiquitous power lines, a constant in this stretch of Santa Barbara–area trails). Jameson Lake can also be made out in the distance from this vantage point.

Continue along the drainage down another set of switchbacks and past another gap (this one marked by an incongruous Aleppo pine) into a north-facing **slope** (**1.4 miles, 2,600', 257989E 3820223N**) populated by a cluster of Pacific madrones and then down through some mature live oaks to the **junction** (**1.7 miles, 2,425', 257864E 3820446N**) leading to Forbush Flat and the camp.

CAMP :: FORBUSH

ELEVATION:	2,375'
MAP:	USGS *Santa Barbara*
UTM:	257770E 3820421N

Established by the US Forest Service (USFS) in 1934 and named for homesteader and pioneer Fred Forbush, Forbush Flat is situated right along the Santa Ynez fault, and the resultant uplifting in the area has left many exposed fossil-laden layers (and makes this spot a prime destination for those interested in geology). The camp still bears some of the apple and pear trees Mr. Forbush nurtured in the early 1900s.

The upper camp (where the Forbush Cabin once stood) also features a smattering of incense cedars. Huge live oaks dominate the immediate camp area, and a handful of madrones supplant their smaller manzanita cousins along the camp's perimeter.

The lower (main) camp beside the creek and flats is shaded by more mature oaks, a stand of pines, and the thick alders along the creek. Upper Gidney Creek can be dry here, but even in the driest months water can usually be found in some pools along the creek.

From the junction to Forbush Flat, it's a quick drop down a short set of switchbacks into the boulder-dotted gap that is the **Mono-Forbush Junction** (**1.8 miles, 2,340', 257882E 3820492N**); see *Route 15* for the trail heading east.

From the junction, a fossil-strewn stretch of trail leads up and around a rocky outcrop to a **gap** (**2 miles, 2,520', 258042E 3820565N**) with commanding views of the local drainage. The trail drops steeply along a series of long chaparral switchbacks (often choked with poison oak) before crossing the **creek** (**2.8 miles, 1,840', 258166E 3821200N**). Now oaks, alders, sycamores, and the occasional big-leaf maple shade much of your route as you cross the creek a handful of times. Note especially the magnificent fern-draped pools formed by the unusually heavy mineral content of the creek along the steep drainage. The most impressive of these is known as the Lower Emerald Pool.

Numerous flowers—among them more Humboldt's spotted lilies and scarlet bugler penstemon—dot the trailside to the junction with the **Gibraltar Trail (3.1 miles, 1,650', 258391E 3821608N)**. Here the quality of trail diminishes noticeably. As you drop into a sandy wash along the creek, USFS-placed Carsonite signs indicate a **designated route (3.6 miles, 1,450', 258587E 3822059N)** leading left (west) just before you reach the Santa Ynez riverbed. This rerouting of parts of the trail in an effort to protect a number of the Los Padres' most endangered species (e.g., California red-legged frogs, arroyo toads, southwestern pond turtles, and steelhead trout) has resulted in numerous use trails fanning out once the trail reaches the **Santa Ynez River**. This designated route is often choked with growth and can be slowgoing, but it leads you quickly to the river's edge.

As a result of these factors—along with whatever flow and debris is present—the crossing of the river here, while not technical nor usually even entailing wet feet, isn't always at the same spot. But **cross** you will (**at approximately 3.7 miles, 1,450'**), to eventually gain the trail along the other side. Keep high on your right (north, and then east) here to keep the route into Mono Creek, especially in years when Gibraltar Reservoir (**spillway elevation 1,399'**) is at or near capacity. *Note:* The trail can be intermittent, and to reach Mono Camp (the formal terminus of the trail) requires a degree of route-finding; if navigating with a GPS receiver, it's advisable to record a waypoint of your destination before you set out.

You'll leave the cottonwood- and willow-covered riverbed for a stretch of chaparral **trail (3.8 miles, 1,575', 258268E 3822471N)**, which will lead you around a knoll and toward the confluence of Mono Creek and the Santa Ynez River near the head of the reservoir. On the other side, after some progress through willow and riparian cover, another rocky ascent leads you out of the drainage and through some oaks up and over into what is known colloquially as the "Mono Jungle." Your route now is upstream along the sandy beds of Mono Creek; shale from the Juncal formation overlays exposed limestone strata on your left (south). Along with heavy cover of white alders and the usual suspects of flora along the perimeter of the creek, thick-pod milk vetches bloom here and there.

Watch for a spur trail coming in from your right (north); this is the route back to the Mono Campground **parking area (5.3 miles, 1,450', 258814E 3823850N)**. If you reach the debris dam, you've overshot the turnoff; simply keep to the east and backtrack a few hundred yards to gain Mono Campground.

■ ■ ■ ■ ■ ■ ■ ■ ■ ■ ■ ■ MONO DEBRIS DAM

An easy destination for day hikers based along Camuesa Road and its campgrounds, the Mono Debris Dam offers an interesting glimpse into the watershed management for Gibraltar Reservoir (one of Santa Barbara's primary sources of water).

Built in 1933 by the Civilian Conservation Corps, the dam was one of two such barriers constructed in response to the increasing sediment (particularly postfire) from certain tributaries into the reservoir (the other was the Agua Caliente Dam to the east, completed in 1937). Built of reinforced concrete, it rises 35 feet above the streambed and spans 192 feet wide. It is a buttress dam (also called an Ambursen dam after the engineer who made frequent use of the design in the early 20th century), meaning the structure is supported at intervals by numerous buttresses. U.S. Department of Agriculture reports from the 1936–37 and 1937–38 runoff seasons indicate the dam's basin was entirely filled with coarse sediment, with the load backing up a half mile upstream.

The dam doesn't offer any official access, and one has to scale onto the lower catwalk to gain access to the structure.

■ ■ ■ ■ ■ ■ ■ ■ ■ ■ ■ ■ ■ ■ ■ ■ ■ ■ ■ ■

Route 15

FORBUSH and BLUE CANYONS

LENGTH AND TYPE:	7.8-mile out-and-back from Blue Canyon Pass to Cottam Camp;
	7.5-mile one-way from Blue Canyon Pass to Cold Spring Saddle trailhead;
	5.8-mile one-way from Blue Canyon Pass to Forbush Camp
RATING:	Easy to moderate
TRAIL CONDITION:	Clear
MAP(S):	USGS *Santa Barbara, Carpinteria,* and *Hildreth Peak;* Conant's *Matilija & Dick Smith Wilderness*
CAMP(S):	Upper Blue Canyon, Blue Canyon, Cottam, and Forbush
HIGHLIGHTS:	Riparian and arroyo willow trekking; serpentine formations in Blue Canyon

TO REACH THE TRAILHEAD(S): Use the Upper Blue Canyon Trailhead for this route.

TRIP SUMMARY: This popular route traverses the drainages of Escondido Creek (named Blue Canyon for its serpentine rock outcrops) and Forbush Canyon through oak-shaded trail and grassy meadows. It's hot in the summer but otherwise a great year-round destination.

Trip Description

From the **Upper Blue Canyon Trailhead (2,125', 264961E 3819093N)**, follow the trail down into the Escondido Creek drainage along crumbling shale and the occasional sandstone exposure. Flowers are pleasant here in the spring, but come summer this stretch is often choked with star thistle and various burr-bearing growth, so pants or gaiters are worth considering.

After a mile of easy and gradual descent, you'll reach the first **crossing** (**1 mile, 1,940',
263678E 3819236N**), a cool and verdant refuge lined with mint, berry brambles, and (of
course) poison oak. You'll continue another 0.5 mile along the alder- and oak-shaded route
until you cross an intermittent tributary and rather unexpectedly walk into **Upper Blue
Canyon Camp** (**1.6 miles, 1,900', 263021E 3819574N**).

CAMP :: UPPER BLUE CANYON

ELEVATION:	1,900'
MAP:	USGS *Carpinteria*
UTM:	263021E 3819574N

A small site set beside Escondido Creek, this camp is beneath a cluster of oaks and
features a fairly new wooden table. Poison oak rings the creekside perimeter, and
there is really only room for one tent. While the Blue Canyon Trail is not heavily
traveled, this site does have the disadvantage of being right on the trail; the fire ring
(sans stove) and table are mere feet from the trail. It makes a better picnic or lunch
spot than an overnight destination. Water can usually be pulled from the creek just
beyond camp.

From camp, follow the trail westward rather steeply into the ravine and up the other side.
Here your route embarks among the namesake blue rock formations, crisscrossing the creek
numerous times along willow arroyo terrain en route to the Upper Romero Trail **junction**
(**2.5 miles, 1,750', 261796E 3819707N**). Large conglomerate boulders also dot the hillsides at
points, and a seasonal tributary to Escondido Creek is just beyond this junction if you wish
to replenish your water supply before endeavoring up the steep slope here; see sidebar in
Route 30 for the route back to Romero-Camuesa Road.

If continuing along Blue Canyon, after a few minutes' walk from the Romero
junction—and a pair of stream crossings—you'll encounter a **spur trail** (**2.8 miles, 1,690',
261473E 3818149N**), where on the north side of the trail a small clearing opens to reveal an
old steel sign indicating **Blue Canyon Camp** just beyond.

CAMP :: BLUE CANYON

ELEVATION:	1,680'
MAP:	USGS *Carpinteria*
UTM:	261516E 3820028N

Sometimes referred to as Lower Blue Canyon Camp, this relatively spacious camp
is likely the nicest along the Blue Canyon route, with a wooden table, three old ice

can stoves, and a fire ring with stove. The Coyote Fire that tore through the region in 1964 didn't reach this area, so it's managed to retain much of its original charm. There is room enough for a few tents, and it even features an old metal privy just west of camp. The creek is easily reached via a use trail to the north (be mindful of poison oak here and around the edges of camp in general).

A number of the canyon's namesake serpentine formations can be seen especially well from the creek bed.

Note: Blue Canyon is incorrectly shown on the south side of the trail on the 1995 *Carpinteria* quad.

From Blue Canyon Camp, continue westward to leave the drainage and ascend a low **gap** (**3.75 miles, 1,620', 260356E 3820200N**). With a view of the huge power lines, drop into the wide field and skirt its eastern edge, rejoining Escondido Creek once again as you enter **Cottam Camp (3.9 miles, 1,550', 260226E 3820321N)**.

CAMP :: COTTAM

ELEVATION:	1,550'
MAP:	USGS *Carpinteria*
UTM:	260226E 3820321N

A barren but well-shaded spot at the northeast edge of the field, this camp—especially beautiful in the spring and fall—is the site of a cabin built by Albert Cottam (among others) in 1915. Evidence of structures nearby are from Camp Ynez, once operated as a guest facility. A table and fire ring (no stove) are available, and space to pitch tents can be had beneath some trees to the south.

Note: Cottam Camp is shown several hundred yards southwest of its actual location on the 1995 *Carpinteria* quad; it is set at the confluence of Forbush and Escondido Creeks.

At Cottam Camp, the Blue Canyon (26W12) and Forbush Canyon (26W13) Trails converge; see the "Lower Blue Canyon" sidebar opposite for the north route along the remainder of Escondido Canyon to the Santa Ynez River and Camuesa Road.

Continuing westward into Forbush Canyon, you'll pass beneath the power lines and climb under cover of more live oaks, gradually climbing for most of the trek but rather steeply along a series of switchbacks as the canyon narrows. In place of the serpentine formations, note the fossils inlaid in much of the exposed rock along the trail. These remnants of ancient seabeds seem especially heavy with various bivalves.

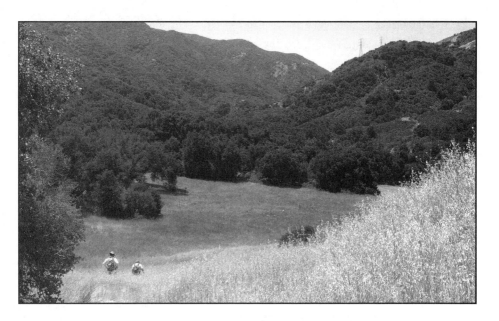

Dropping in on Cottam Camp

In a boulder-dotted gap you'll reach the **Mono-Forbush Junction (5.7 miles, 2,340',
257882E 3820492N)** on the edge of the Gidney Creek drainage. It's a quick hike left (south)
up the curve from this junction to another junction leading to Forbush Flat and **Forbush
Camp (5.8 miles, 2,400', 257770E 3820421N)**.

See *Route 14* if ascending this portion of the trail to Cold Spring Saddle for a shuttle or
if heading south from here toward Mono Campground.

■ ■ ■ ■ ■ ■ ■ ■ ■ ■ ■ ■ **LOWER BLUE CANYON**

If heading for the Santa Ynez or the lower stretch of Romero-Camuesa Road from
Cottam, your route heads out from the north of the campsite, down into the ravine,
and back up to the trail on the other side. Be sure to follow the little dogleg to the
right (east) on the other side and not simply follow the creek to its confluence with
Forbush Creek. The 1995 *Carpinteria* 7.5-minute quad shows a veritable spiderweb
of trails here—some long gone and others since rerouted. But the route in its current configuration follows a well-groomed and often well-shaded trail just above
the creek and heads north for 0.5 mile, reentering the streambed at a wide, cobble-
strewn **bend (0.5 mile from Cottam Camp, 1,490', 260366E 3820854N)** and then again
on the other side of the **bend (0.6 mile, 1,490', 260448E 3821116N)**, gaining the old

road after passing through an old fence and hiking easily eastward to the **Santa Ynez River (1 mile, 1,500', 260767E 3821462N)**.

Usually this crossing can be done with some deft rock-hopping to avoid wet feet; other years it's bone-dry, and still others you will be resigned to a soggy exit. Head for the coppice of mature sycamores on the other side, and you'll again find yourself walking through bucolic fields on the old doubletrack, with stately live oaks along either side. As the route again approaches the Santa Ynez, you'll keep to your left (the river's eastern banks) through a willow-choked and recently rerouted stretch up to the lower **"Cottam" trailhead (1.5 miles, 1,570', 261251E 3822136N)** beside Romero-Camuesa Road beneath a lone live oak.

Route 16

UPPER FRANKLIN TRAIL (25W09)

LENGTH AND TYPE:	10-mile out-and-back from Juncal to Alder Creek Camp; 5.8-mile one-way from Juncal to Franklin/Divide Peak OHV junction
RATING:	Moderately strenuous (climb along last portion)
TRAIL CONDITION:	Well maintained (service road) to passable (unmaintained trail)
MAP(S):	USGS *Carpinteria* and *White Ledge Peak*; Conant's *Matilija & Dick Smith Wilderness*
CAMP(S):	Alder Creek
HIGHLIGHTS:	Views of Juncal Dam and Jameson Lake; lush riparian trekking along Alder Creek

TO REACH THE TRAILHEAD(S): Use the Juncal Trailhead to access this route.

TRIP SUMMARY: This pleasant hike explores a stretch of the forest not often visited, despite its proximity to Montecito and Santa Barbara, passing Jameson Lake and following a nearly forgotten route along verdant Alder Creek. There is very little shade for the first 3.5 miles along Juncal Road; water (filter or purify) can typically be found at creek crossings.

Trip Description

From the gate at the junction (**1,800', 266738E 3819092N**) of Juncal and Romero-Camuesa Roads, walk around the gate and follow Juncal Road past the old Juncal (formerly Bear) Campground on your left (north). This old spot—now little more than a pleasant oak-lined flat suitable for picnicking—was a Civilian Conservation Corps camp in 1935–1936, and the campground featured six sites, a pair of barbecue pits, and tables for its campers. Footings of the double latrine and an incongruous western red cedar near the eastern edge of the flat are really all that is left to bear testament to its former use. It was closed in 2000 as part of larger efforts to protect the habitat of the arroyo toad.

Follow the road easily to a second **gate (0.1 mile, 1,800', 266768E 3819105N)** on the other side of camp, crossing the creek just beyond and endeavoring eastward along the service road. This stretch follows a very gradual upstream grade; it can be hot and dusty in the summer but most times is a lovely stroll beside the river wash, accompanied by sporadic oak and sycamore cover.

After the road crosses the **Santa Ynez River (1.6 miles, 1,920', 268905E 3819295N)**, you'll begin a fairly steep 0.5-mile stretch of road, switchbacking up and away from the river and through a gap where you'll get your first **views of Jameson Lake (2.1 miles, 2,200', 269411E 3819362N)** and the southern half of the dam (not the spillway). Continue along the road, staying right/straight at the next junction (here the numerous NO TRESPASSING signs posted by the Montecito Water District (MWD) begin to appear; stay to the road and you'll be fine), continuing to gain elevation as you work around the southern perimeter of the MWD's holding. Once south of the lake, the road levels out and then descends to a signed

A little paint, some new tires . . .

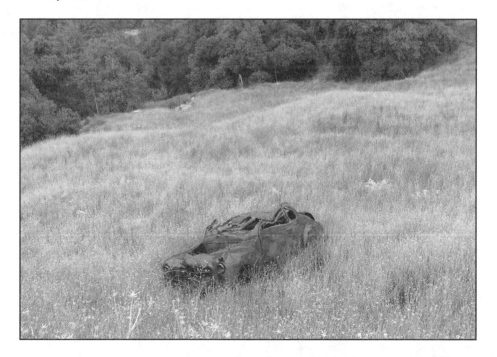

junction (3.5 miles, 2,275', 270515E 3818921N); the sign here is extremely outdated and a curious piece of forest history. Your route (the old Franklin Trail) follows the spur road on the right (south) heading down toward Alder Creek; the left continues up toward the headwaters of the Santa Ynez River and the Murietta Divide.

Follow this road easily downward (note the abandoned 1940s-era car on the slope to your right just as you continue), and as you approach the creek you'll find yourself walking beneath the sluice built to feed Alder Creek's water to the lake. At another split in the road here, veer right into the **clearing** and turnaround (**3.8 miles, 2,240', 270814E 3818682N**), where a massive live oak on the southern end marks the start of the singletrack.

From the clearing, the route immediately grows lush, shaded by the namesake white alders and narrow canyon walls.

Note: The 1995 *White Ledge* 7.5-minute quad shows a markedly different (historical) route from this junction than what is in current use. As volunteers' efforts on the southern half of the Franklin Trail slowly increase the route's popularity, it's possible the old route will be reborn—check with the ranger to confirm.

The trail will curve briefly to the left (east) and then cross the creek, directly below the sluice. Cross the creek here and then follow the sluice toward the old **weir (3.9 miles, 2,240', 270835E 3818515N)**, splitting left and crossing the creek again. A cold and rather foul-smelling sulfur spring sits just beside this slope, which when not maintained can be choked with poison oak. Bays, oaks, and sycamores join the alders here and provide shade on even the clearest of summer days, and a smattering of bigcone Douglas-firs hem the creek's banks high above you.

Follow the lush route twice more across the creek, all the while steadily climbing alongside good cover and some surprisingly large fern specimens, another mile to **Alder Creek Camp (5 miles, 2,700', 270595E 3817740N)**.

CAMP :: ALDER CREEK

ELEVATION:	2,700'
MAPS:	USGS *White Ledge Peak*; Conant's *Matilija & Dick Smith Wilderness*
UTM:	270595E 3817740N

This site is seldom used but a target destination for some hard-core local hikers. Marked simply "Alder" on many maps over the past few decades (perhaps to avoid confusion with Alder Creek campsite in the Sespe Wilderness), this little site situated in a very small clearing contains an old rock fire ring and space enough for a tent or two. It is well shaded by oaks and bays, and water is available most months from the creek.

From Alder Creek campsite, you have the option to either return the way you came or continue up the trail along the ridge for a steep ascent southward, following the ridge toward one of the ubiquitous **power pylons (5.5 miles, 3,500', 270307E 3817005N)** before topping out at the **Divide Peak OHV route (5.8 miles, 3,620', 270217E 3816720N)**. From the road—formerly Trail 24W08, now Forest Road 5N12—views of Carpinteria, the Pacific, and surrounding features in all directions (including the valley through which you just labored) are some of the best to be had.

From the road (and with some prior planning), you have a few options—the Divide Peak Trailhead some 8 miles to your west, Noon Peak and Divide Peak (2.1 miles and 4.1 miles to the east, respectively; see *Route 50: Divide Peak* for the approach to Divide Peak via the Murietta Divide and the Monte Arido Trail). There is also a small **pond (3,680', 269552E 3816919N)** at the head of Sutton Creek drainage about 0.3 mile to your west if you need to restock; another near the headwaters of Fox Creek (though less reliable) also avails itself to you some 1.7 miles west of the Franklin junction. There is no water to speak of to your east until over the Murietta Divide.

■ ■ ■ ■ ■ ■ ■ ■ ■ ■ **FRIENDS OF FRANKLIN TRAIL**

The southern portion of the Franklin Trail is not a viable route as of this writing, but a volunteer group (Friends of Franklin Trail) is working to reestablish the old southern half of this trail, which over the past few decades has been closed to the public as it crosses several privately owned properties. Visit **franklintrail.org** for more information.

■ ■

CHAPTER five

Santa Barbara Frontcountry

This chapter details the trails of the Santa Barbara and Montecito/ Carpinteria frontcountry, up to East Camino Cielo.

BUILT AROUND WHAT MANY CONSIDER to be "the Queen of the Missions," Santa Barbara is a vibrant city of about 90,000 with a sprawling unincorporated area encompassing some 220,000 souls. Steeped in Chumash, mission-era, and Californio history, the area is often called the American Riviera for its climate, lifestyle, and affluence. It is hemmed in by the Pacific at its southern edge and the Santa Ynez ridge on the north.

Day hiking opportunities here are quite possibly the finest in the state for a city this size, with the marine influence, soaring ocean and mountain views, fern-clad grottoes, and numerous routes only minutes from the mission and downtown.

Santa Barbara/Montecito Trailheads

Cater Water Treatment Plant (530', 249321E 3815921N)

From US 101 in Santa Barbara, take the Las Positas Road exit (Exit 100). If coming from the south/east, follow Calle Real for 0.33 mile before reaching Las Positas Road. Follow Las Positas Road (it becomes San Roque Road along the way) north 1.4 miles to the intersection with Foothill Road (CA 192). Cross Foothill Road and continue along San Roque Road another 0.5 mile (past the Cater Water Treatment Plant) to a small parking area. Parking is available on either side of the road; the trail begins at the north end of the left (eastern) parking area. There are no facilities here.

Tunnel Trailhead (980', 250848E 3816964N)

From US 101 in Santa Barbara, take the Mission Street exit (Exit 99) and follow Mission Street northeast for approximately 1 mile to Laguna Street. Turn left (northwest) here and

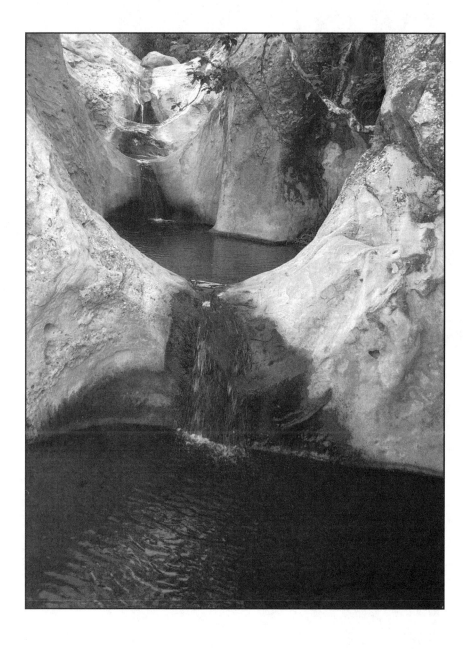

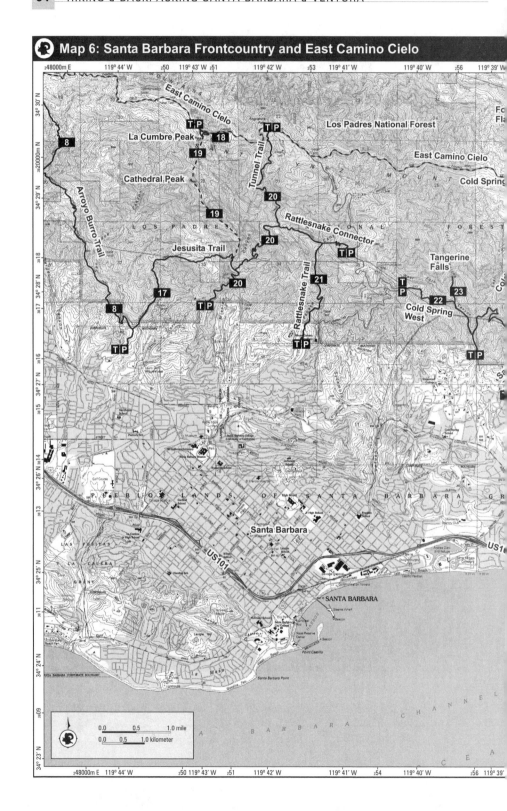

Map 6: Santa Barbara Frontcountry and East Camino Cielo

East Camino Cielo

La Cumbre Peak

Los Padres National Forest

East Camino Cielo

Cold Spring

Cathedral Peak

Arroyo Burro Trail

Tunnel Trail

Jesusita Trail

Rattlesnake Connector

Tangerine Falls

Rattlesnake Trail

Cold Spring West

LOS PADRES

Santa Barbara

US101

SANTA BARBARA

PUEBLO LANDS OF SANTA BARBARA

LAS POSITAS

LA CALERA

Golf Course

Point Castillo

Santa Barbara Point

SANTA BARBARA CHANNEL

0.0   0.5   1.0 mile
0.0   0.5   1.0 kilometer

MAP 6 Santa Barbara Frontcountry and East Camino Cielo   95

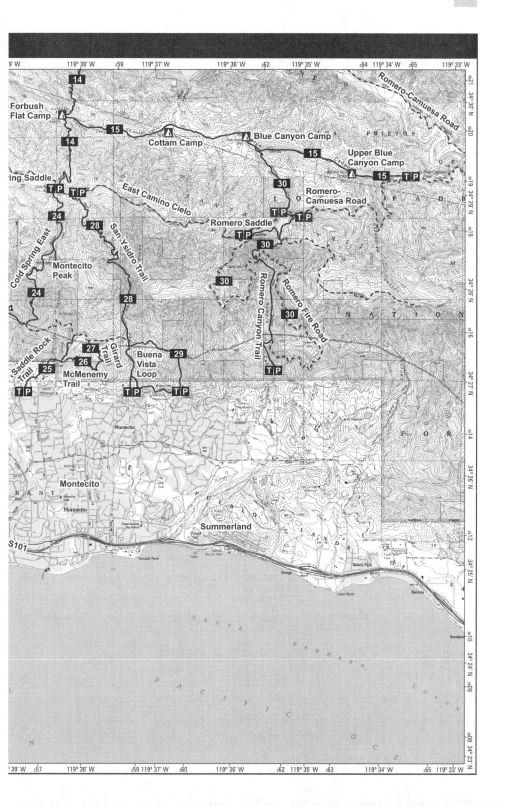

follow Laguna 3 blocks to the Mission Santa Barbara grounds. Turn right at the four-way stop to follow East Los Olivos Street (which becomes Mission Canyon Road) for 0.7 mile to Foothill Road. Turn right (east) here and follow Foothill Road 0.25 mile to a three-way stop in front of the fire station. Turn left (north) here and follow Mission Canyon Road approximately 0.3 mile. At the Y with Tunnel Road, stay left (onto Tunnel Road). Follow Tunnel Road into a winding residential area for another mile to the parking area. Ensure that your vehicle is within the white lines as stated on the various signs, as local law enforcement has been known to ticket errant vehicles. There are no facilities here.

Rattlesnake Canyon (910', 252671E 3816185N)

From the intersection of Mission Canyon Road and Foothill Road (CA 192) in Santa Barbara, follow Foothill Road (here both roads follow the same path) 0.2 mile east to the stop sign and intersection where Mission Canyon Road splits away again to head north. Turn left (north) and follow Mission Canyon Road 0.3 mile to the intersection with Las Canoas Road, making a sharp right (southeast) onto Las Canoas. Follow Las Canoas east 1.2 miles to the small parking area on the left (north) side of the road, just past a large boulder beside the road and just before the stone bridge begins. There is room enough for two cars here; if those spots are already taken, there are numerous spots both back along the road and farther past the bridge where one may park. There is a large wooden sign at the trailhead here marking the SKOFIELD PARK RATTLESNAKE CANYON WILDERNESS AREA. There are no facilities here.

Cold Spring Canyon Trailhead (780', 256269E 3815901N)

From US 101 in Montecito, take Exit 94A (Olive Mill Road) and drive north along Olive Mill Road (turning into Hot Springs Road) for approximately 3 miles to East Mountain Drive. Turn left (west) on East Mountain Drive and continue 1.1 miles to the trailhead. Parking is available on the side of the road either side of the water crossing, as well as in an overflow area just east of the main parking areas. There is signage on both sides of the creek; the easiest route to follow is that on the east side of the creek. There are no facilities here.

Saddle Rock Trailhead (600', 257034E 3815087N)

From US 101 in Montecito, take Exit 94A (Olive Mill Road) and drive north along Olive Mill Road (turning into Hot Springs Road) for approximately 3 miles to East Mountain Drive. Turn left (west) on East Mountain Drive and continue 0.2 mile to the Saddle Rock parking area on the right (north) side of the road. The trailhead is on the east end of the parking area; there are no facilities here.

San Ysidro Canyon Trailhead (420', 259098E 3814727N)

From US 101 in Montecito, take Exit 93 (San Ysidro Road) and drive north along San Ysidro Road approximately 1 mile to East Valley Road/CA 192. Turn right (east) here and continue 0.9 mile to Park Lane (the turnoff to Park Lane is easy to miss; it's just as the road begins to rise after passing the Knowlwood Tennis Club and crossing San Ysidro Creek). Turn left (north) on Park Lane and proceed 0.4 mile until the split; stay left and continue another 0.5 mile to the parking area; parking is available on either side of the road. The trailhead is at the end of the parking area, on the north side of the road. There are no facilities here.

Note: Several online mapping sites indicate that two segments of East Mountain Drive either side of San Ysdiro Ranch connect; this is not the case in a practical sense. San Ysidro Ranch is a privately held resort property, and motor traffic is not allowed to use the private road to connect the roads; please bear this in mind if planning a shuttle between two trailheads in the Montecito frontcountry.

Buena Vista Trailhead (665', 260133E 3815007N)

From US 101 in Montecito, take Exit 93 (San Ysidro Road) and drive north along San Ysidro Road approximately 1 mile to East Valley Road/CA 192. Turn right (east) here and continue 0.9 mile to Park Lane (the turnoff to Park Lane is easy to miss; it's just as the road begins to rise after passing the Knowlwood Tennis Club). Turn left (north) onto Park Lane and proceed 0.4 mile until the split; stay right at the split and continue another 0.6 mile northeast to a small parking area on the left (north) side of the road. The trailhead is at the east end of the parking area; there are no facilities here.

Romero Canyon Trailhead (985', 262008E 3815429N)

From Carpinteria and Points South: From US 101 N in Carpinteria, take Exit 88 (Padaro Lane) and turn right at the end of the ramp toward Via Real. Turn left at Via Real and continue 0.6 mile to Nidever Road. Turn right (north) onto Nidever Road (it becomes Foothill Road and CA 192 after 0.1 mile) and travel 2.1 miles until your route bends into Toro Canyon Road at a stop sign. Turn right and continue along Toro Canyon (which likewise becomes CA 192) for 1.1 miles until you reach Ladera Lane. Turn right (north) onto Ladera Lane and drive 1 mile north to Bella Vista Drive. Turn left (west) here and continue another 0.7 mile to the parking area and trailhead on your right (just before the water crossing where Romero Creek pours across the road).

From Santa Barbara and Points North: From US 101 S in Montecito, take Exit 92 (Sheffield Road). This is a left-hand exit, so note you'll need to be in the left (passing) lane. Turn left off the exit toward Jameson Lane, and then turn right onto Jameson, following signage for Sheffield Road (stay left at the split with Sheffield and Ortega Hill Road). Continue northeast along Sheffield Drive 1.3 miles until you reach East Valley Road (CA 192). Turn left here and make an almost immediate right (north) onto Romero Canyon Road. Follow Romero Canyon Road 1.5 miles (staying right at the split with Lilac Way at 0.4 mile) until you reach Bella Vista Drive. Turn right onto Bella Vista and continue 0.3 mile to the parking area and trailhead on your left (just after the water crossing where Romero Creek pours across the road).

There is room enough in the parking area for three or four vehicles, but typically you'll need to find roadside parking somewhere along Bella Vista Drive. There are no facilities here.

Camino Cielo Trailheads

Knapp's Castle/Upper Snyder Trailhead (2,960', 243582E 3823200N)

From the junction of US 101 and CA 154 in Santa Barbara, follow CA 154 (also San Marcos Pass Road) north 7.8 miles to East Camino Cielo Road (also Forest Road 5N12). Turn right (east) here and continue along East Camino Cielo 3 miles to a small parking area on the left (north) side of the road. There is also space along the road in both directions. There are no facilities here.

La Cumbre Peak Trailhead (3,825', 250779E 3820443N)

From the junction of US 101 and CA 154 in Santa Barbara, follow CA 154 (also San Marcos Pass Road) north 7.8 miles to East Camino Cielo Road (also Forest Road 5N12). Turn right (east) here and continue along East Camino Cielo 9.3 miles to the La Cumbre Peak turnoff and parking space.

Alternately, from the junction of CA 192 and Mountain Drive in Santa Barbara, follow Mountain Drive north 0.2 mile to the junction with Gibraltar Road. Turn left (north) at this dogleg and continue along Gibraltar Road 7.3 miles (this is a slow and winding route) to its intersection with East Camino Cielo Road (also Forest Road 5N12). Stay straight (west) here and continue another mile to the La Cumbre Peak turnoff and parking space.

There are no facilities here, but there is a single restroom atop La Cumbre Peak (no water available).

Angostura Pass (3,370', 252164E 3820489N)

From the junction of US 101 and CA 154 in Santa Barbara, follow CA 154 (also San Marcos Pass Road) north 7.8 miles to East Camino Cielo Road (also Forest Road 5N12). Turn right (east) here and continue along East Camino Cielo 10.4 miles to the Angostura Pass parking area (on the left/north side). Be sure not to block the gate.

Alternately, from the junction of CA 192 and Mountain Drive in Santa Barbara, follow Mountain Drive north 0.2 mile to the junction with Gibraltar Road. Turn left (north) at this dogleg and continue along Gibraltar Road 7.3 miles (this is a slow and winding route) to its intersection with East Camino Cielo Road (also Forest Road 5N12). Stay straight (west) here and continue another 0.6 mile to the Angostura Pass parking area (on the right/north side). Be sure not to block the gate. There are no facilities here.

Cold Spring Saddle (3,400', 257657E 3818995N)

From the junction of US 101 and CA 154 in Santa Barbara, follow CA 154 (also San Marcos Pass Road) north 7.8 miles to East Camino Cielo Road (also Forest Road 5N12). Turn right (east) here and continue along East Camino Cielo 14.7 miles to the Cold Spring Saddle parking area.

Alternately, from the junction of CA 192 and Mountain Drive in Santa Barbara, follow Mountain Drive north 0.2 mile to the junction with Gibraltar Road. Turn left (north) at this dogleg and continue along Gibraltar Road 7.3 miles (this is a slow and winding route) to its intersection with East Camino Cielo Road (also Forest Road 5N12). Turn right (east) here and continue along East Camino Cielo 3.6 miles to the Cold Spring Saddle parking area.

Upper San Ysidro Trailhead (3,455', 258006E 3818912N)

From the junction of US 101 and CA 154 in Santa Barbara, follow CA 154 (also San Marcos Pass Road) north 7.8 miles to East Camino Cielo Road (also Forest Road 5N12). Turn right (east) here and continue along East Camino Cielo 14.9 miles to the Upper San Ysidro Trailhead (just past Cold Spring Saddle).

Alternately, from the junction of CA 192 and Mountain Drive in Santa Barbara, follow Mountain Drive north 0.2 mile to the junction with Gibraltar Road. Turn left (north) at this dogleg and continue along Gibraltar Road 7.3 miles (this is a slow and winding route) to its intersection with East Camino Cielo Road (also Forest Road 5N12). Turn right (east) here and continue along East Camino Cielo 3.8 miles to the Upper San Ysidro Trailhead (just past Cold Spring Saddle).

Romero Saddle (3,015', 261588E 3817974N)

From the junction of US 101 and CA 154 in Santa Barbara, follow CA 154 (also San Marcos Pass Road) north 7.8 miles to East Camino Cielo Road (also Forest Road 5N12). Turn right (east) here and continue along East Camino Cielo 17.8 miles to Romero Saddle.

Alternately, from the junction of CA 192 and Mountain Drive in Santa Barbara, follow Mountain Drive north 0.2 mile to the junction with Gibraltar Road. Turn left (north) at this dogleg and continue along Gibraltar Road 7.3 miles (this is a slow and winding route) to its intersection with East Camino Cielo Road (also Forest Road 5N12). Turn right (east) here and continue along East Camino Cielo 6.7 miles to Romero Saddle.

Route 17

JESUSITA TRAIL (27W17) and INSPIRATION POINT

LENGTH AND TYPE:	6.8-mile out-and-back to Inspiration Point; 4.4-mile one-way to junction with Tunnel Trail
RATING:	Moderate (climb; steep at times)
TRAIL CONDITION:	Clear
MAP(S):	USGS *Santa Barbara*; Conant's *Matilija & Dick Smith Wilderness*
CAMP(S):	—
HIGHLIGHTS:	Riparian trekking; great views from Inspiration Point

TO REACH THE TRAILHEAD(S): Use the Cater Water Treatment Plant trailhead for this route.

TRIP SUMMARY: From the suburbs along lower San Roque Creek, the Jesusita Trail climbs into the Los Padres frontcountry to head east along well-cut trails and service roads to Inspiration Point and then down into Mission Canyon. Burned during the Jesusita Fire that engulfed the area in May 2009 and consumed nearly 9,000 acres, the route still remains popular on the weekends and is heavily frequented by trail runners. Watch out for poison oak.

Note: Like many of the trails in the region, this route is also frequently traveled by mountain bikers, so do exercise caution (especially at blind corners).

The first leg of the trip is outside the Los Padres; instead you'll be along property managed by the County of Santa Barbara Parks Department for the first 0.5 mile or so (though technically the City of Santa Barbara, County of Santa Barbara, and the Los Padres National Forest share jurisdictional oversight of this and other Santa Barbara frontcountry trails). Noted local outdoor writer Ray Ford points out that unlike most of the local trails, the Jesusita wasn't a historical mission-era or Chumash path, but rather a project developed by the State Division of Beaches and Parks in the mid-1960s.

Trip Description

From the **trailhead/parking area** (**530', 249321E 3815921N**), follow the trail (and old service road) northward and down under cover of coast live oaks and scrub. Follow the right fork at the first **junction** (**0.1 mile, 490', 249296E 3816039N**) to continue heading upstream. A number of spur trails—some tempting and well cut—provide alternatives, but stay low (left) to follow the course of San Roque Creek, through thistle- and fennel-lined trail, climbing very easily (and at times closely) along the stream's edge. Pass some avocado orchards on your right before coming to a very pleasant picnic area set beneath massive live oaks and with easy access to the creek. This spot is easily identified by the landmark wooden **table (0.4 mile, 510', 249397E 3816539N)**.

From the table, continue through the well-shaded riparian cover of oaks and sycamores to the **junction (0.6 mile, 660', 249274E 3816623N)** of the Arroyo Burro and Jesusita Trails. Follow the right fork (see *Route 8* for the route heading left) and climb briefly away from the main San Roque drainage into a wide pair of fields; these grassy expanses are beautiful and dotted with wildflowers in the spring.

After the second field you'll drop briefly into a western tributary drainage—skirting a private road along a stretch well shaded by sycamores, oaks, bays, and the occasional cluster of cottonwoods—crossing the creek thrice before coming out onto the **private road (1.2 miles, 780', 249040E 3817431N)** at its intersection with a smaller route to your right (east).

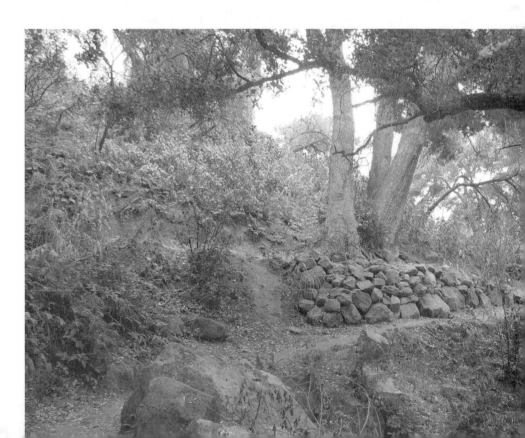

Follow the main road along the left edge of a small grassy field, and then take the right fork up a slope toward the gates of the **Moreno Ranch (1.3 miles, 800', 249102E 3817483N)**. There are chairs, a water fountain, and usually even a bowl for your canine companions just past the entrance here.

The trail follows the right edge of the road here, passing onto private property briefly and dropping into the drainage again—numerous trail signs direct you (as do numerous NO TRESPASSING signs) to the **split (1.4 miles, 850', 249222E 3817552N)** where the trail leaves the dirt road and continues up the canyon beneath mature riparian cover. Once you've hiked off the main ranch property, the canyon will narrow and the red sandstone of the Vaqueros formation comes into view, mixing with the lighter sandstone that has dominated much of your route. Soon a series of switchbacks—bisected by an old and occasionally overgrown **service road (2.1 miles, 1,340', 249808E 3818341N)**—will lead you to a **gap (2.4 miles, 1,490', 249877E 3818247N)** with views of the canyon and water tanks below (many of the rocks at the small lookout to your south are inlaid with marine fossils).

Follow a fairly level portion of trail along the head of this small canyon and then pass through a small grotto before climbing another series of switchbacks. These switchbacks top out and then drop you on an Edison **service road (2.8 miles, 1,675', 250304E 3818069N)** used to serve the power lines above. Follow this road up its winding course—the inspiring Mission Crags come into view here, as does Cathedral Peak high above—to the trail marked with an old **wooden post (3.1 miles, 1,700', 250366E 3817913N)**. This thin trail parallels the service road to lead up toward a **vista (3.4 miles, 1,750', 250642E 3817853N)** often mistakenly taken to be Inspiration Point.

Rather, continue along the trail (or—to be fair—the road, which will also get you there, only without some of the views en route) to a **junction (3.6 miles, 1,800', 250689E 3817848N)** just short of the service road. Follow the trail west to **Inspiration Point (3.7 miles, 1,800', 250454E 3817892N)**, where you'll enjoy expansive views of the community below, as well as the Santa Barbara Channel and Channel Islands.

From Inspiration Point you can either retrace your steps, or with a shuttle vehicle in place, make a loop by continuing east to cross the **service road (3.8 miles, 1,780', 250714E 3817858N)**, which leads toward the eastern stretch of the Jesusita Trail.

The trail will lead you beneath the power lines along an easy grade and into a **gap (4 miles, 1,720', 250808E 3817938N)** with excellent lateral views of the Santa Ynez foothills before you descend a series of switchbacks toward Mission Canyon (the gap marks the end of the real climbing for those coming from Mission Canyon). Especially after the Jesusita Fire, there are only a few spots of shade here during the day until you reach the canyon floor. Two intermittent creek crossings are punctuated by excellent views of Santa Barbara and

Montecito and the ocean beyond every time the trail hangs on the south edges of this drainage; the views succumb to the mountainous terrain just as you cross another **tributary (4.4 miles, 1,350', 251360E 3817951N)**, round a corner, and drop down into the Mission Creek crossing **(4.6 miles, 1,330', 251364E 3817902N)**.

From this crossing, you have numerous options in addition to the 1-mile trek down to the Tunnel Trailhead (see the opening passages of *Route 20* for those details). You may wish to consider the off-trail but relatively easy rock-hop up to 7 Falls and 3 Pools, or—again, if you've planned ahead—an ascent of the Tunnel Trail to Angostura Pass/Camino Cielo. An unofficial route upstream along Mission Canyon also leads to Cathedral Peak (see *Route 19*).

Route 18

LA CUMBRE PEAK

LENGTH AND TYPE:	0.3-mile round-trip
RATING:	Easy
TRAIL CONDITION:	Clear
MAP(S):	USGS *Santa Barbara*; Conant's *Matilija & Dick Smith Wilderness*
CAMP(S):	—
HIGHLIGHTS:	Easy access; picnic sites; panoramic views of the Santa Ynez River Valley; great walk for small children

TO REACH THE TRAILHEAD(S): Use the La Cumbre Peak Trailhead for this route.

TRIP SUMMARY: This very easy walk from East Camino Cielo Road follows the old road to sweeping vistas of both the southern and northern slopes—and arguably the best views of Santa Barbara to be had anywhere—from 3,985-foot-high La Cumbre Peak. The peak is the highest point in the Santa Barbara Ranger District accessible by passenger cars.

Trip Description

From the parking area, follow the service road past the gate and to the junction. Follow the right fork (against the road's prescribed direction of traffic) for a few hundred feet past a pair of radio transmitter dishes to the first hairpin in the road, where there are a number of benches and truly spectacular views of all points south. Cathedral Peak and Arlington Peak are easily identified, to the right and left, respectively, along La Cumbre's southern flank. The unofficial but popular route to Cathedral Peak starts here from the bench **(0.1 mile, 3,910', 250801E 3820327N)**; see *Route 19* for that route.

Also easily noted here is damage from the 2009 Jesusita Fire, which advanced right up to the base of the peak and scorched most of the nearby slopes. Numerous trees were killed and have since been cut or trimmed by US Forest Service crews and/or volunteers.

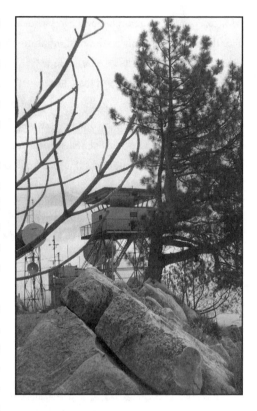

Continue following the road to the left, where it climbs easily to deposit you along the top of the ridge and where you'll get a good idea of what the peak was like when day-trippers could park and picnic here. This area is often called Lookout Park by local trail runners and hikers.

At the eastern edge of the flat is the old La Cumbre Peak **fire lookout (0.2 mile, 3,975', 250908E 3820334N**), originally built in 1923 but replaced in 1945 with an innovative and experimental design that included sloped windows reminiscent of an airport control tower, supported by a steel frame and girders. It was considered quite expensive for its time, costing $6,500—few other such ambitious lookouts were subsequently built, as budgets and the Civilian Conservation Corp's scope both diminished significantly in the postwar years. Now the lookout—shuttered in 1982—is surrounded by a chain-link fence and closed-circuit TV cameras, and the lower 10 feet of the old steel ladders have been cut to discourage trespassers. Just behind the old lookout are the satellite transmitter arrays (constructed in 1962 and subsequently operated by Cox Cable under a special use permit). The actual peak is to the immediate southeast of the tower and arrays along the orange boulders.

There is a group of sandstone boulders and a rock wall popular with local climbers about a 5-minute walk southwest of the peak and arrays. Hang-gliding enthusiasts are also known to frequent the peak, so you may witness a few takeoffs during your visit.

Continue left past the tower and transmitter equipment and follow the road as it curves to return to the parking area. Along this straight stretch you'll often be shaded by Coulter pines and a few incongruous cypresses. Far down the northern slope, the Gibraltar Dam and Gibraltar Reservoir are easily identified. Continue back to the gate and **parking area (0.3 mile, 3,825', 250779E 3820443N**) to complete this easy loop.

Route 19

CATHEDRAL PEAK

LENGTH AND TYPE:	1.8-mile round-trip from La Cumbre Peak; 5.4-mile round-trip from Tunnel Trailhead; 12.6-mile round-trip from Jesusita Trailhead
RATING:	Strenuous
TRAIL CONDITION:	Passable to difficult since the Jesusita Fire; there has been some subsequent trail work but also a great deal of postfire erosion; could return to difficult quickly if not regularly traveled
MAP(S):	USGS *Santa Barbara*; Conant's *Matilija & Dick Smith Wilderness* *Note:* Route not shown on either map
CAMP(S):	—
HIGHLIGHTS:	Panoramic views of Santa Barbara and Ventura Counties and the Pacific

TO REACH THE TRAILHEAD(S): Use the La Cumbre Peak Trailhead (if approaching from the north) or Tunnel Trailhead (if approaching from the south) for this route.

Note: Cathedral Peak can also be accessed from far below by following the Jesusita Trail or the lower Tunnel Trail (see *Routes 17* and *20*, respectively), and then climbing from Mission Creek (strenuous), but it is highly recommended you hike not only with a buddy but also with one who has done the route before! The ascent to Arlington and Cathedral Peaks from Mission Canyon is deceiving and takes longer and is often more difficult to navigate than it appears.

TRIP SUMMARY: From the lower La Cumbre Peak vista point, this route follows a thin spur trail—well cleared by crews defending against the 2009 Jesusita Fire—to the rock outcrops that form Cathedral Peak. Give yourself plenty of time to make the trip, whatever route you choose. The distances are deceptive, as both directions entail a great deal of slow clambering, scrambling, and route-finding. Dogs are not recommended (but a hiking companion who has done the trip is!), and those with a fear of heights should avoid the actual summit of Cathedral Peak.

Note: This is not an official US Forest Service (USFS) trail.

Trip Description

La Cumbre Peak to Cathedral Peak

From the parking area, follow the service road past the gate and to the first road split. Follow the right fork (against the old road's prescribed direction of traffic) for a few hundred feet—past a pair of radio transmitter dishes—to the first hairpin in the road. There are a number of benches and truly spectacular views of all points south here. Cathedral Peak and Arlington

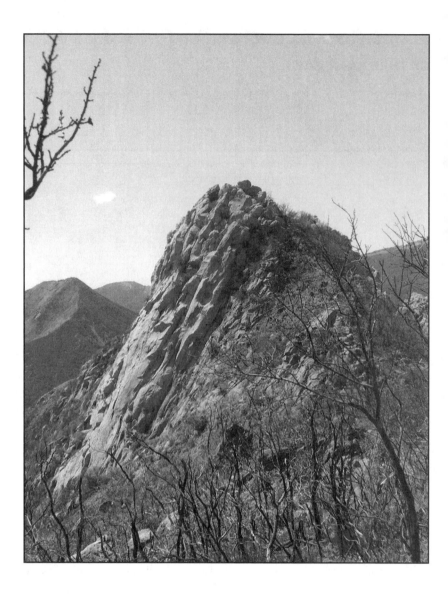

Peak are easily identified, to the right and left, respectively, along La Cumbre's southern flank. The trail to Cathedral Peak starts here from the bench (**3,920', 250801E 3820322N**); continuing along the road will lead you to the top of the old La Cumbre Peak picnic area (see *Route 18*). Also easily noted here is damage from the 2009 Jesusita Fire, which advanced right up to the base of the peak and scorched most of the nearby slopes. Numerous trees were killed and have since been cut or trimmed by USFS crews and/or volunteers.

Follow the clear trail southward from the bench, dropping easily toward a large outcrop of Matilija sandstone **boulders** (**100 yards, 3,870', 250799E 3820270N**), popular with local climbers and day-trippers. Cut right (west) from the boulders and follow the drainage toward the thread of a trail visible below. The route entails a great deal of scrambling and route-finding; since the fires it's easier to navigate in many regards, but still be aware of snags, burnt stumps, exposed roots, and loose rocks.

The route toward Cathedral Peak crosses several different geologic layers, beginning with the middle-to-late Eocene-age Matilija sandstone of which La Cumbre Peak is composed. From that starting point, you'll soon pass across the dark gray late-Eocene Cozy Dell shale and then into the hard, orange (and quite abrasive and unforgiving) Coldwater sandstone, as well as greenish gray siltstone with interbeds of that sandstone. It makes for fascinating hiking and amateur field geology, but the sandstone especially can be hard on gear (and skin), so dress and scramble appropriately.

The main route curves toward the southwest through sandstone boulders and manzanita and down several very steep stretches that will require trekking poles or use of all fours to safely descend before reaching the **trail (0.25 mile, 3,460', 250616E 3820179N)** at the base of a rock face, a short portion of which you've just slid/climbed down. The route here is a navigable—and after the scramble down, quite pleasant—path through grass, classic "elfin forest" chaparral canopy, and scrub. This section of your route was spared from the Jesusita Fire and features some very mature growth all the way up to the lower ridge just north of Cathedral Peak.

Continue the easy descent toward the saddle between La Cumbre and Cathedral Peaks, and at a trail **junction (0.45 mile, 3,210', 250616E 3820179N)** bear left (east). Be certain you do not find yourself on the right (west) fork, which skirts the north and west flanks of Cathedral Peak: this is an old, long out-of-use trail that once led far down into San Roque Canyon.

Follow the left trail to a small rock outcrop before dropping down through a thickly wooded and fern-ensconced ravine (often so choked you might think you've gone off-route), eventually coming to a clearing of thick reeds and then another stretch of eerie, mossy limb-covered trail before the vegetation abruptly changes back to "classic" chaparral and you begin the climb up the north slope of Cathedral Peak. It's a short but fairly steep stretch here, with some poison oak and low-hanging branches.

With very little view of where the trail is leading, it's quite abruptly that you find yourself at a fantastic **vista (0.75 mile, 3,285', 250454E 3819502N)** with commanding views of the Channel Islands and the communities below. The trail makes a sharp left (east) turn here; follow the ridge toward a small saddle, where the Jesusita Fire consumed most of the south-facing slopes, to the **junction (0.85 mile, 3,290', 250517E 3819457N)** with the trail from Arlington Peak.

Follow the short trail up to **Cathedral Peak (0.9 mile, 3,333', 250509E 3819445N)**. The short east-to-west ridgeline atop the peak is narrow and drops precipitously off both faces, so do exercise caution if you venture westward to the actual peak. There is a summit register stored beneath the last set of boulders.

Retrace your steps to return, or with prior planning you can eschew the return ascent for a longer (but only marginally more exerting) rock-hopping descent along Arlington Ridge and then the Dragon's Back toward Mission Canyon (see below).

From the Tunnel Trail

The route ascending the Dragon's Back forks from the Tunnel Trail just downstream from the gorge: follow the trip description for *Route 20*, and at the creek **crossing (1 mile, 1,330', 251364E 3817902N)** follow the thin use trail 0.25 mile upstream to the Cathedral Peak **turn-off (1.3 miles, 1,560', 251470E 3818077N)**, which splits off to the left (northwest) from the main trail. There is a distinct rock jutting out over the canyon on your right (east) here.

Note: For those following this description in reverse coming from La Cumbre, be certain as you approach Tunnel Canyon to stay on the south slopes of the last portion of Dragon's Back. Do not follow the trails others have trod dropping down the north slope; that ravine is steep and choked with poison oak, and it creates more work for you than is necessary.

Since the Jesusita Fire, what was once an exercise in bushwhacking has become an exercise in climbing through eroded, debris-ridden tread to ascend the slope and gain the top of the Dragon's Back and the long ridge of gear-shredding sandstone boulders lining your route.

Follow the route up to the first stony **ridge (1.4 miles, 1,800', 251463E 3818194N)**, cutting left (west) to follow the rift for a short time and then climbing another fire-damaged slope to the main ridge, where you'll head left (west) along the rocky outcrop, following sections of trail and wear along the at-times huge boulders. Passage through a small **tunnel (2 miles, 2,575', 250976E 3818757N)** beneath two massive boulders leaning against one another confirms your route and comes about two-thirds of the way up the Dragon's Back, but it can be easy to miss and the route can be a matter of picking a line. A smattering of Coulter pines dot the landscape as you continue the steep climb, eventually topping out at **Arlington Peak (2.4 miles, 3,250', 250719E 3819041N)**, a jumble of sandstone boulders and very little vegetation.

Enjoy the views and the respite the remainder of the route brings, and pick your way through the boulders to a much clearer track that leads you northwest along a ridge burned by the Jesusita Fire. You'll skirt the southern face of a few large rock faces and then climb quickly to the trail **junction (2.6 miles, 3,290', 250517E 3819457N)** beneath the north-facing approach to Cathedral Peak.

From the junction, follow the short trail up to **Cathedral Peak (2.7 miles, 3,333', 250509E 3819445N)**. The short east-to-west ridgeline atop the peak is narrow and drops precipitously off both faces, so do exercise caution if you venture westward to the actual peak. There is a summit register stored beneath the last set of boulders.

Route 20

MISSION CANYON/TUNNEL TRAIL (27W14)

LENGTH AND TYPE:	8.2-mile out-and-back to East Camino Cielo; 2.3-mile one-way to Rattlesnake Connector; 5.8-mile out-and-back to Mission Falls; 2-mile out-and-back to Mission Creek (partially along Jesusita Trail); 2.5-mile out-and-back to 7 Falls/3 Pools (partially along Jesusita Trail)
RATING:	Moderate to Mission Creek (moderate elevation gain); strenuous from Jesusita-Tunnel Junction to East Camino Cielo (steep climb)
TRAIL CONDITION:	Clear
MAP(S):	USGS *Santa Barbara*; Conant's *Matilija & Dick Smith Wilderness*
CAMP(S):	—
HIGHLIGHTS:	Fantastic views of La Cumbre, Cathedral, and Arlington Peaks, the Santa Ynez range and Santa Barbara Channel, 7 Falls, and Mission Falls

TO REACH THE TRAILHEAD(S): Use the Tunnel Trailhead for this route. The start of the route is another 0.8 mile up the road (mileages are marked from the gate at the start of the service road). There are no facilities here, but there are a few trash receptacles set beside the gate.

Note: Like many of the trails in the region, this popular route is also frequently traveled by mountain bikers, so do exercise caution (especially at blind corners).

TRIP SUMMARY: From the mouth of Mission Canyon, the Tunnel Trail climbs the south face of the Santa Ynez range to East Camino Cielo along the old water tunnel route. You'll encounter Mission Falls and several trail junctions en route.

Trip Description

From the **parking area (980', 250848E 3816964N)**, hike past a water tank and around the **gate (1,030', 250861E 3817625N)** and head up the coarse but still-paved Edison service road. Views of the nearby neighborhoods—and the damage wrought by the 2009 Jesusita Fire—are laid out to your right (east and south). La Cumbre and Cathedral Peaks are both easy to pick out on the western ridge during your brief but steady climb before you enter a more riparian setting and, with a slight drop, approach the South Portal engine house set beside the creek. Fern Falls—a venerable destination that typically flows in winter and spring—can be accessed just downstream

Cross the **bridge (0.7 mile, 1,220', 251353E 3817578N)** here and continue up the road as it turns to dirt and brings you to the **junction (0.8 mile, 1,270', 251461E 3817609N)** with the Jesusita (left/west) and Tunnel (right/east) trails. Heading left gives several options, including Inspiration Point and Cathedral Peak (see *Routes 17* and *19*, respectively) as well as 7 Falls (see page 111); heading right here gives the option to continue the Tunnel Trail up to the Rattlesnake Trail, Mission Falls, and—eventually—through Angostura Pass to East Camino Cielo.

To East Camino Cielo (Angostura Pass)

From the junction, bear right (northeast) onto the singletrack, climbing steadily along the sandstone and boulder-strewn route with views of one of Mission Creek's eastern tributaries. You'll pass beneath the ubiquitous **power lines (1.1 miles, 1,600', 251747E 3817858N)** and cross the service road used to access them; views of the Mission Crags use trail(s) are high on your northeast. On the southeast-facing rocks up the canyon, you'll spot a large and long-standing peace sign constructed of sandstone cobbles before reaching a (by this point) welcome set of switchbacks that will lead you somewhat more easily toward great views of Mission Canyon and its accompanying peaks: Arlington, Cathedral, and La Cumbre all loom along the western edge of the ravine.

Small clusters of charred Coulter pines join the rest of the charred vegetation wrought by the Jesusita Fire as you reach a **saddle (1.8 miles, 2,190', 252051E 3818245N)** affording views of both the main and eastern forks of the drainage. Work your way clockwise around a knoll (just as you begin to head east again, a use trail heads off toward the crags) to gain

Rattlesnake Connector–Tunnel Trail junction

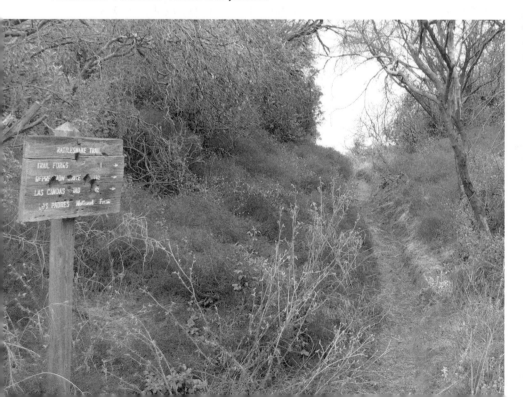

the **junction (2.3 miles, 2,485', 252292E 3818494N)** with the Rattlesnake Connector (see *Route 21*). This little corner of the forest was spared the ravages of the recent fires (as evidenced by the decades-old and worm-chewed wooden US Forest Service signs), and you'll enjoy a short section of unburned terrain before continuing upward to a **crossing (2.7 miles, 2,620', 252272E 3819021N)** along a far more gradual ascent now, hiking beneath some huge slabs of stone and arcing westward toward the vista above **Mission Falls (2.9 miles, 2,675', 252053E 3819213N)**.

The falls, visible from the city, are often dry in summer but make for an impressive cascade over the sandstone in the wetter seasons. From this vantage point, the trail heads up the creek a very short way between some very large boulders under cover of large oaks that survived the fires. This is a great rest/picnic spot before continuing farther up-canyon.

From the falls, the final stretch can almost feel like a long staircase as you curve toward the north and follow the rocky, sand- and sandstone-dominated route. Near the end of your ascent, you'll reach a final creek **crossing (3.7 miles, 3,300', 252181E 3819934N)** into a shale- and talus-covered bowl popular with dirt bikers. (And while the trail is clearly closed to motorcycles at a certain point, you'll often find riders or their tracks along the very upper stretch of the trail, so do mind the corners.)

Follow the main route directly to **East Camino Cielo (4.1 miles, 3,425', 252209E 3820405N)**.

If inclined, you can follow the road left (westward) up the grade for another 1.2 miles to La Cumbre Peak (see *Route 18*).

To 7 Falls

From the Jesusita/Tunnel junction, bear left (northwest) to stay on the road, keeping left to follow the Jesusita Trail as it leads toward the canyon. You'll cross the **creek (1 mile, 1,330', 251364E 3817902N)**; upon reaching the creek head directly upstream along the drainage (heading across along the main trail here will lead up the Jesusita Trail toward Inspiration Point; the use trail that heads upstream along the creek's side leads toward Arlington and Cathedral Peaks) and follow the watershed upstream. It's a fairly easy 0.25-mile rock-hop along the Mission Creek watershed to reach the base of the lowest **fall (1.25 miles, 1,450', 251547E 3818090N)**. An old citrus tree is on the west side of the canyon between the first and second pools; each fall cascades over especially hardy Coldwater sandstone layers and forms a series of pools in the weaker spots.

A number of use trails higher above the canyon lead farther upstream, but use them with caution, as they are not officially maintained nor always easy to follow.

To Cathedral Peak: See *Route 19*.

RUN TO THE HILLS ▧ ▧ ▧ ▧ ▧ ▧ ▧ ▧ ▧ ▧ ▧ ▧

In the midafternoon of February 21, 1824, Chumash neophytes revolted at the Mission Santa Inés and burned much of the mission and grounds. Word spread and soon uprisings were under way at La Purísima Concepción (Mexican forces did not retake the mission for nearly a month) and then—most notably—at the Mission Santa Barbara to the south. There, the Chumash disarmed the Mexican soldiers and sent them back to the presidio before taking flight up what is now Mission Canyon, through the present-day San Rafael Wilderness, and into the San Joaquin Valley.

A military expedition under the command of Pablo de la Portilla secured a peace with and return of the Chumash, and the revolt was resolved without further (immediate) conflict.

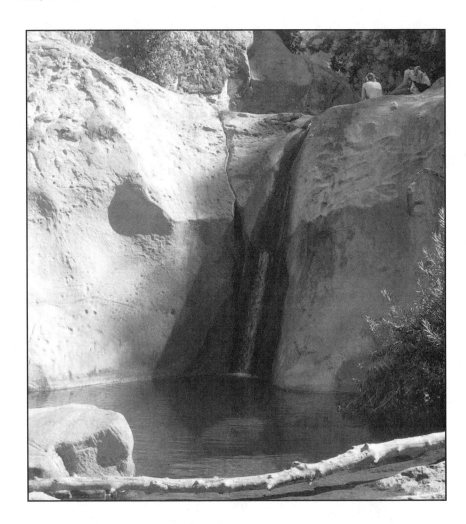

■ ■ ■ ■ ■ ■ ■ ■ ■ ■ ■ ■ ■ **WHAT'S IN A NAME?**

The Tunnel Trail is named for the water projects that brought water from the Santa Ynez River on the other side of the mountains up and over to the growing (and therefore increasingly thirsty) Santa Barbara populace. The first water tunnel devised by city engineers was the Cold Spring Tunnel (see *Route 22*), contributing approximately 290 acre-feet to the city's reserves. After a series of droughts in years immediately following, it became clear that far more water would be necessary to sate the growing population, and the USGS's head of hydrology made the recommendation to construct a tunnel from Mission Canyon to the Santa Ynez River.

An arduous, obstacle-laden process commenced in 1904, and for eight years workers toiled to complete the project (their supplies were brought into the tunnel— and material shipped out—via a small rail system). The tunnel extends 19,540 feet (3.7 miles) and currently delivers an average of 1,348 acre-feet per year (AFY; one acre-foot equals 326,000 gallons). A major rehabilitation project was completed in December 1994.

With the completion of the Gibraltar Dam in 1921, the tunnel's workload increased dramatically, as it also delivered the Gibraltar Reservoir's water to Santa Barbara. The Gibraltar Dam was raised to its current height in 1949 and delivers approximately 4,600 AFY to Santa Barbara. In conjunction with the Bureau of Reclamation's massive Lake Cachuma project—completed in the 1950s—the old Mission Tunnel continues to play a key role in sustaining Santa Barbara (now with a population nearing 100,000).

■ ■

Route 21

RATTLESNAKE CANYON (27W15)

LENGTH AND TYPE:	1.8-mile one-way to Tunnel/Rattlesnake Connector; 4.8-mile out-and-back to Gibraltar Road
RATING:	Moderate (climb at end)
TRAIL CONDITION:	Clear
MAP(S):	USGS *Santa Barbara*; Conant's *Matilija & Dick Smith Wilderness*
CAMP(S):	—
HIGHLIGHTS:	Expansive views of Santa Barbara Channel; riparian trekking; meadow and fantastic wildflower displays in spring

TO REACH THE TRAILHEAD(S): Use the Rattlesnake Canyon Trailhead for this route.

TRIP SUMMARY: A very popular destination named for the fact the canyon snakes through the Santa Barbara frontcountry, the Rattlesnake Trail passes through lush riparian stretches toward a meadow before meeting with the Tunnel Trail Connector and then climbs to Gibraltar Road.

Trip Description

From the **trailhead (890', 252671E 3816185N)**, the wide and well-maintained trail almost immediately leads you over the perennial **creek (<0.1 mile, 890', 252680E 3816240N)**. This is typically an exercise in easy rock-hopping along the large cobbles, but do mind wet rocks before and after rains, as they can be slippery here. From the creek, follow the track up a ways to the junction with the **fire road (0.1 mile, 950', 252749E 3816318N)** and head left (north). In addition to the coastal live oak and sycamore coverage, (introduced) rockroses sometimes line your progress here. (As an aside, these flowers are capable of recovering well in postfire landscapes and also can thrive in relatively poor soil due to symbiotic relationships with moisture-supplying fungi underground. In light of the Tea Fire of November 2008, they are well suited to this stretch.)

After walking along the road a short way, you'll approach a junction with an older **equestrian trail (0.5 mile, 1,175', 252952E 3816847N)**; stay left (low) here as the route levels out a bit and continue to follow the drainage toward a series of steep rock cliffs on your right (east), which you'll hike around to the right to again cross the **creek (0.6 mile, 1,175', 253033E 3816890N)**. On both sides of the trail as you climb into one of the areas clearly burned by the fires, you'll pass through a coppice of Aleppo pines planted by the Santa Barbara chapter of the Sierra Club in 1966 to replace those lost in the Coyote Fire of 1964.

Continue along the trail back into the lush riparian drainage; this stretch is magnificent and a cool place to laze beneath large trees or upon the many huge boulders, or to soak your feet in the many available pools. Mature live oaks, sycamores, big-leaf maples, and bays provide all the shade you need—even at noon most stretches are still cast in shadow. Make your way across a pair of **crossings (first at 1.3 miles, 1,550', 253032E 3817615N)** with massive rock clefts looming beside the creek, and then climb gently but steadily along the west bank of the creek for a time until you enter the beautiful **Tin Cabin meadow (1.7 miles, 1,850', 253165E 3818113N)** that in the spring can boast a very impressive wildflower display. This glade was named for the cabin partially built of 5-gallon kerosene cans by William O'Connor. The cabin burned in 1925.

Just beyond the meadow is the junction with the **connector trail (1.8 miles, 1,900', 253204E 3818136N)**. A collection of large boulders set beneath a very mature coast live oak makes this junction nearly impossible to miss.

From the junction, go right/east (heading left/west will lead toward the Tunnel Trail; see sidebar below); most of your views of the Santa Barbara Channel and points south are lost, but you'll gain a great vista of Gibraltar Rock and upper Rattlesnake Canyon to your left (northward). Around the first bend from the junction is a **tributary (1.8 miles, 1,875', 253237E 3818169N)** to the main Rattlesnake drainage on your left (north); even in dry years this little ravine tends to have water. In little time you'll cross the **wash (1.9 miles, 1,875', 253360E 3818237N)** of the main drainage. This is typically dry save for the spring season and after rains, but is well shaded by bays, sycamores, and huge oaks and makes for a fine rest area. From the cool of the wash you'll then embark upon a series of switchbacks; the north-facing slopes are dotted by sword ferns and reeds, where in the wetter months the hillside seeps keep things moist, and the more exposed stretches are rocky and rough. Your ascent here is a relatively steep affair, 0.5 mile of often-rutted trail (eroded after the recent fires) climbing to **Gibraltar Road (2.4 miles, 2,475', 253747E 3818007N)**.

■ ■ ■ ■ ■ ■ ■ ■ ■ **RATTLESNAKE CONNECTOR**

The connector route linking the Tunnel and Rattlesnake Trails is a marginally steep climb westward. As of this writing, the erosion and gullying that occurred post–Jesusita Fire makes for a fairly poor tread, but despite some brushy and washed-over spots it's a simple enough matter to navigate the trail 0.75 mile to the **gap and junction (2.4 miles from Skofield trailhead, 2,485', 252292E 3818494N)** with the Tunnel Trail (see *Route 20* for your options here along Mission Canyon).

■ ■ ■ ■ ■ ■ ■ ■ ■ ■ ■ ■ ■ ■ ■ ■ ■ ■ ■ ■

Route 22

COLD SPRING CANYON WEST (27W16)

LENGTH AND TYPE:	4.4-mile out-and-back to Gibraltar Road
RATING:	Moderately strenuous (climb)
TRAIL CONDITION:	Clear to Cold Spring Tunnel; passable between tunnel and Gibraltar Road (fire damage); poison oak
MAP(S):	USGS *Santa Barbara*; Conant's *Matilija & Dick Smith Wilderness*
CAMP(S):	—
HIGHLIGHTS:	Views of Montecito and the Pacific

TO REACH THE TRAILHEAD(S): Use the Cold Spring Canyon Trailhead for this route.

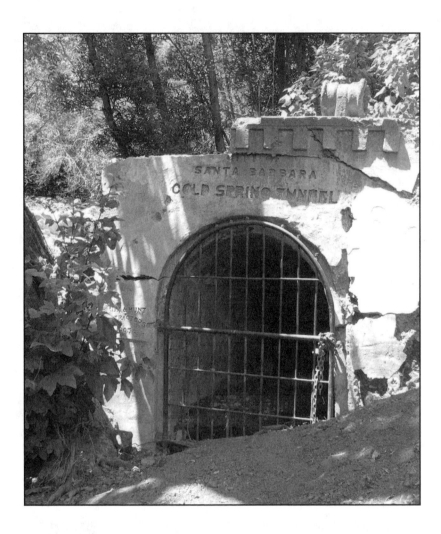

TRIP SUMMARY: This moderately strenuous ascent along the West Fork of Cold Spring Creek leads through lush riparian trail and then climbs rather steeply through the bare and fire-scarred slopes of Hill 2317 to Gibraltar Road.

Trip Description

From the **trailhead (780', 256269E 3815901N)**, follow the trail northward along the well-shaded path 0.25 mile to the junction with **West Fork Cold Spring Trail (0.25 mile, 865', 256163E 3816269N)**; a bench marks this junction. Follow the West Fork trail, crossing the creek once and continuing northward. You'll climb moderately under the cover of live oaks and sycamores, passing some unique rock formations and following a series of iron and PVC water pipes, until you reach the junction to **Tangerine Falls (0.8 mile, 1,190', 255815E 3816925N)**, marked by two large boulders on the right side of the trail. Bear left here (see *Route 23* for the route that leads to the right and into the middle fork).

Ascend the trail a short distance to the first crossing where the water pipe crosses the creek bed; damage from 2008's Tea Fire slowly begins to make itself apparent. At the fourth and final crossing is the gate of the **Cold Spring Tunnel (1.2 miles, 1,370', 255437E 3817195N)**, constructed in 1896 to tap the nearby spring and bring water into Santa Barbara before more ambitious methods were pursued (e.g., the Mission Tunnel and Lake Cachuma).

After crossing the creek bed from the tunnel, your ascent of the upper drainage begins, and here is where damage from the Tea Fire is blatant. While hardier trees and growth survived in the lower riparian areas and in select draws, most everything else was decimated. The trail has eroded in several places and would be a difficult navigation but for the efforts of local volunteers.

After a short period of climbing, you'll reach a **crest (1.4 miles, 1,470', 255407E 3817048N)** along a low ridge with a view of another drainage to your west; follow the better-traveled track to your left (south) and not the use track to your right. Drop approximately 50 vertical feet into the drainage, and then begin the steady ascent along the switchbacks (passing numerous US Forest Service DESIGNATED ROUTE signs), gaining better views of Cold Spring Canyon and eventually a slice of the Santa Barbara Channel, before reaching a gap near the top. The trail will level a bit and lead west to deposit you at the hairpin along **Gibraltar Road (2.2 miles, 1,900', 254855E 3817223N)**.

Route 23

TANGERINE FALLS

LENGTH AND TYPE:	2.6-mile out-and-back to base of falls; 3-mile out-and-back to top of falls
RATING:	Moderate to base of falls; moderately strenuous to top of falls
TRAIL CONDITION:	Clear to top of falls; some scrambling required at the very end to base of falls; poison oak
MAP(S):	USGS *Santa Barbara*; Conant's *Matilija & Dick Smith Wilderness*
CAMP(S):	—
HIGHLIGHTS:	Waterfall; numerous pools; views of Montecito and the Pacific

TO REACH THE TRAILHEAD(S): Use the Cold Spring Canyon Trailhead for this route.

TRIP SUMMARY: This popular and moderate hike leads to the base of Tangerine Falls through the very lush riparian trail along Cold Spring Creek. Some scrambling is required at the very end of the route. An alternate route leads to the creek area above the falls.

Trip Description

From the **trailhead** (**780', 256269E 3815901N**), follow the trail northward along the well-shaded route 0.25 mile to the junction with the **West Fork Cold Spring Trail** (**0.25 mile, 865', 256163E 3816269N**); a bench marks this junction. Follow the West Fork trail, crossing the creek once and continuing northward. You'll climb moderately under the cover of live oaks and sycamores, passing some unique rock formations and following a series of iron and PVC water pipes, until you reach the junction to **Tangerine Falls** (**0.8 mile, 1,190', 255815E 3816925N**), marked by two large boulders on the right side of the trail. Bear right here (see *Route 22* for the route that leads straight) along a well-worn trail and cross the West Fork once, climbing steadily but not over-aggressively to the next **junction** (**1.1 miles, 1,225', 255817E 3817012N**), where you've the option to continue straight (northward) toward the base of the falls (stepping over or around a large metal pipe that almost obscures the fact the trail continues up-creek; this trail is easily missed) or bear left and climb along the west ridge to the area above the falls.

Route to the Base

From the **junction** (**1.1 miles, 1,225', 255817E 3817012N**), continue straight along the trail to the next crossing, this being the main fork of Cold Spring Creek. The trail here begins to not only steepen but also get slick, as the packed soil, combined with the limited sun this narrow canyon receives, stays cool and quite moist. For portions of the hike exposed oak, sycamore, and bay tree roots and saplings avail themselves to navigating the more difficult stretches. Continue along this route, crossing the creek again to gain the west bank for the remainder of the hike, until the trail is reduced to a series of enjoyable scrambles along rocks and around trees (while avoiding the increasing poison oak) to the base of **Tangerine Falls** (**1.3 miles, 1,625', 255795E 3817455N**). This area is popular with local rock climbers, and you may spot anchors, bolts, and other climbing hardware along certain routes on the rock faces on the left (west) of the falls proper.

Route to Above the Falls

From the **junction** (**1.1 miles, 1,225', 255817E 3817012N**), bear left along the fern-lined track, which is often choked with grass. Several sets of short but steep switchbacks lead you to a ridge between the main and west forks of Cold Spring Creek; washed-out stretches of trail and debris are common in the years after 2008's Tea Fire (the origin of which is only a ridge away). Follow this ridge with an intermittent view of Tangerine Falls to the north, climbing steadily with little shade until the trail curves eastward, following the line of the fault to the **bend** (**1.4 miles, 1,890', 255732E 3817510N**), at which point the trail makes a sharp left (north) to rejoin the creek, making an abrupt return to the cool riparian cover of the alder- and sycamore-shaded canyon.

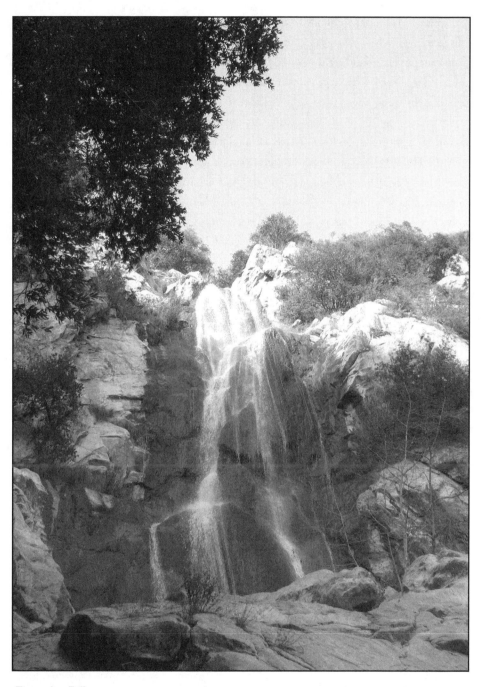

Tangerine Falls

From this bend there are two ways by which you can access the final few pools above the falls (one, especially, is ideal for wading). The first option is to follow the thin thread of a trail from your vantage point here and continue eastward toward the falls, picking your way through the boulders and trees and then dropping down the left (north) face of the steep embankment, rejoining the creek just as it begins to narrow. The other option, which can prove easier to navigate after rains or in the spring after undergrowth makes some of the banks thick with poison oak and brush, is to follow the trail from the bend to the next **crossing (1.5 miles, 1,850', 255697E 3817561N)** and then rock-hop your way along the creek for a few hundred feet.

Both options lead you along the creek until you reach a deep **pool (1,840', 255795E 3817509N)** that is held back by a very large boulder jammed in the narrowed canyon. Descending to the next set of smaller pools can prove tricky, though there is usually a rope or two you can use to scramble down (just be sure you can make the climb back up!). From there you can rock-hop beneath a few bay saplings through where the creek has cut the harder rock to the very skirts of the falls' drop; do exercise extreme caution here. While the actual falls are not visible from this point, the cascade's sound is proof enough you've reached the top.

Farther along the thin thread of trail that continues upstream from the bend described above, you can continue another 0.5 mile or so to the remains of the old Romero homestead. This seldom-visited destination makes a pleasant picnic spot. Finding a path much farther beyond the old stone foundations of the homestead is sketchy at best, as the terrain not only becomes quite steep but also the brush and growth less forgiving as you continue up-canyon.

Route 24

EAST FORK COLD SPRING (26W10) and MONTECITO PEAK

LENGTH AND TYPE:	9.2-mile out-and-back to Camino Cielo from Cold Spring Trailhead; 7.6-mile out-and-back to Montecito Peak from Cold Spring Trailhead
RATING:	Moderately strenuous
TRAIL CONDITION:	Clear
MAP(S):	USGS *Santa Barbara*; Conant's *Matilija & Dick Smith Wilderness*
CAMP(S):	—
HIGHLIGHTS:	Numerous wading pools; fantastic views of Montecito and the Pacific; side trail to Montecito Peak

TO REACH THE TRAILHEAD(S): Use the Cold Spring Canyon Trailhead for this route.

TRIP SUMMARY: From the Cold Spring Trailhead, this moderately strenuous trek follows the cool riparian trail alongside the main and east fork of Cold Spring Creek, and then ascends the southwest flank of Montecito Peak and beyond to Camino Cielo. Fantastic views.

Trip Description

From the **trailhead** (**780', 256269E 3815901N**), follow the trail northward, passing the junction with **West Fork Cold Spring Trail** (**0.25 mile, 865', 256163E 3816269N**) and climbing easily beneath alders, oaks, and sycamores. Cross the stream twice as you wind toward the junction with what is known locally as the **Hippie House Trail** (**1.5 miles, 1,425', 256515E 3816520N**). Bear left here, continuing along a lush stretch of trail to the junction with the Edison **road** (**1.6 miles, 1,650', 256976E 3816418N**), keeping left and continuing along the road approximately 100 yards to rejoin the trail on your left (north).

Upon leaving the road, your climb begins in earnest. In short time you'll come upon the **junction** (**1.9 miles, 1,820', 257230E 3816496N**) to the closed Hot Springs Trail (see sidebar on the next page), marked by a metal private property sign. Continue climbing as the trail becomes increasingly rocky and the tree cover diminishes to ceanothus and scrub, making for a warm, exposed ascent in the summer months. Follow a series of switchbacks up onto a ridge along the southwest skirts of Montecito Peak, eventually curving toward a pair of incongruous **eucalyptus trees** (**2.8 miles, 2,475', 257087E 3817353N**), which make for an ideal rest spot (and is the turnaround spot for many) on an otherwise exposed stretch. By this point your views of Montecito and the Pacific are expansive; as you continue climbing, the Channel Islands continue to spread out before you. Much of the route below, as well as Santa Barbara Harbor, are well framed by the eucalypti at this vantage point.

Continuing to climb, the cobbles and boulders make for slow going at points but eventually yield to the higher portion of the trail where the tread improves and regains a degree of vegetation. This portion of the ascent is much less exposed and provides some shade. Watch for the **turnoff** (**3.5 miles, 2,880', 257609E 3817844N**) to Montecito Peak on your right (east), as the narrow unmarked trail is neither an official route nor maintained with any regularity and is easy to miss.

■ ■ ■ ■ ■ ■ ■ ■ ■ ■ ■ ■ ■ ■ **MONTECITO PEAK**

Montecito Peak can be accessed easily from the parking area at the terminus of the Cold Spring East Trail atop Camino Cielo or by following the more difficult ascent from the Cold Spring Trailhead along East Mountain Drive.

Something of a scramble at points, the short (0.25-mile) ascent to **Montecito Peak** (**3.8 miles, 3,214', 257611E 3817648N**) is an exercise in basic route-finding and some easy scrambling. A register at the peak (maintained for the last several years by the students at the Montecito Montessori school) provides the opportunity to document your ascent for posterity; it's located among the sandstone boulders gathered at the southwest corner of the little scrub-covered plateau. There is also an Aleppo pine, known as the "Montecito Peak Pine," which local hikers planted in 1997 and hope will become something of a shade-providing landmark atop this barren peak top in the years to come. Views from the summit stretch from the Santa Ynez ridgeline along Camino Cielo to the north, Santa Barbara, Montecito, Carpinteria, and other communities, and far-reaching views of the Channel Islands and Santa Barbara Channel up and down the coast.

■ ■ ■ ■ ■ ■ ■ ■ ■ ■ ■ ■ ■ ■ ■ ■ ■ ■ ■ ■

From the junction, continue another (at times steep) mile to the north. The tread improves a great deal north of Montecito Peak, eschewing the rock- and cobble-strewn terrain of the previous stretches for well-packed shale and soil. After a few twists, the trail hooks to the west before climbing to the trailhead at **Camino Cielo Road (4.6 miles, 3,400', 257657E 3818995N)**. The concrete water tank here is a common reference point.

In addition to returning the way you came, your position here grants you numerous opportunities. Directly across the road is the trail leading down the north slope to Forbush Camp (see *Route 14*). An easy 0.2-mile stroll east along Camino Cielo will put you at the top trailhead for the San Ysidro trail (see *Route 28*) on your right (south).

Additional trails can be accessed along the road in both directions; see Map 6.

MONTECITO HOT SPRINGS ■ ■ ■ ■ ■ ■ ■ ■ ■ ■ ■ ■

The Montecito Hot Springs has developed something of a mythic, near-urban legend status among Santa Barbara hikers. This mystique has made the springs all the more enticing by its being made (legally) off-limits in recent years.

There are at least four hot springs ranging 99°–122°F in the stretch of Hot Springs Canyon typically referred to simply as "the Hot Springs," or—on some older maps— Hot Spring Club. These springs flow at an estimated rate of 74 gallons per minute (approximately 100,000 gallons per day) and have very low salinity. Owners of the property over the last 150 years have included Wilbur Curtiss, the man accredited with introducing the springs to the public, as well as such entities as the Santa Barbara Hot Springs Hotel, the La Parra Grande Hot Springs Company, and the uberexclusive Hot Springs Club.

In 1855, Curtiss—an ailing '49er who by many reports had been given a life expectancy of six months—arrived in Santa Barbara. There, a Canalino (Chumash) native named El Viejo—referred to as the "ancient one" and reputed to be more than 100 years old—led him up the canyon to the hot springs, the virtues of which had been extolled by various American soldiers toward the end of the 1846–1848 Mexican-American War. Curtiss's ailments left him, and sometime between 1857 and 1862 he filed a homestead claim in Hot Springs Canyon, by some accounts becoming Montecito's first American settler, and began developing the springs and immediate surroundings for commercial gain (and the healthful benefits, of course). He built the first of four wooden hotels at the springs; fires took each in turn.

In the 1880s, ownership of the hot springs transferred to a handful of well-to-do Montecito residents, who built a hotel on the grounds. In 1908, the site was put up for sale and purchased by local investors (members/directors of the Montecito Water Company). The hotel was lost in the 1920 fire but soon replaced by a private resort. This super-exclusive "clubhouse" was in turn lost in the Coyote Fire of 1964.

You'll likely note the huge growths of Arundo (*Arundo donax,* also known as giant reed) beginning near the abandoned gardens near the Hot Springs Hotel ruins. This naturalized cane, commonly planted around hot springs areas, has become extremely invasive from this point down into and beyond where Hot Springs and Cold Spring Creeks meet to form lower Montecito Creek.

Route 25

SADDLE ROCK LOOP

LENGTH AND TYPE:	2-mile loop utilizing a portion of the Girard Trail; 2.4-mile out-and-back to Edison Catway
RATING:	Moderate (for a short but steep climb up Saddle Rock)
TRAIL CONDITION:	Clear
MAP(S):	USGS *Santa Barbara*; Conant's *Matilija & Dick Smith Wilderness* *Note:* Route only partially shown on USGS map
CAMP(S):	—
HIGHLIGHTS:	Sandstone formations; excellent views of Montecito and surroundings

TO REACH THE TRAILHEAD(S): Use the Saddle Rock Trailhead for this route.

TRIP SUMMARY: From East Mountain Drive, this popular day trip ascends the southern flank of Saddle Rock to the Edison service road through riparian and then chaparral-covered sandstone trail, topping out with fantastic views at Saddle Rock.

Trip Description

From the **parking area (600', 257034E 3815087N)**, follow the trail northward along an easy and well-worn track shaded by numerous sycamores and live oaks and skirted by poison oak. The trail progresses behind numerous private properties and along a number of fence lines; be sure to stay to the trail and respect private property. Some nonnative plants (fennel, along with some that are landscaped) creep into the mix here, and soon you'll cross a marginally residential stretch of **Hot Springs Road (0.2 mile, 720', 257132E 3815338N)**; cross the first street and then stay left as the track parallels the road northward for a short spell before cutting onto the road proper.

Follow the road, crossing the **creek (0.25 mile, 720', 257178E 3815420N)** and continuing on the narrow road until reaching a large driveway **gate (0.3 mile, 750', 257218E 3815484N)**. The trail follows this private drive along the right (east) side of the property before passing it and joining a dirt service road. Continue northward here until a Montecito Trails Foundation sign **(0.45 mile, 850', 257415E 3815691N)**

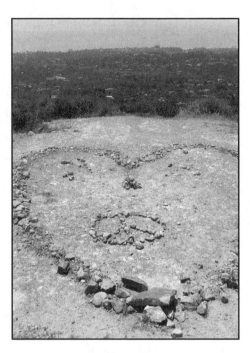

Plein Air Rock Art

directs you to the right (east) off the road to follow a small stretch of trail that then curves right to rejoin the road rather quickly and then cross **Hot Springs Creek (0.5 mile, 860', 257448E 3815684N)**.

From the creek, follow the stone steps up and to your left, again following private property fences as you continue up the increasingly rock-strewn service road. Soon you'll spot a large gate across the road—clearly indicating private property lays beyond—and it's just before this gate that the **trail (0.6 mile, 925', 257540E 3815685N)** forks off to your right (east). Follow the trail up the erosion bars (not the deep-cut drainage on your left, which is an old and now abandoned route to the once-accessible hot springs), and from here you'll climb somewhat steeply at points alternately beneath the shade of oaks or rocky, exposed trail for a brief stretch until you reach a **gap (0.7 mile, 1,090', 257717E 3815640N)** under cover of a mature live oak. Here the McMenemy Trail cuts down to your right (north); follow the left fork to continue up the Saddle Rock route.

From the gap, the route becomes steep and very rocky, leveling out at the **Saddle Rock formation (0.75 mile, 1,120', 257760E 3815695N)**, a series of sandstone outcrops that curve above Oak Creek and provide some fairly mild but worthwhile opportunities for bouldering and scrambling. Bush monkeyflower is often the easiest-identified flower along this stretch of trail, but also common on this route are sage, nonnative fennel, gooseberry, and brodiaea.

Continue following the trail up along the exposed rock while you're hemmed in by high chaparral (heavy on the chamise and laurel sumac) on both sides for another steep 0.25 mile—gaining impressive views rather quickly en route—until you crest the **hill** (**1 mile, 1,400', 257853E 3815939N**). Most hikers turn around here, the bulk of the work done, but consider continuing beyond the north slopes, where the trail continues, dropping into a saddle along which the well-known power lines travel. Follow the trail down into this gap, then climb again, passing beneath the power lines before gaining the service road, known locally as the **Edison Catway** (**1.2 miles, 1,300', 257988E 257988N**).

Here you have a few options. You can either return the way you came or follow the service road a very easy 0.3 mile right (eastward) to the junction with the **Girard Trail** (**1.8 miles, 1,450', 258285E 3816066N**), which you can follow for a nice loop to the upper McMenemy and back to the junction with the Saddle Rock Trail (see Map 6 and *Routes 26* and *27*).

You may also wish to follow the service road left (west) from the junction, climbing 1.5 miles to the road's intersection of the East Fork Cold Spring Trail (see *Route 24*).

Route 26

McMENEMY

LENGTH AND TYPE:	2.1-mile one-way
RATING:	Moderate (elevation gain)
TRAIL CONDITION:	Clear
MAP(S):	USGS *Carpinteria* and *Santa Barbara*; Conant's *Matilija & Dick Smith Wilderness* *Note:* Route only partially shown on USGS map
CAMP(S):	—
HIGHLIGHTS:	Excellent views of Montecito, Santa Barbara Channel, Channel Islands, and surroundings

TO REACH THE TRAILHEAD(S): Use the San Ysidro Canyon Trailhead for this route.

TRIP SUMMARY: From the San Ysidro Trail, the McMenemy Trail cuts westward across the foothills of Montecito, connecting with the Girard and Saddle Rock Trails.

Trip Description

From the **trailhead** (**420', 259098E, 3814727N**), follow the shaded and well-maintained trail between slices of private property to the upper stretch of West Park Lane and the residences there. Continue following the trail as it parallels the left (west) side of the street before cutting around the perimeter of a large property to find yourself at the start of the dirt service road along which you'll be hiking for the next stretch. Continue along the main road where the road gate marks the junction for the **Old Pueblo Trail (0.4 mile, 640', 259115E 3815261N)** on your right (east). The road continues climbing easily under cover of large live oaks and sycamores to the McMenemy Trail **junction (0.5 mile, 675', 259140E 3815438N)** on your left (west).

Follow this down into the San Ysidro ravine, where even in drier years the creek typically has water collected here. The pool on the far (west) side of the crossing is especially deep and is quite popular with little hikers and any four-legged companions; however, the trail typically receives a bit too much traffic to make it a very restful wading area. Continue following the trail southwest through a mix of alder-, oak-, and blue gum–shaded stretch of trail. The introduced eucalypti planted here can give one the brief impression of hiking in the Australian bush; in the heat and after rains the trees are especially fragrant. At a **junction (0.7 mile, 655', 259005E 259005N)** beside a gravel service road, head right (north) into a draw.

Follow the track up the creek and then along a long, arcing switchback that leads you back out of the riparian zones into the scrub and oak woodland above some of the more secluded private properties of the Montecito foothills. Views of the local communities, Santa Barbara Channel, and the Channel Islands immediately avail themselves to you. The trail leads up a steep, grassy slope across which numerous switchbacks zigzag—recent volunteer efforts have attempted to minimize the damage and erosion wrought by those who cut the switchbacks, so please be sure to adhere to the prescribed trail. The switchbacks continue into the bush before topping out at a **sharp right** (west) **(1.2 miles, 985', 258644E 3815323N)**. Follow the trail up along the ridge at a much easier grade to the **top (1.4 miles, 1,125', 258469E 3815454N)**, where on your left (south) you'll spy the bench commemorating Colonel McMenemy, placed here shortly after his death in 1972 by the Montecito Trails Foundation.

Just beyond the bench is the **junction (1.4 miles, 1,080', 258449E 3815473N)** with the Girard Trail (see *Route 27*), which heads to the right (north) and climbs to the Edison Catway. Stay left (west) here to drop easily through the rock-bottomed trail bordered by grasses and low chaparral and still with excellent views of Montecito below. Soon you'll pass a water tank on your left (south) and continue easily downhill until you reach **Oak Creek (1.8 miles, 940', 258065E 3815736N)**. Climb out of the drainage here, and views of the rock formations along the Saddle Rock Trail come into view as you navigate some larger sandstone boulders along your route. Ascend easily to the junction with the **Saddle Rock Trail (2.1 miles, 1,090', 257717E 3815640N)** under a mature live oak.

Here you have the option to return the way you came or make a longer loop up the Saddle Rock Trail, along a portion of the Edison Catway, and down the Girard Trail (rejoining the McMenemy at the saddle near the bench you passed less than a mile ago). See *Routes 25* and *27* for information detailing those options.

■ ■ ■ ■ ■ ■ ■ ■ ■ **COLONEL LOGAN T. McMENEMY**

Colonel Logan T. McMenemy deeded the trail that bears his name to the public (via the Santa Barbara Parks Department) in 1962, and the Montecito Trails Association (a precursor of the Montecito Trails Foundation) constructed the current trail in 1964.

Colonel McMenemy served as an ambulance driver in France, as well as an officer with the aviation branch of the United States Signal Corps during both World Wars, and was a prominent businessman in Chicago before retiring to Santa Barbara, where he purchased the Oak Creek Ranch in Montecito in 1947 (the ranch has since been sold and subdivided). A lower trail once ran along the lower stretches of the Oak Creek property, and as a result the current trail is often still referred to as the Upper McMenemy Trail.

■ ■ ■ ■ ■ ■ ■ ■ ■ ■ ■ ■ ■ ■ ■ ■ ■ ■

Route 27

GIRARD TRAIL

LENGTH AND TYPE:	0.6-mile one-way (connect either via McMenemy or from Edison Catway)
RATING:	Easy north-to-south; easy to moderate south-to-north
TRAIL CONDITION:	Clear
MAP(S):	USGS *Santa Barbara*; Conant's *Matilija & Dick Smith Wilderness*
CAMP(S):	—
HIGHLIGHTS:	Excellent views of Montecito and surroundings

TO REACH THE TRAILHEAD(S): Use either the San Ysidro Canyon or Saddle Rock Trailheads for this route.

TRIP SUMMARY: Named for local trails and preservation advocate Edward "Bud" Girard, the Girard Trail descends from the Edison Catway to the McMenemy Junction along a pleasant oak- and chaparral-shaded track along the northeastern flank of the knoll immediately east of Oak Creek's headwaters. The trail was established in 2000 by the Montecito Trails Foundation, and a nice lookout is about two-thirds of the way down.

Trip Description

The trip is described from north to south, beginning at its upper junction with the Girard Trail and ending at the McMenemy Junction.

From the junction service road known locally as the Edison Catway and the upper Girard **trailhead (1,450', 258285E 3816066N)**, head south along the wide spur road toward the power lines, and then cut right along the singletrack just before the first tower. Here the trail curves slowly to the left (eastward) beneath the tower to follow an old road base, long since abandoned but providing a very nice grade for the trail. Because this stretch is better shaded than much of the surrounding area, poison oak and ferns reappear for a stretch.

Follow the trail down, eventually curving back toward the south as you skirt the knoll. As the trail begins to curve farther right and lead you westward, you'll come to the **junction (0.4 mile, 1,185', 258588E 3815642N)** for the spur trail leading to a lookout where there are a handful of plaques, as well as stone benches for enjoying the fine views both up-canyon but especially those toward the ocean. A number of large sandstone boulders jut from this location, making it an ideal spot for youngsters to practice their scrambling skills.

To continue from the lookout junction, follow the trail westward for a short stretch and then south toward the **junction (0.6 mile, 1,080', 258449E 3815473N)** with the upper stretch of the McMenemy Trail. See *Route 26* for a full description of the McMenemy Trail, but in short heading right (west) from here will lead you to the Saddle Rock Trail (see *Route 25*); proceeding left (east) here will first take you to a stone bench commemorating Colonel McMenemy and then down toward the San Ysidro Trail (see *Route 28*).

Route 28

SAN YSIDRO CANYON (26W15)

LENGTH AND TYPE:	3.7-mile out-and-back to San Ysidro Falls; 9-mile out-and-back to Camino Cielo
RATING:	Moderate to base of San Ysidro Falls; strenuous to top of falls (climb)
TRAIL CONDITION:	Clear
MAP(S):	USGS *Carpinteria* and *Santa Barbara*; Conant's *Matilija & Dick Smith Wilderness*
CAMP(S):	—
HIGHLIGHTS:	Waterfall; numerous pools en route; fantastic views of Montecito and the Pacific

TO REACH THE TRAILHEAD(S): Use the San Ysidro Trailhead for this route.

TRIP SUMMARY: This route leads along San Ysidro Canyon to San Ysidro Falls (passing numerous fantastic wading pools along the way), and then climbs steeply out of the drainage along exposed chaparral some 3,000 vertical feet to Camino Cielo Road atop the Santa Ynez mountain range.

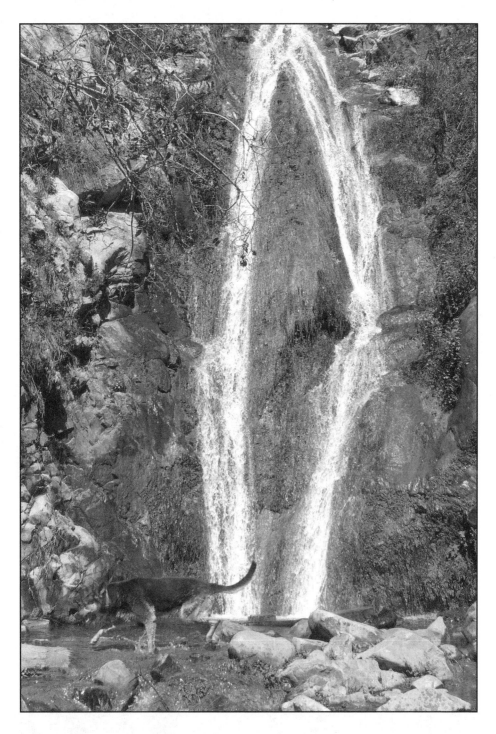

San Ysidro Falls

Trip Description

From the **trailhead** (**420', 259098E, 3814727N**), follow the shaded and well-maintained trail along a corridor through sections of private property to the upper stretch of West Park Lane and the residences there. Continue following the trail as it parallels the left (west) side of the street before cutting around the perimeter of a large property to find yourself at the start of the dirt service road along which you'll be hiking for the next stretch. Continue along the main road where the road gate marks the junction for the **Old Pueblo Trail** (**0.4 mile, 640', 259115E 3815261N**) on your right (east). The road continues climbing easily under cover of large live oaks and sycamores past the McMenemy Trail **junction** (**0.5 mile, 675', 259140E 3815438N;** see *Route 26*) on your left (west).

After nearly a mile of easy hiking, follow the Montecito Trails Association sign to bear right to leave the road for the **singletrack** (**0.9 mile, 880', 259079E 3816058N**), climbing steadily in well-shaded stretches at times heavy with poison oak. Along the creekside, stretches of the trail climb along rock faces of the canyon, and you'll note several fine pools that are sure to invite waders on warmer days. Cross the **creek** (**1.7 miles, 1,475', 259081E 3817253N**) just before climbing a final stretch to the **turnoff** to San Ysidro Falls (**1.8 miles, 1,500', 259036E 3817296N**). Retaining walls built by local Eagle Scout candidates help keep the shale from overrunning portions of the trail as you approach the falls.

Climbers work out problems along San Ysidro's canyon walls.

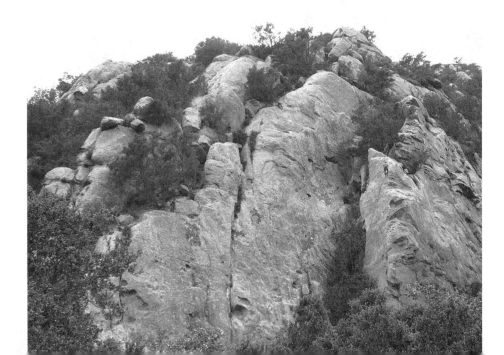

To continue toward Camino Cielo, return to the fork and follow the trail up along the canyon along an exposed track through chaparral with heavy vegetation but little shade another 2.5 miles. Along the way, views of Camino Cielo and the lower stretches of San Ysidro Canyon open, as do eventually breathtaking vistas of Montecito, the Channel Islands, and the Pacific. Finally, the trail levels slightly and curves around a final bend to bring you to **Camino Cielo (4.5 miles, 3,455', 258006E 3818912N).**

In addition to savoring the views and simply returning the way you came, there are numerous options available to you with some planning. An easy 0.2-mile stroll west along Camino Cielo will put you at the top trailhead for both sections of the East Fork Cold Spring Canyon trail.

The Romero Canyon Trailhead lies 1.5 miles to the east and forms the other entry point for the San Ysidro–to–Romero Canyon loop, popular especially among mountain bikers.

Route 29

BUENA VISTA LOOP

LENGTH AND TYPE:	2.8-mile loop
RATING:	Moderate (climb)
TRAIL CONDITION:	Clear; some well-maintained portions (Edison service road); poison oak
MAP(S):	USGS *Carpinteria*; Conant's *Matilija & Dick Smith Wilderness*
CAMP(S):	—
HIGHLIGHTS:	Views of Montecito and the Pacific; riparian trekking in multiple watersheds

TO REACH THE TRAILHEAD(S): Use the Buena Vista Trailhead for this route.

TRIP SUMMARY: This loop trip links several shorter Montecito trails in a counterclockwise direction through riparian trails and dirt service roads.

Trip Description

From the **Buena Vista Trailhead (665', 260133E 3815007N)**, follow the usually well-maintained trail through an easement, climbing easily toward a coppice of acacia trees and into a stretch of creekside hiking lined with huge sandstone boulders, crossing the creek twice before gaining the **junction (0.5 mile, 1,000', 260084E 3815702N)** with the Buena Vista Trail and the Romero Catway. Continue left (westward) here and climb out of the drainage, roughly following the landmark high-voltage power lines that traverse the area. Short views of the ocean soon avail themselves, and after a few well-cut switchbacks in the shale-lined trail to a trio of **power line towers** (**0.9 mile, 1,330', 259719E 3815823N**), you'll reach the terminus of an Edison service road.

Follow the largely shale road (at times steeply) down into San Ysidro Canyon; the split at 1.3 miles rejoins shortly on the other side of the knob, but it's typically easiest to follow the upper (right) route as it receives better maintenance from the utility. Soon the sounds of San Ysidro Falls and the creek below will reach you in all but the driest years. Beneath a cluster of live oaks is the junction with the San Ysidro **service road** (**1.5 miles, 831', 259071E 3815923N**); head left (south) here and follow the road down-canyon (see *Route 28* for the route up-canyon). Soon you'll pass an outcrop of Cold Spring sandstone well regarded by rock climbers. More often than not you'll spot climbers there on weekends.

Continue the easy descent under cover of large live oaks and sycamores past the **McMenemy Trail junction** (**1.8 miles, 675', 259140E 3815438N;** see *Route 26*) on your right (west). Just beyond you'll come to the main gate, which also marks the junction for the **Old Pueblo Trail** (**0.4 mile, 640', 259115E 3815261N**). Yet another left here will lead you along a well-maintained trail that scythes through a few plots of private property; please be respectful of the local landowners and stay on the trail. Because of the trail's proximity to private homes and the landscaping those typically entail, numerous introduced species (most notably eucalypti and more acacia trees, as well as oleander, nasturtium, and other hardy species) line this stretch of your hike. You'll parallel a private road and then cross the upper section of **Park Hill Lane** (**2.3 miles, 660', 259478E 3815061N**) to return to the trail along the drainages on the other side.

Soon the junction with the **Wiman Trail** (**2.5 miles, 650', 259625E 3814925N**) will come in on your right (south); stay left again and climb easily above more homes to meet a **side road** (**2.7 miles, 700', 259901E 3814936N**). Follow the drive some 400 feet down to the intersection with Park Lane; another 100 yards to your left (east) is the **trailhead** (**2.8 miles, 665', 260133E 3815007N**) from which you began this hike.

WIMAN TRAIL

The Wiman Trail is a very short (0.3-mile) spur trail that provides an easy shortcut to the Old Pueblo Trail. The **Wiman Trailhead** (**440', 259383E 3814647N**) is situated between both the San Ysidro and Buena Vista Trailheads, though small enough to be easily missed. From the intersection of Park Lane and CA 192 (East Valley Road) in Montecito, turn left (north) onto Park Lane and proceed 0.4 mile until the split; stay left and continue another 100 feet northeast along East Mountain Drive to a small parking area on the right (north) side of the road.

From the trailhead, you can follow this easy route northward along a well-shaded trail, vegetated by various introduced species. Plants the likes of which can thrive without much human tending (English ivy, nasturtium, palms, etc.) line the route alongside the native oaks and sycamores. The route climbs quickly around the (covered) Park Lane Reservoir to join the **Old Pueblo Trail (0.3 mile, 650', 259625E 3814925N)** alongside a chain-link fence. From here you can design a route of your own, and with the network of connected routes in the Montecito foothills, that could entail as long a day as you wish.

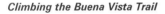

Climbing the Buena Vista Trail

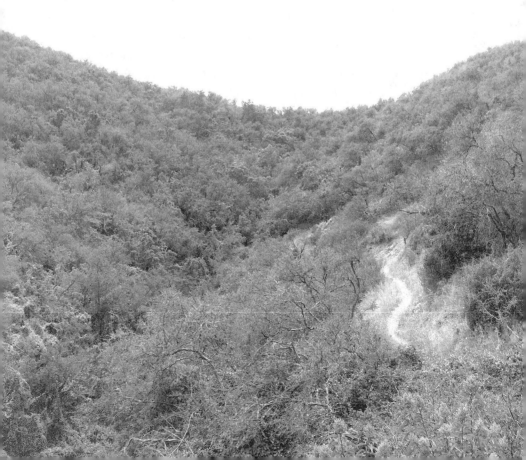

Route 30

ROMERO CANYON

LENGTH AND TYPE:	7.1-mile out-and-back to Camino Cielo via Romero Trail (26W14);
	3.8-mile out-and-back to second intersection with trail and fire road;
	10.3-mile figure eight (up Romero Trail and back via Romero Fire Road);
	4.9-mile up-and-over (one-way) to Blue Canyon trail junction
RATING:	Moderately strenuous
TRAIL CONDITION:	Clear (Romero Trail) and well maintained (old Romero Fire Road)
MAP(S):	USGS *Carpinteria*; Conant's *Matilija & Dick Smith Wilderness*
CAMP(S):	—
HIGHLIGHTS:	Classic riparian (and then chaparral) trekking; excellent views from Montecito to the Channel Islands to the south and from Camino Cielo to the San Rafael and Dick Smith Wildernesses to the north

TO REACH THE TRAILHEAD(S): Use the Romero Canyon Trailhead for this route.

TRIP SUMMARY: This fairly strenuous transect of Romero Canyon climbs 3.5 miles along the lush riparian Romero Trail, topping out at the east end of Camino Cielo Road, and then makes a long S-shaped drop back to the bottom of the canyon.

Note: The trails of Romero Canyon are quite possibly the most popular in the Santa Barbara frontcountry, so you'll seldom have the trail(s) to yourself. It is also heavily frequented by mountain bikers (and even the occasional mountain unicyclist!), so do be mindful of their presence. Most bikers doing the entire route tend to climb the road and descend along the technical singletrack. The local Santa Barbara Mountain Bike Trail Volunteers association (**sbmtv.org**) provides bells for bikes in small metal boxes posted at both the top and bottom of this trail and others along Camino Cielo and through the county. (A vast majority of the bikers who use the Romero Trail are exceedingly polite and courteous—it will be that one-off, less-considerate or less-attentive rider for whom you should be alert.)

Trip Description

Ascent via Romero Trail (26W14)

From the **parking area and trailhead** (985', 262008E 3815429N), walk around the large metal gate; pedestrian access is on the left (creek) side. Hike up the dirt road along the creek's east bank until the concrete **bridge** (0.25 mile, 1,040', 261882E 3815798N), at which point you'll cross to the other side and continue toward the junction with the Romero Catway (Edison) **service road** (0.3 mile, 1,060', 261847E 3815876N). Bear right here and continue along the main road; it's fenced on the creekside here and huge live oaks reach over to shade your route. Soon you'll reach the road's stream **crossing (0.5 mile, 1,120', 261993E 3815968N)**; just beyond on the left is the trail **junction (0.5 mile, 1,130', 262004E 3815986N)**.

Follow this singletrack along Romero Creek, progressing over a moderate but consistent ascent through fern-dappled track under cover of sycamores, bays, and oaks. Large boulders frame many stretches of the trail, which stays shaded for a majority of the climb toward the first crossing with the fire road. The few spots that do receive regular sun put on impressive wildflower displays in the spring, with lupines and golden poppies especially colorful during the blooms. Over the course of the first mile of singletrack, you'll cross the creek three times—the **second crossing (1.25 miles, 1,685', 261977E 3815171N)** especially makes a very nice lunch spot, with a pool ideal for wading right at the trailside and a handful of other tempting options just down the ravine from the crossing.

After the third crossing you'll begin a series of looping switchbacks, which during the course of climbing you'll cross the **Romero Fire Road (1.9 miles, 2,280', 261807E 3817606N)**. An old wooden sign directly across the road, wound within the exposed roots of a gnarled

Approaching Romero Saddle

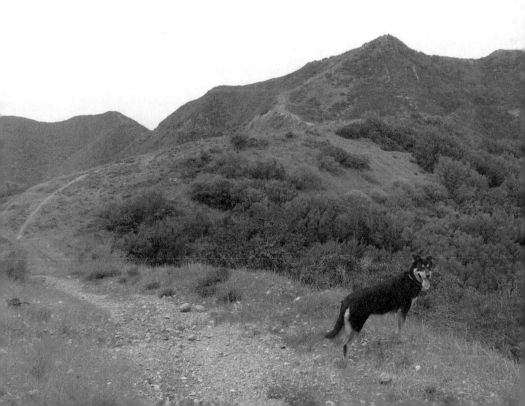

bay tree, marks another mile to the old (East) Ocean View Trail, and 3 to the Blue Canyon Trail. If this junction is your target high-point, from here you have the option to return to the parking area either by a direct turnaround or by following the road to your right (eastward) about 4 miles back to the parking area. See the *Romero Fire Road* description below, and follow the route from where this junction is mentioned again.

If your target is the top of the ridge, cross the road and continue along the switchbacks until the trail begins a long arc toward the east, culminating in another series of steep switchbacks that will deposit you among the grassy fields and expansive views of Montecito and the coast below. Stay left/straight at the **junction (3 miles, 3,075', 262212E 3817930N)**, following the old upper portion of the Romero Trail and the old Ocean View Trail (see sidebar for the portion of the Romero Trail on this side of the road and *Route 15* for the portion connecting Camino Cielo Road to Blue Canyon).

Continue north, wrapping left (eastward) around the back side of a knoll carved by mountain bikers and the occasional errant motorcyclist. As you progress, views of the Santa Ynez River Valley and the San Rafael and Dick Smith Wildernesses lay out before you. The trail drops a bit steeply at the very end to deposit you at the junction with Camino Cielo Road's asphalt and the graded dirt Romero-Camuesa Road. It's a quick walk westward to the water tank at **Romero Saddle (3.5 miles, 3,015', 261588E 3817974N)**, once the site of a USFS guard station.

From this vantage point, you have numerous options for exploring other routes along this ridgeline. The drop-in points for San Ysidro Canyon and East Fork Cold Spring (along with Montecito Peak) are both within walking distance of Romero Saddle.

Descent via Romero Fire Road

From Romero Saddle, follow the gated service road leading southwest from the water tank. Follow this former road and enjoy the downhill, as you certainly earned it in the ascent from the lower trailhead. (Once a viable dirt road, it was closed permanently after heavy rains in 1978 and is littered with detritus and rockfall in the winter and spring after the seasons' storms.) Though this portion of the route requires very little exertion compared to the ascent through the canyon, you'll notice the sun and heat far more here, as it is exposed to the south and there is little to no shade for more than 5 miles of road.

After 0.5 mile of easy hiking, you'll enter a **gap (4 miles, 3,080', 261106E 3817459N)** where views open on both sides of the road. Here the road wraps around the outer periphery of a lower knoll, and you begin the first long arc eastward. Bird's-eye views of various Montecito estates and the outlying communities stretch out before you, and after nearly 2 miles the first of a few **springs (5.9 miles, 2,415', 261526E 3817362N)** wedged in the crux of this stretch are marked by a small clusters of big-leaf maples nestled in this north-facing slope.

Soon you'll cross the **singletrack (6.3 miles, 2,280', 261807E 3817606N)** that led you across this road 4 miles ago. You have the option here, of course, to cut right (south) back onto the track and make the 2-mile return along the cooler riparian route, or you can continue along the road, crossing a tributary after another 100 feet and over the next few miles crossing numerous concrete runoffs in various states of cover as the road curves now toward the south again and eventually westward.

Another 2 miles and you'll approach another gap and then the junction with the upper stretches of the Toro Canyon **fire road (8.4 miles, 1,800', 262827E 3815932N)** on your left (east); the road is blocked by a metal gate and NO TRESPASSING signs. Follow the road's curve as it stretches westward again, eventually reconnecting with the first trail split and your earlier stream **crossing (9.8 miles, 1,120', 261993E 3815968N)**.

Retrace your earlier route down the road to return to the **parking area and trailhead (10.3 miles, 985', 262008E 3815429N)**.

MAKING THE CONNECTION ▓ ▓ ▓ ▓ ▓ ▓ ▓ ▓ ▓

From the **junction (3 miles, 3,075', 262212E 3817930N)** with the Ocean View Trail just southeast of the Romero Saddle, that little thread of a trail that drops down through the meadow and disappears from view is the actual continuation of the Romero Trail, as formally designated by the US Forest Service; the route most often taken these days follows the firebreak to the saddle and water tower and makes for the easiest access (especially because it allows drivers to park their vehicle on asphalt rather than venture down a sometimes-questionable dirt service road).

For the purists or completists, the final 0.75 mile down this oft-forgotten stretch is a nice (and often shadier) option from the exposed and heavily traveled usual route.

From the junction, head down into the field, quickly giving up the views of the ocean for a narrow trail lined with classic chaparral, thistles, and scrub oaks, and—very soon—expansive views of Blue Canyon and the greater Santa Ynez River Valley. Mind the poison oak as you follow a drainage lined with thick clusters of bays and live oaks—crossing the creek and a second tributary a few times—before a **sharp left** (west) **(3.4 miles, 2,850', 262571E 3818338N)** leads you to parallel the dirt Romero-Camuesa Road below. *Note:* The 1995 *Carpinteria* quad shows the trail cutting down to the road here. While there is an old cut leading to the road near the turn, the proper trail continues northwest as described here. Conant's *Matilija & Dick Smith Wilderness* map portrays the current route.

Oaks, manzanita, and a handful of ferns dot your easy descent toward the road. You'll cross an old **trail cut (3.6 miles, 2,820', 262346E 3818456N)** before entering a coppice of Pacific madrones, which usher you out onto the **Romero-Camuesa Road**

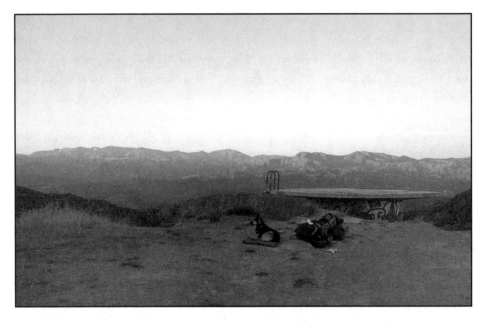

Romero Saddle at dusk

(3.7 miles, 2,790', 262259E 3818440N). From here, you can hike up the road about 0.5 mile to Romero Saddle if you have a vehicle there, or (with planning and provisions) continue down the Upper Romero Trail, the trailhead of which is just yards down the road on the right (north) side.

To continue toward Blue Canyon, head down the road perhaps 20 yards to where the opposite **trailhead (3.7 miles, 2,900', 262287E 3818453N)** leads northward. Follow this trail as it descends steadily, passing alternately through chaparral- and oak-hedged trail and wide grass meadows. This route is a long-retired service road used during the construction of the power lines you'll see spanning the length of Blue Canyon. After a 0.5-mile descent, you'll reach a **gap (4.2 miles, 2,220', 262264E 3819086N)** beside an intermittent stream, and from there climb very briefly to gain a low, rounded ridge, along which you'll hike and slowly triangulate toward one of the massive power pylons. Pass beneath the **power lines (4.6 miles, 2,060', 261976E 3819445N)** and then shortly afterward follow a brief series of switchbacks down to the junction with **Blue Canyon Trail (4.9 miles, 1,750', 261796E 3819707N)**. See *Route 15* for this route.

■ ■ ■ ■ ■ ■ ■ ■ ■ ■ ■ ■ ■ ■ ■ ■ **KRYPTOR**

If you're interested in seeing one of the serpentine rock formations that give Blue Canyon its name, one such outcrop is far more accessible than those now laid out far below you along the Escondido Creek drainage.

From the true Romero trailhead's parking area (some 0.6 mile along the dirt road east of Romero Saddle), there is a thin **use trail (2,860', 262183E 3818427N)** that begins at the upper stretch of the parking area. While you'll likely need to duck to get under some of the surrounding brush (a fellow hiker was heard lamenting that the trail "was built for Frodo [expletive] Baggins!"), the tread is usually in very good condition and leads you along a moderately steep trail to **Kryptor (0.15 mile, 2,700', 262127E 3818600N)**, a well-known and well-respected climbing spot composed of the namesake blue-green serpentine. Views of the canyon from here are just as spectacular as those from the road above (if not better).

■ ■ ■ ■ ■ ■ ■ ■ ■ ■ ■ ■ **OCEAN VIEW TRAIL**

The Ocean View Trail is a historical route that has been cut, dozed, and altered over the last century as to barely resemble the route described in a 1910s guidebook as "one of the most beautiful of all the [Santa Barbara] trails." Many of the changes are due to fire lines being cut along the ridgelines east of Romero Saddle, as well as some expansions in OHV routes (the Divide Peak OHV Route now constitutes a large portion of the former Ocean View route). The far western portion that remains a foot trail is still a nice stretch with magnificent views.

From the **junction (3,075', 262212E 3817930N)** with the Romero Trail just southeast of the Romero Saddle (see *Route 30* for details), the route heads east along the old fire road, climbing the first (and fairly steep) rise to a hilltop where stands Island View Trail **signpost No. 3 (0.1 mile, 3,050', 262341E 3817947N)**.

From here continue eastward, undulating up and down the alternately gentle and then rather steep sections to the gate intended to separate this earlier route with the network of motorcycle and ATV trails along the western drainage of upper Escondido Canyon. Follow the trail down to the junction, staying left (east) and following the track just less than a mile down to its junction with the **Divide Peak OHV Route (0.9 mile, 3,320', 263319E 3817571N)**.

■ ■ ■ ■ ■ ■ ■ ■ ■ ■ ■ ■ ■ ■ ■ ■ ■ ■ ■

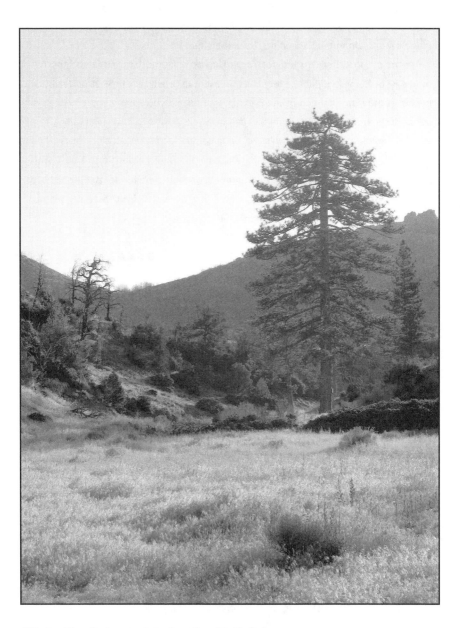

Mission Pine Basin; courtesy Jonathan M. McCabe

Santa Barbara Backcountry and Southern San Rafael Wilderness

This chapter details routes in the Santa Barbara backcountry and the southern San Rafael Wilderness within the Santa Barbara Ranger District (Mission Pine Ridge and points south).

THE SAN RAFAEL WILDERNESS, originally 75,000 acres established as a primitive area by US Forest Service Chief Robert Y. Stuart in 1932, was in 1968 (and at more than 110,000 acres) the first federally designated wilderness area established under the 1964 Wilderness Act. Subsequent legislation in 1984 and 1991 expanded the wilderness to 197,319 acres, making it second only to the Sespe (established in 1992) in size among the Los Padres wildernesses.

The "San Raf" hosts the Sisquoc Condor Sanctuary (established in 1937) and plays a critical role in the bird's recovery. Long-inhabited by humans, the wilderness hosts numerous Chumash rock art sites (those along the Sierra Madre ridge are still the source of heated debate, as many believe that stretch of the forest should be included in the wilderness), abandoned homesteads, hunters' camps, and historical trails. In recent years, nearly three-fourths of the San Rafael Wilderness has burned, in either the 2007 Zaca Fire or the 2009 La Brea Fire. And while a veritable army of volunteers has helped the US Forest Service (USFS) rebuild many of the trails, much of the trail network is still suffering from those fires' lasting effects.

The wilderness is administered by the Santa Barbara Ranger District in the south and by the Santa Lucia Ranger District in the north. This guide details those sections within the Santa Barbara RD; several popular routes—including the Sisquoc River and Hurricane Deck—are under the administration of the Santa Lucia RD and therefore not detailed herein.

As with other backcountry regions in the forest, summers can be dry and mercilessly hot; winter snows often make most high-elevation routes impassable. Plan accordingly.

See individual entries for trailhead specifics.

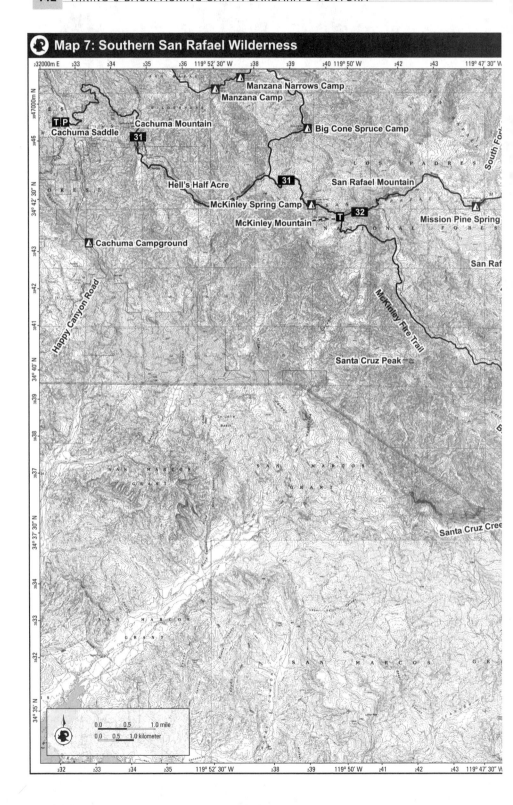

Map 7: Southern San Rafael Wilderness

Manzana Narrows Camp

Manzana Camp

Cachuma Mountain

Cachuma Saddle

31

Big Cone Spruce Camp

Hell's Half Acre

31

San Rafael Mountain

McKinley Spring Camp

Mission Pine Spring

McKinley Mountain

T **32**

Cachuma Campground

San Raf

Happy Canyon Road

McKinley Fire Trail

Santa Cruz Peak

Santa Cruz Cree

Santa Cruz Creek

0.0   0.5   1.0 mile

0.0   0.5   1.0 kilometer

MAP 7 Southern San Rafael Wilderness 143

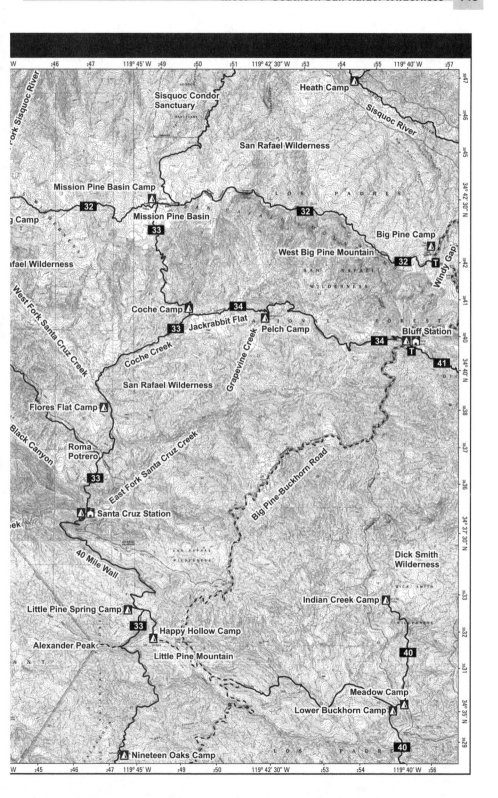

Route 31

MCKINLEY SPRING (28W01) and MCKINLEY MOUNTAIN

LENGTH AND TYPE:	9.1-mile one-way to McKinley Saddle; 16.8-mile out-and-back to McKinley Spring Camp; 19.4-mile out-and-back to McKinley Mountain
RATING:	Moderate
TRAIL CONDITION:	Well maintained (fire road); passable from McKinley Saddle to McKinley Mountain (old route and fire line)
MAP(S):	USGS *Figueroa Mountain* and *San Rafael Mountain*; Conant's *San Rafael Wilderness*
CAMP(S):	McKinley Spring
HIGHLIGHTS:	Views spanning from the Sierra Nevada to the Pacific

TO REACH THE TRAILHEAD(S): From the intersection of Armour Ranch Road and CA 154 (San Marcos Pass Road) just west of Lake Cachuma, head north along Armour Ranch Road approximately 1.25 miles to the intersection with Happy Canyon Road. Turn right (east) onto Happy Canyon Road (which will become Forest Road 7N07 upon entering the forest) and follow this approximately 13.75 miles to **Cachuma Saddle (3,050', 232636E 3846640N)**, just inside the Santa Lucia Ranger District boundary. Parts of this road are dirt and can prove rather mucky when wet. Four-wheel drive isn't typically necessary, but high clearance helps.

The Cachuma Saddle Guard Station once stood on the west of the road here. Parking is available on either side of Forest Road 7N07, but there is also a **flat (3,070', 232740E 3846608N)** up the McKinley Fire Road (Forest Road 8N08) just short of the gate.

TRIP SUMMARY: This pleasant hike along a service road climbs steadily from Cachuma Saddle eastward toward McKinley Spring, McKinley Saddle, and the edge of the San Rafael Wilderness.

Trip Description

From the McKinley **parking area (3,070', 232740E 3846608N)**, head east along the dirt road. The road—designated both Trail 28W01 and Forest Road 8N08 and lined with Coulter pines for many stretches—curves through the drainages of numerous upper tributaries of Fish Creek before reaching a concrete **water tank (2.5 miles, 4,110', 233992E 3846928N)**. From here and onward, views of the Sisquoc and Manzana drainages, Hurricane Deck, and the Sierra Madre to the north; Ranger Peak and Figueroa Mountain to the west; and Lake Cachuma, the Santa Ynez Valley, and the Pacific to your south prove near-constant companions.

Your route parallels the San Rafael Wilderness boundary once on the eastern flanks of Cachuma Mountain. Near here, the road and the Santa Lucia–Santa Barbara Ranger

District line are effectively one. After climbing to another saddle on the eastern shoulder of Cachuma Mountain and an easy descent, you'll pass a second water tank and **picnic area** (**3.8 miles, 4,150', 234714E 3845769N**) with a hitching post, trough, and table. Your route will lead southeast along the south-facing slopes of the ridge—returning to your excellent views of Lake Cachuma and beyond—and then through **Hell's Half-Acre** (**4.9 miles, 4,430', 235689E 3844876N**), a stretch punctuated on its eastern edge by outcrops of boulders.

From here the road ushers you along the more strenuous climb of McKinley Mountain's western and then northern flanks to the **junction** (**7.7 miles, 5,330', 238957E 3844969N**) with the Big Cone Spruce Trail 28W04 (which leads down into the Sisquoc). There is a table here.

Continue climbing another 0.5 mile along the road to **McKinley Spring Camp** (**8.4 miles, 5,620', 239343E 3844179N**).

Formations along Hell's Half-Acre

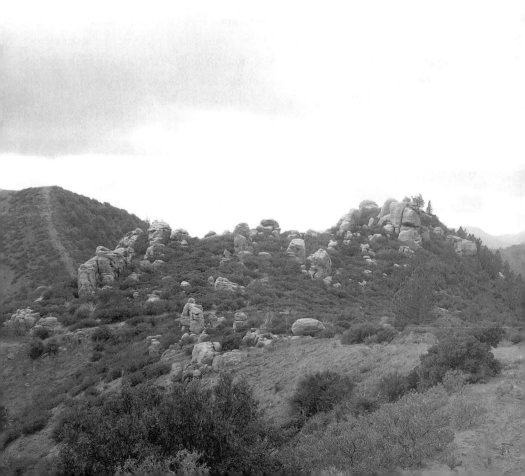

CAMP :: MCKINLEY SPRING

ELEVATION:	5,620'
MAP:	USGS *San Rafael Mountain*
UTM:	239343E 3844179N

This site remains in good repair and features two picnic tables, a hitching post, a fire ring with stove, and a spring trough. (Despite the camp's name, the spring here is Cold Spring. McKinley's namesake spring is a bit farther west back down the road.) This site also has a latrine.

It's another 0.5 mile to **McKinley Saddle** (**9.1 miles, 5,780', 240224E 3843830N**), where the Mission Pine Trail (see *Route 32*) and the McKinley Fire Road depart to your east.

For those inclined, the non-system trail heading west up McKinley Mountain departs from the southwest corner of the saddle. It's another 0.5 mile to the sandstone outcrops atop **McKinley Mountain** (**9.7 miles, 6,182', 239351E 3843738N**). The mountain was named for President McKinley, who, at the close of the 19th century, set aside the Pine Mountain and Zaca Lake Forest Reserve, which in subsequent decades proved the foundation of the Los Padres.

In a sandstone-hemmed clearing just east of the peak, there once stood an **Aircraft Warning Service station** (**239378E 3843736N**). Records indicate the hut built in 1935 (which might indicate plane spotting was not its initial role) and was removed by the US Forest Service in 1974, following the station's destruction by high winds.

Route 32

MISSION PINE TRAIL (28W01)

LENGTH AND TYPE:	3.4-mile out-and-back from McKinley Saddle to San Rafael Mountain;
	5.2-mile out-and-back from McKinley Saddle to Mission Pine Spring;
	12.8-mile out-and-back from McKinley Saddle to Mission Pine Basin;
	6.6-mile one-way from McKinley Saddle to Santa Cruz Trail Junction;
	6.9-mile one-way from McKinley Saddle to Falls Canyon Trail Junction;
	13.8-mile one-way from McKinley Saddle to Windy Gap
RATING:	Moderate
TRAIL CONDITION:	Clear to passable (considerable tree fall in the years post–Zaca Fire)
MAP(S):	USGS *San Rafael Mountain* and *Big Pine Mountain*; Conant's *San Rafael Wilderness*
CAMP(S):	Mission Pine Spring and Mission Pine Basin
HIGHLIGHTS:	Several peak-bagging opportunities; sweeping views of the Sisquoc River drainage and Hurricane Deck and out toward the Pacific

TO REACH THE TRAILHEAD(S): See directions for Cachuma Saddle trailhead in *Route 31*.

TRIP SUMMARY: Also called the "Santa Barbara high route" by die-hard local trekkers, Mission Pine Ridge is one of the Los Padres' crown jewels, crossing through heavy conifer stands and sandstone rock formations toward Windy Gap at Big Pine–Buckhorn Road. The route is described west to east from McKinley Saddle to Windy Gap, but both the start and end points are several miles from the nearest vehicle-accessible trailhead—plan your trek accordingly. This route follows the spine of the San Rafael Mountains, the ridgeline of which forms the boundary between the Santa Barbara and Santa Lucia Ranger Districts.

Trip Description

Note: This route begins along the eastern flank of McKinley Mountain at the end of Forest Road 8N08. See *Route 31* for the first 9.1 miles of this route.

From **McKinley Saddle (5,780', 240224E 3843830N)**, follow the singletrack starting at the northeast corner of the saddle, almost immediately entering the San Rafael Wilderness. The route climbs steadily but not overly steeply here. The first half of your climb was spared the ravages of the 2007 Zaca Fire; you'll note the stark contrast when entering the burned area as you approach the gap and spur trail leading to **San Rafael Mountain (1.7 miles, 6,593', 242276E 3844603N)**. San Rafael Mountain is the second-highest point in Santa Barbara County (the highest being Big Pine Mountain).

From San Rafael, descend easily beneath the Coulter, ponderosa, and incense cedar forest and fascinating rock formations through several drainages. The Mission Pine appellation is derived from tales of many of the timbers used in the Missions Santa Barbara and Santa Ynez, harvested here and hauled down Peachtree Canyon. A final drop brings you to a lily-clad glade marking **Mission Pine Spring (2.6 miles, 5,840', 244267E 3844001N)**. The camp is just yards to your right (east).

CAMP :: MISSION PINE SPRING

ELEVATION:	5,840'
MAP:	USGS *San Rafael Mountain*
UTM:	244273E 3843975N

This site, effectively the last reliable water as one heads eastward toward Windy Gap, features a table, rock fire ring, and a few well-worn tent flats. Oaks and conifers mingle here, and views a bit farther south from the rock formations are impressive. The meadow at the junction seems to yield an unusually high number of the relatively rare Humboldt's spotted lily (*Lilium humboldtii*) in spring and early summer.

The piped spring is accessible upslope from the meadow, southwest of the campsite.

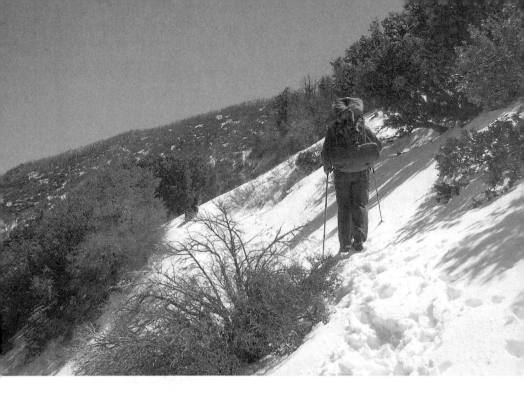

Approaching San Rafael Mountain

From Mission Pine Spring, continue eastward to drop into a lush fern- and lily-clad drainage, and then climb again through the pleasant boulder- and pine-dotted terrain. While your mean elevation change from Mission Pine Spring to the Mission Pine Basin is nominal, don't let that deceive you: the 4 miles between the two points is a constant seesaw of ridge ascents and drops into unnamed drainages. Some stretches of the trail here, damaged in the fires and consisting largely of decomposed granite, can at times feel like hiking in sand.

You work through several stretches of rerouted and severely fire-damaged trail to arrive at the **rocky wash (6.3 miles, 5,370', 248229E 3843889N)**. Follow the trail to the edge of the grassy meadow that marks **Mission Pine Basin (6.4 miles, 5,325', 248523E 3844041N)**.

Turning to your left (north) and then proceeding west up the shallow drainage 0.25 mile will lead you to **Mission Pine Basin Camp (5,350', 248352E 3844084)**.

CAMP :: **MISSION PINE BASIN**

ELEVATION:	5,350'
MAP:	USGS *Big Pine Mountain*

UTM: 248352E 3844084N

This site, nearly obliterated by the Zaca Fire, is now surrounded by burnt and failing Coulter pines—be mindful of tree fall (and those cones!) when camping here. Despite the fire damage, the camp enjoys a nice setting and still retains the old fire ring, some makeshift benches, abandoned ice can stoves, and some old accoutrements from camping days long gone. The site was originally established in the 1920s by a trail crew, and later served as a spike camp for deer hunters before World War II.

This is usually a dry camp, though water can *sometimes* be found 0.5 mile down along the Falls Canyon Trail, near the old Cooper site.

From the basin, it's a quick 0.25 mile across the grass to the **junction** (**6.6 miles, 5,300', 248708E 3844070N**) with the Santa Cruz National Recreation Trail (see *Route 33*), and then another 0.33 mile to the **junction** (**6.9 miles, 5,370', 249050E 3844226N**) with the Falls Canyon Trail, which drops north into the Sisquoc River drainage.

Beyond the Falls Canyon junction, your route continues eastward, very easily for a few miles and then somewhat more steeply along the uppermost headwaters of Coche Creek. A final set of switchbacks gets you up onto the ridge for the last stretch toward **West Big Pine Mountain** (**12.4 miles, 6,490', 254752E 3842556N**), the site of a former fire lookout. Some signs of the lookout, notably the concrete footings, remain. The abrupt drop-off along this excellent lunch spot's southern edge is sheer and quite long, so do mind your step.

From West Big Pine, it's an easy and gentle 1.5-mile descent through scrub and across shale barrens toward the former lookout service road to **Windy Gap** (**13.8 miles, 6,320', 256472E 3842190N**) along the Big Pine–Buckhorn Road.

Note: If you are heading north from here and need a good spot for the night or require water, seldom-used Big Pine Camp is 0.5 mile north along the road and a short spur trail. If heading south and short on water, there is a water tank (cistern) from which you can sometimes pull water 0.5 mile south along the road. See "A Road Runs Through It" on page 177 for information regarding the Big Pine–Buckhorn Road and the camps alongside the historical road.

Route 33

SANTA CRUZ NATIONAL RECREATION TRAIL (27W09)

LENGTH AND TYPE:	5.3-mile one-way from Upper Oso to Alexander Saddle; 6.5-mile one-way to Little Pine Spring; 10.8-mile one-way to Santa Cruz Station and camp; 13.7-mile one-way to Flores Flat; 16.8-mile one-way to Coche campsite; 21.5-mile one-way to Mission Pine Basin
RATING:	Moderate to strenuous
TRAIL CONDITION:	Clear to passable
MAP(S):	USGS *San Marcos Pass*, *Little Pine Mountain*, *San Rafael Mountain*, and *Big Pine Mountain*; Conant's *San Rafael Wilderness*
CAMP(S):	Nineteen Oaks (see description in *Route 7*), Little Pine Spring, Santa Cruz, Flores Flat, Coche, and Mission Pine Basin (see description in *Route 32*).

HIGHLIGHTS:	Wildflower displays; excellent views from numerous vantage points; historical Santa Cruz Guard Station; Mission Pine Ridge

TO REACH THE TRAILHEAD(S): Use the Upper Oso Trailhead for this trip.

TRIP SUMMARY: Whether you have a weekend or full week at your disposal, the Santa Cruz National Recreational Trail can likely accommodate—or at least factor in—your plans. This venerable 21-mile route begins after a short walk on an OHV route, and climbs and drops and then climbs some more all the way to Mission Pine Ridge. In the spring, wildflower displays (lupine, golden poppy, mariposa lily, peony, chocolate lily, coreopsis, and a host of others) en route to Alexander Saddle are a botanist's dream.

Trip Description

Note: Follow the description provided in *Route 7* for the first 1.7 miles of this route. Mileage, however, is calculated from the start at Upper Oso.

From the **upper Nineteen Oaks junction (1,620', 247195E 3829150N)** on the trail, cross **Oso Creek (1.8 miles, 1,600', 247212E 3829178N)** almost immediately; this is often the last water for several miles.

From the crossing, you embark on a long and steady stretch of switchbacks, first through exposed sections of sparse scrub and serpentine outcrops, and then into chaparral and scrub oaks. Shade is at a premium here as you ascend along the almost-infamous cribwall section and reach the easy-to-miss **spur trail (4.4 miles, 2,950', 248141E 3831315N)** leading to a stock trough that usually has water even in summer. (Keep an eye out for a cluster of bays and sycamores shortly before the turnoff.) The water can often be still, so take the necessary precautions and treat accordingly.

Continuing, you'll break into wide grassy stretches shortly after the stock trough and continue steeply toward **Alexander Saddle (5.3 miles, 3,960', 247349E 3832018N)**. From here, you have as good a view of the Santa Ynez River Valley and points south as you've had the entire climb, and now Santa Cruz and the San Rafael Wilderness are laid out before you to the north. It's a unique vantage point for one so close to the clamor and chaos of the recreation area below. The junction here effectively splits four ways: to the left (west) is the use trail to Alexander Peak; to the right (northeast) is the trail heading up to Happy Hollow camp (and the former guard station site) atop Little Pine Mountain; straight on (north) is the next stretch of the Santa Cruz trail.

And now you drop.

Follow the fire-scarred and often-overgrown but mercifully better-shaded trail down the slope of Little Pine Mountain's northern flanks, dropping into a stretch of Coulter pines, serpentine rock, and marshy seeps. Across the chasm that is the unnamed tributary to Santa

Cruz Creek to the north, you'll see the long line of trail that disappears around the valley; that is the 40 Mile Wall and one of your upcoming stretches. To reach that exposed stretch, continue past the **lower Happy Hollow junction** (**6.2 miles, 3,700', 247879E 3833032N**) out to the upper edge of the potrero and the **Little Pine Spring junction** (**6.3 miles, 3,620', 247858E 3833031N**). To reach the Little Pine Spring campsite, follow the trail skirting the edge of the potrero westward 0.25 mile.

CAMP :: LITTLE PINE SPRING

ELEVATION:	3,420'
MAP:	USGS *San Marcos Pass*
UTM:	247403E 3833111N

Though caught in the Zaca Fire, this site—hemmed in by live oaks and some brush— still features a wooden table and is a pleasant spot for a weekend trek. The stock trough is usually a reliable source of water (treat first), and there is enough space to pick a good spot to throw down the bedroll.

From the Little Pine Spring junction, the trail leads you down a pleasant potrero and then into another stretch of trail often brushed-over in the years since the Zaca Fire. A mile of avoiding the poison oak here will position you at the upper drainage (marked by thick bays,

40 Mile Wall

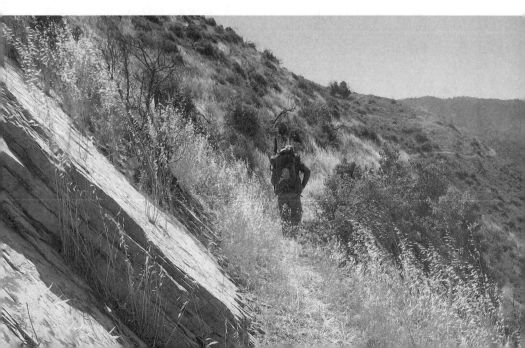

blackberries, and ferns) and the start of the **40 Mile Wall** (**7 miles, 3,200', 248278E 3833511N**). Here you won't have to push through encroaching trees, brush, or poison oak, but neither will you have any real shade for the next 2.5 miles. This stretch suffers from scree slides and rutting after storms, as most of its vegetation was lost in the fires. Volunteers and California Conservation Corps crews continue to work the trail in an effort to return it to its former glory, but be prepared for subpar conditions.

Descend this long section along the easy grade to the **bend** (**9.4 miles, 2,625', 245726E 3835395N**) overlooking the Santa Cruz drainage, and then cut north and drop into the shady mixed oak–conifer switchbacks to the **creek crossing** (**10.5 miles, 1,950', 246471E 3835733N**). From here it's a quick walk to the **junction** (**10.6 miles, 1,960', 246462E 3835774N**) with the trail and the doubletrack heading into Black Canyon. Head right (east) here along an increasingly improving route, passing one overflow site and up into the **Santa Cruz Guard Station** grounds (**10.8 miles, 1,980', 246664E 3835712N**).

CAMP :: SANTA CRUZ

ELEVATION:	1,980'
MAP:	USGS *San Rafael Mountain*
UTM:	246664E 3835712N

The Santa Cruz Guard Station area features camping spots, most with tables and good fire rings. Numerous old car campground–style concrete stoves with cast-iron plates still exist, forgotten in the brush or used as a flat spot for a backpacking stove. There is an old outhouse just east along the service road, and water can be retrieved from the alder- and maple-shaded creek just to the south. Several species of oak shade the area.

The route continues from the steel sign and trail register directly across from the main camping area, heading up the eastern slopes above Black Canyon and through a corner of Roma Potrero to the **junction** (**12.4 miles, 2,900', 246874E 3837146N**) with the McKinley Fire Trail. Continue east along the singletrack here, passing into the San Rafael Wilderness and through a final upper stretch of grassland before starting the descent back toward Santa Cruz Creek. While the trail bed has kept in good stead in recent years, this section can be overgrown with mustard, thistle, and other opportunistic weeds, so watch your step for snakes and be mindful of ticks.

Finally off the winding hillside, cross the **creek** (**13.4 miles, 2,350', 247265E 3838213N**) and continue to Flores Flat, a wide grassy meadow. The **camp** (**13.7 miles, 2,400', 247186E 3838594N**) is set beneath a massive live oak on your left (west), just above the creek.

▪ ▪ ▪ ▪ ▪ ▪ ▪ ▪ ▪ SANTA CRUZ GUARD STATION

Built in 1938, the guard station at Santa Cruz is one of the few such remaining structures in the forest (other notable guard stations still in existence include the South
Fork station along the Sisquoc River, Bluff along the Big Pine–Buckhorn Road, and
the dilapidated structure at Thorn Meadow). It is currently tended to and maintained
largely by volunteers, and the environs include a horse barn and paddock. It is seldom occupied and therefore usually closed to visitors.

▪ ▪ ▪ ▪ ▪ ▪ ▪ ▪ ▪ ▪ ▪ ▪ ▪ ▪ ▪ ▪ ▪ ▪

CAMP :: FLORES FLAT

ELEVATION:	2,400'
MAP:	USGS *San Rafael Mountain*
UTM:	247186E 3838594N

This campsite is situated on the edge of the grass meadow that was once the
homestead of José Flores. Camping guides from a half century ago relate how
Flores grazed cattle and raised some crops here; little evidence of the cabin that was
situated near the current camp remains. The campsite proper is situated beneath a
gargantuan live oak and has a fire pit. Water is available from the generally reliable

Santa Cruz Creek

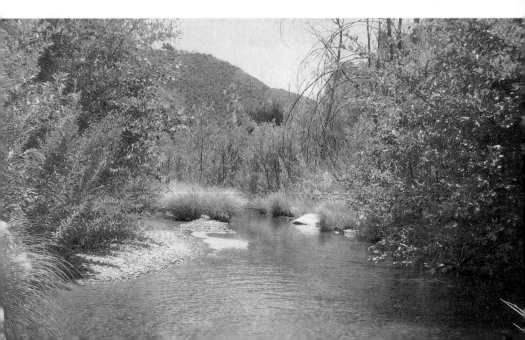

Santa Cruz Creek (which also features some excellent swimming holes). Be mindful of poison oak when dropping into the creek.

From Flores Flat, continue upstream to a gap with fine views of the west fork's drainage, and then make your way rather easily up the Coche drainage. The crossings are thick with alders and sycamores; the stretches out of the immediate drainage are lined by oaks and scrub. It's an easy 3 miles to reach the **junction (16.6 miles, 3,300', 249509E 3840959N)** with the Grapevine Trail. Take the left (north) fork here; see *Route 34* for the route up to Bluff Station.

It's an easy 0.25 mile through the oaks along the banks of Coche Creek to **Coche Camp (16.8 miles, 3,350', 249584E 3841240N)**.

CAMP :: COCHE

ELEVATION:	3,350'
MAP:	USGS *Big Pine Mountain*
UTM:	249584E 3841240N

Said to have been named for wild or feral pigs that once inhabited the area, Coche Camp is a nearly forgotten spot with a fire ring and shade provided by a cluster of fire-scarred live oaks. Water is available most times of the year in the creek below camp.

From camp, follow the trail upstream to the lush creek **crossing (16.9 miles, 3,870', 249570E 3841392N)**; the pools just up from the crossing are also great spots for a dip when water levels allow.

From here, your route is largely shade-free and quite strenuous. Much of the upper Santa Cruz National Recreation Trail has suffered from erosion postfire, and despite volunteer and official trail work (including a reroute around a slide about 0.5 mile from this crossing), it can still be rough going. Follow the trail as it winds westward above the Coche drainage, crossing the last marginally reliable water at a small oak-shaded spring the next drainage over, and then climbing steadily through a route hemmed in by charred manzanitas and aggressive yerba santa (there are worse plants to push through, granted).

Toward the end of the long, exposed climb, you'll note the trail bed effectively vanishes, lost among the smooth sandstone washes; navigate carefully here and watch for the cairns that usually mark the route. These will lead you to a small **saddle (20.3 miles, 5,350', 248689E 3842703N)** marking the southern edge of Mission Pine Basin. Continue a much easier final mile to a towering ponderosa, under which you'll find the junction with **Mission Pine Trail (21.5 miles, 5,300', 248708E 3844070N)**; see *Route 32* for the description. Mission Pine Basin Camp is 0.25 mile to your left (west).

Route 34

GRAPEVINE TRAIL (27W10)

LENGTH AND TYPE:	5.5-mile one-way from Grapevine/Santa Cruz junction to Bluff Station
RATING:	Moderate
TRAIL CONDITION:	Clear to passable
MAP(S):	USGS *San Rafael Mountain*; Conant's *San Rafael Wilderness*
CAMP(S):	Lower Grapevine (abandoned), Pelch, and Bluff
HIGHLIGHTS:	Bluff Guard Station

TO REACH THE TRAILHEAD(S): This route is a remote trail; see Map 7 to design your best approach.

TRIP SUMMARY: From the Grapevine/Santa Cruz junction, this short stretch climbs out of the eastern drainage of Santa Cruz Creek to Big Pine–Buckhorn Road and the Bluff Guard Station.

Trip Description

This area was burned in the 2007 Zaca Fire, and as a result there can be some washouts or brushed-in sections of trail. Most of the widely distributed oaks are recovering fairly well, and it's a pleasant ascent toward the Big Pine–Buckhorn Road to the old Bluff Guard Station.

From the **Grapevine/Santa Cruz junction (3,300', 249509E 3840959N)** at Jackrabbit Flat, follow the right (east) fork easily along a fairly level stretch through brush and grasses, passing to the north of a short knoll. Cross an intermittent **tributary (0.5 mile, 3,365', 250155E 3841014N)** before reaching **Grapevine Creek (1 mile, 3,375', 250250E 3841029N)** proper. A short walk upstream is the site of the abandoned **Lower Grapevine campsite (3,420', 250916E 3841283N)**.

From Lower Grapevine, continue easily eastward through a section that can be a bit thick with grass to the **junction (1.4 miles, 3,650', 251480E 3841134N)** with the spur trail leading to Pelch Camp. The junction still features a very old porcelain-and-steel sign. It's an easy 0.25 mile to **Pelch Camp (1.6 miles, 3,320', 251584E 3840890N)** from here.

CAMP :: PELCH

ELEVATION:	3,320'
MAP:	USGS *San Rafael Mountain*
UTM:	251584E 3840890N

Named for half of the Pelch/Pinkham partnership who in the 1930s often hunted in this area, Pelch is surrounded by live oaks and brush. There is a table, as well as numerous old steel relics from its use a century ago as a hunters' camp. It sees little use.

Back at the trail junction, a short set of switchbacks leads you to a gap and then down into the upper eastern drainage, only to cross again and climb toward a second gap, this one being the divide between the upper Grapevine drainage and the eastern fork of Santa Cruz Creek. Follow this drainage easily downstream to the base of a **low ridge (3.7 miles, 3,700', 253858E 3840157N)** amid the confluences of numerous tributaries, and then climb the final 2 miles along the ridge's north flanks to **Big Pine–Buckhorn Road (5.5 miles, 4,480', 255488E 3840140N)**.

Bluff Camp and the guard station are a few hundred yards due east along the spur road. (See page 185 for Bluff Camp description.)

Sierra Madre Ridge

This chapter details routes along the Sierra Madre ridge, from McPherson Peak eastward to Santa Barbara Canyon.

A HOTLY CONTESTED STRETCH OF FOREST due to its concentration of Chumash rock art juxtaposed with numerous grazing leases, the Sierra Madre ridge is the dividing line between the Sisquoc and Cuyama Rivers. Like most in the Transverse Ranges, the mountains run east-west rather than north-south, and much of the ridge detailed in this guide is covered by a series of grassy pastures (potreros).

The western portion of the Sierra Madre—from CA 166 to McPherson Peak—is administered by the Santa Lucia Ranger District and is not detailed in this guide.

Sierra Madre Trailheads

Alamo Canyon Trailhead (3,478', 263324E 3851071N)

From CA 33 in the Cuyama Valley, head west along Foothill Road just south of the Santa Barbara/San Luis Obispo County line for 2.1 miles—crossing the Cuyama River en route—to Santa Barbara Canyon Road. Turn left (south) here and follow Santa Barbara Canyon Road 3 miles to the private property boundary. Turn right (south) here to follow Santa Barbara Canyon Road/Forest Route 9N11 another 4.4 miles to the split near Santa Barbara Canyon Ranch. Follow the right fork onto the dirt road and continue 4.9 miles (keep right at the split with Dry Canyon Road/Forest Route 8N19), passing through Cox Flat to the gate at the end of the road. There's plenty of room in the turnaround for parking. There are no facilities here.

If coming from Santa Maria or points farther north—or if the Cuyama presents too great an obstacle for your vehicle (either due to your vehicle's clearance or capabilities or due to the river's level)—you can also access Santa Barbara Canyon through a series of surface roads from the town of Cuyama along CA 166 (thereby utilizing the state highway to cross the river). From CA 166 just east of Cuyama, follow Kirschenmann Road southward approximately 2.4 miles to Foothill Road. Turn left (east) onto Foothill Road and follow it

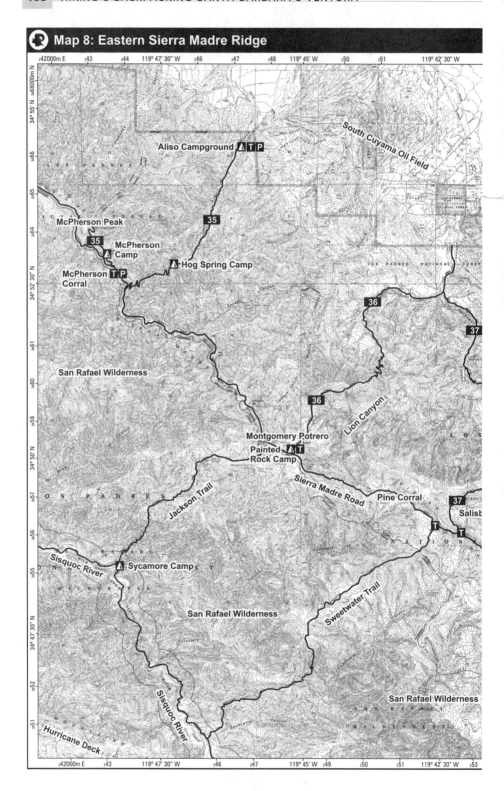

Map 8: Eastern Sierra Madre Ridge

Aliso Campground

McPherson Peak

McPherson Camp

Hog Spring Camp

McPherson Corral

South Cuyama Oil Field

San Rafael Wilderness

Lion Canyon

Montgomery Potrero

Painted Rock Camp

Sierra Madre Road

Pine Corral

Jackson Trail

Salisb...

Sisquoc River

Sycamore Camp

San Rafael Wilderness

Sweetwater Trail

Sisquoc River

Hurricane Deck

San Rafael Wilderness

MAP 8 Eastern Sierra Madre Ridge 159

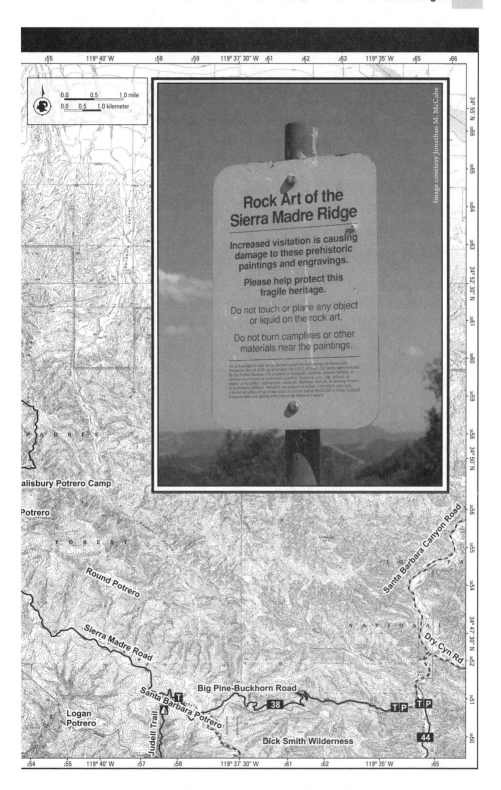

for 3 miles to Santa Barbara Canyon Road, turning right (south) here. Follow the directions described above from that point.

Note: The trailhead is slightly farther west along the road from where it is shown on the 1995 *Fox Mountain* quad.

Aliso Park Campground (2,900', 246983E 3866236N)

From Santa Maria, follow CA 166 eastward approximately 49 miles to the turnoff for Aliso Canyon Road. Turn right (south) here and follow the signage approximately 6 miles to the campground.

Alternately, from the junction of CA 166 and CA 33 east of Cuyama, follow CA 166 westward approximately 12.5 miles to the turnoff for Aliso Canyon Road. Turn left (south) here and follow the signage approximately 6 miles to the campground.

McPherson Corral (5,050', 243499E 3863195N)

From CA 166, approximately 39 miles east of Santa Maria (or 13 miles west of New Cuyama), follow Cottonwood Canyon Road southward approximately 4.4 miles to Foothill Road. Head right (west) here and stay left as the road becomes Bates Canyon Road (Forest Route 11N01) and heads southward toward the Sierra Madre Ridge, passing Bates Canyon Campground at about 6.6 miles. The road meets Sierra Madre Road (Forest Route 32S13) 12.5 miles from CA 166. From this junction, continue left (east) 8.5 miles along Sierra Madre Road (Forest Road 32S13) to the corral. Passenger cars are not recommended.

Note: When Bates Canyon Road is closed, it is a slow and often rough 32 miles starting from CA 166 approximately 26 miles east of Santa Maria.

Route 35

McPHERSON PEAK (27W01 and 27W02)

LENGTH AND TYPE:	6.3-mile one-way via Aliso Canyon (27W01) and Sierra Madre Road; 3.8-mile one-way via McPherson Peak Trail (27W02); 10.1-mile loop
RATING:	Moderate to strenuous
TRAIL CONDITION:	Well maintained (service roads) to passable (unmaintained route)
MAP(S):	USGS *Peak Mountain* and *Hurricane Deck*; Conant's *San Rafael Wilderness*
CAMP(S):	Hog Pen Spring and McPherson (abandoned)
HIGHLIGHTS:	Fantastic views from along the Sierra Madre ridge and McPherson Peak

TO REACH THE TRAILHEAD(S): Use the Aliso Park Campground Trailhead to access this route.

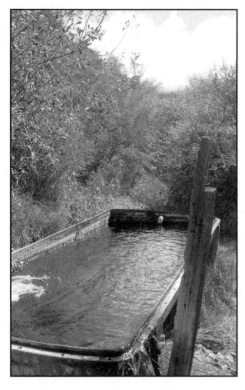

Hog Pen Spring

TRIP SUMMARY: From Aliso Park Campground, this hike climbs out of the Aliso Canyon drainage to the Sierra Madre ridge, and then heads west along the service road to McPherson Peak. You also have the option to return via an older route for a loop.

Trip Description

From **Aliso Park Campground (2,900', 246983E 3866236N)** follow the semiretired stretch of Forest Road 10N04 southward along Aliso Creek, crossing the creek almost immediately. Your progress here is beside (and beneath) massive old live oaks, and in short time you'll spot corrals and a small **camp (0.2 mile, 2,920', 246840E 3866013N)** off the spur road to your left (east); this is an ideal site for those preferring slightly more privacy and solace than the car camp downstream might provide on busy weekends.

The easy road will usher you to the often-locked road **gate (1 mile, 3,155', 246292E 3864852N)** that prevents cattle from getting downstream into camp and beyond. If locked, you'll have to climb over the gate. Continue along the road easily upstream—crossing the creek a few more times—before cutting right (west) to the junction with the old Hog Pen Spring car **camp** on your left (north) (**2.4 miles, 3,650', 245098E 3863201N**), though there is often a fire ring situated in the old pens area as well. **Hog Pen Spring (2.5 miles, 3,700', 244996E 3863336N)** proper can be found up the little westward spur of the road.

CAMP :: HOG PEN SPRING

ELEVATION:	3,650'
MAP:	USGS *Peak Mountain*
UTM:	245098E 3863201N

An old car camp now mostly accessible only on foot, Hog Pen Spring Camp is situated in a small meadow surrounded by massive, mature oaks. There is an old fire ring here but little else. Named for the hogs the McPhersons raised in this area in the

1880s, this site has not appeared on US Forest Service visitor maps for some time, but is shown on Conant's *San Rafael Wilderness.* Water is available in the creek or—more reliably—from the Hog Pen Spring trough 0.1 mile westward up the ravine.

To the left (south) of the old pens' wire your route follows the singletrack and leads southwest up a fairly intimidating ridge, but one made surprisingly easy by the long and generally forgiving switchbacks. Because this stretch of the forest is leased for cattle grazing, expect "obstacles" along the trail, and—after rains—for the trail to be a bit chewed up by bovine hooves. While the tread does take a beating from the cattle, the cattle also help keep this trail (which receives very little maintenance) relatively clear. This stretch of the forest was spared the numerous fires in recent years, and so the flora here is still thick and aged.

Eventually you'll crest the chaparral-covered slope to gain **Sierra Madre Road (4.7 miles, 4,960', 243762E 3862602N)**. Now on the road, head right (west). To the north, you will have great views of the Cuyama Valley, the Caliente Range and Tehachapi Mountains, and the southern end of the Sierra Nevada. Continue climbing 0.5 mile to the locked **gate (5.2 miles, 5,050', 243499E 3863195N)** and corral. (Just short of the gate on the southern ridge you'll spot an interpretive sign detailing features of the San Rafael Wilderness, the boundary of which you are now treading. The sign was placed here in 1989 to coincide with the 25th anniversary of the Wilderness Act.)

Beyond the corral, the roadbed of a long-abandoned route splits right (northwest). Though the lower portion of it has been graded and set with erosion drainages, you'll find you can follow it easily enough past some very old stock pens to finally gain the old roadbed. Follow this less-traveled route to cut nearly a mile from the more circuitous route the current service road takes. You'll pass the old **McPherson Campground (5.6 miles, 5,400', 243165E 3863712N)** along the way.

NAVIGATOR'S NOTE ■ ■ ■ ■ ■ ■ ■ ■ ■ ■ ■ ■ ■

Over the years there has been some discrepancy as to the trail designations in the McPherson Peak area; this narrative describes the route through Aliso Canyon to Sierra Madre Road via Hog Pen Spring as 27W01, the old McPherson Trail as 27W02, and the long-abandoned trail along the eastern ridge of Messenger Canyon as 27W03. This may not match your current Los Padres maps, so bear this in mind when planning and navigating.

■ ■ ■ ■ ■ ■ ■ ■ ■ ■ ■ ■ ■ ■ ■ ■ ■ ■ ■

CAMP :: McPHERSON

ELEVATION:	5,400'
MAP:	USGS *Peak Mountain*
UTM:	243300E 3863765N

Long-abandoned and nearly forgotten, this site is situated in a small clearing along the old road. It has not appeared on any maps for some time, though the 1995 7.5-minute *Peak Mountain* quad did place it after having been excluded from federal maps for some years. Formerly a hunters' camp, it held a quartet of stoves, though only one remains in useable condition as of this writing.

From the old McPherson Campground, continue along the road to its junction with the main peak access **road** (**6 miles, 5,650', 242804E 3864242N**) and then head right (north) along

McPherson Corral and Parking Area

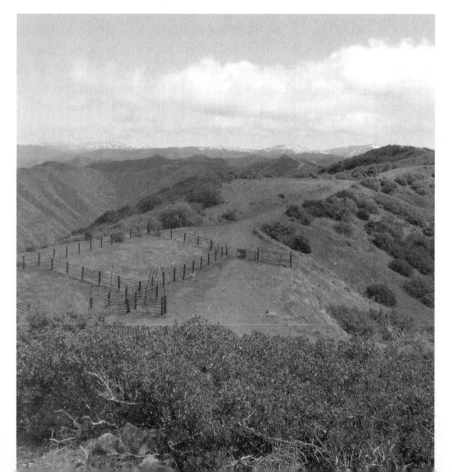

the main road to **McPherson Peak** (**6.3 miles, 5,749', 242959E 3864300N**). The footings near the cistern/water tank are from the old fire lookout, constructed in 1934 and removed by the Forest Service in 1987 to be fully supplanted by the U.S. Air Force communications array and solar panels you see here.

McPherson Trail (27W02)

Another route back to Aliso Park Campground avails itself to the slightly adventurous; this route is a popular approach among Sierra Club peak-baggers, but it's not regularly maintained and can be something of a bushwack depending on recent volunteer efforts. Navigation skills are a must. From McPherson Peak, find the heading northeast from the peak and along the ridge dividing the Messenger Canyon and Aliso Canyon drainages. Though often overgrown for lack of use but still with a fairly stable tread, this McPherson Trail (27W02) effectively marks the boundary between the Santa Lucia and Mt. Pinos Ranger Districts of the forest.

Two miles on, at the saddle just before Hill 4784, the abandoned eastern Messenger Canyon Trail (27W03) cuts left (north) to continue along the district boundary; stay right here and continue toward Aliso Canyon. After another 0.5 mile you may (depending on season) note another thread of a trail heading off to the left again; this is the original tread of this route, which once led due north to an old jeep trail outside the forest boundary. Again, stay right, and you'll note the trail improves significantly along this lower portion as you wind down to the southwesternmost camp in **Aliso Park Campground** (**10.1 miles, 2,900', 246983E 3866236N**).

Route 36

MONTGOMERY POTRERO and ROCKY RIDGE TRAIL (27W04)

LENGTH AND TYPE:	6.2-mile one-way from Painted Rock Camp to Bull Ridge junction (12.4-mile out-and-back); 6.9-mile one-way from Painted Rock Camp to old Lion Canyon Trailhead
RATING:	Moderate to strenuous (climb on return; typically some overgrowth)
TRAIL CONDITION:	Passable (lightly used route)
MAP(S):	USGS *Hurricane Deck* and *Salisbury Potrero*; Conant's *San Rafael Wilderness*
CAMP(S):	Painted Rock
HIGHLIGHTS:	Chumash rock art; fantastic views of Lion Canyon and the Cuyama Valley

TO REACH THE TRAILHEAD(S): To reach the upper trailhead at Painted Rock, either follow the McPherson/Aliso Trail (*Route 35*) to the Sierra Madre Road and then proceed 5.7 miles east to the camp, or (from Santa Barbara Potrero) hike 9 miles west along Sierra Madre Road to the camp.

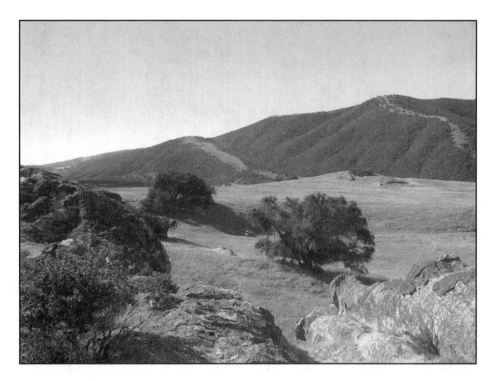

Montgomery Potrero

TRIP SUMMARY: From Painted Rock campsite, this hike drops steeply through fascinating geology to the Newsome/Lion confluence and junction with the Bull Ridge Trail. There is no lower access at present.

Trip Description

Note: This route is described south to north (from the Painted Rock campsite to the Lion Canyon Trailhead).

From **Painted Rock Camp (4,600', 248190E 3858290N)**, follow the marked trail just below the huge fallen oak toward the northeast, easily climbing to the northern edge of the potrero and immediately being rewarded with fantastic views of Lion Canyon, the Cuyama River Valley, the Caliente Range, and points beyond.

The trail enters the **brush and rock formations (0.4 mile, 4,600', 248634E 3858689N)** atop Lion Canyon, winding through the basal sandstone of the Branch Canyon formation and the Monterey formation until breaking out of the brush and back into the more classic **chaparral (1.2 miles, 4,425', 249022E 3859681N)** of the divide between Lion and Branch Canyons (the "Rocky Ridge").

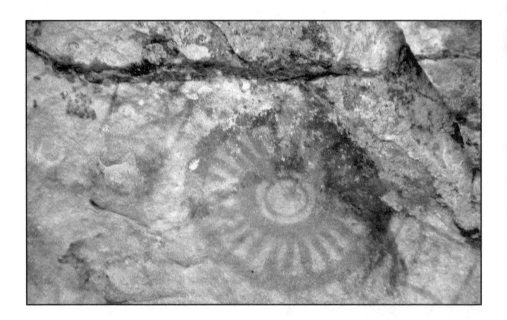

Follow the lightly used switchbacks here as they wind rather steeply down into lower **Lion Canyon (3.2 miles, 3,030', 250764E 3860696N)**, crossing the creek a handful of times as you follow the drainage north and then eastward as it curves toward **Lower Lion Spring (5.6 miles, 2,825', 251184E 3862395N)**. From the spring, the trail down-canyon expands to an old doubletrack for the last mile before you cross the widened watershed and reach the **junction (6.2 miles, 2,620', 252400E 3862317N)** with the Bull Ridge Trail (26W01) at the Newsome/Lion confluence.

From this point, you effectively either have to retrace your steps or ascend Bull Ridge Trail toward Salisbury Potrero, as the lower access of these trails is currently closed due to an impasse between the US Forest Service and the oil leases in the South Cuyama Oil Field.

The old **Lion Canyon Trailhead (6.9 miles, 2,520', 252695E 3863539N)**, once the popular starting point for many routes until the late 1980s, is another 0.75 mile down the dirt road (technically part of this trail) from this junction.

CAMP :: PAINTED ROCK

ELEVATION:	4,600'
MAPS:	USGS *Hurricane Deck*; Conant's *San Rafael Wilderness*
UTM:	248190E 3858290N

This site, surprisingly still maintained given its proximity to the rock art, features a single table, fire ring, and latrine. There is a grazing paddock as well.

One can imagine how much shade the old fallen oak must have provided in decades past, but now the table and fire ring are exposed and receive virtually no shade. This is a hot place to enjoy a meal in the summer.

Just east up the slope from the kitchen area is a small cluster of oaks, beneath which a few tent-size spots have been terraced over the years. These trees provide good cover from the sun virtually all day. Just west of the site is the old latrine.

The best source of water here is the Montgomery No. 1 Spring 0.25 mile west along the road; the spring here is often (in the words of one longtime Los Padres trekker) a "cesspool of bovine 'befoulment,'" but one can usually secure one of the pipes or hoses issuing from the spring and not pull water directly from the hoof-rutted muck. Definitely treat all water.

■ ■ ■ ■ "SET THE CONTROLS FOR THE HEART OF THE SUN"

The white sandstone outcrops just west of the Painted Rock campsite are some of the most accessible and most impressive examples of Chumash rock art most folks will ever see. The Sapaksi, or House of the Sun, cave is the best known.

Signs posted by the forest archaeologist abound, advising visitors to not disturb the art. All the advice is common sense, and yet it's apparently still necessary to remind folks, as signs of abuse are present. Entry of the upper rock shelter is strictly forbidden. Please adhere to these guidelines to ensure future generations have the opportunity to view these unique examples of prehistoric art.

Route 37

SALISBURY POTRERO and BULL RIDGE TRAIL (26W01)

LENGTH AND TYPE:	6.6-mile one-way to the junction with Rocky Ridge Trail (27W04)
RATING:	Moderate to strenuous (climb on return; typically some overgrowth)
TRAIL CONDITION:	Clear (current and semiretired service roads) and passable (lightly used route)
MAP(S):	USGS *Salisbury Potrero*; Conant's *San Rafael Wilderness*
CAMP(S):	Salisbury Potrero
HIGHLIGHTS:	Fantastic views of Cuyama Valley, the Caliente Range, and points beyond

TO REACH THE TRAILHEAD(S): To reach the upper trailhead (the Sierra Madre Road/Salisbury junction), either follow the McPherson/Aliso Trail (*Route 35*) to the Sierra Madre Road and then proceed 9.4 miles east to the junction, or (from Santa Barbara Potrero) hike 5.3 miles west along Sierra Madre Road to the junction.

TRIP SUMMARY: From the Sierra Madre Road/Salisbury junction, this route heads north through Salisbury Potrero and then along Bull Ridge and Newsome Canyon to the Newsome/Lion confluence (and junction with the Rocky Ridge Trail). Much of the route is along current or semiretired dirt roads, making navigation somewhat easier. There is no lower access at present.

Trip Description

Note: This route is described south to north (from the Sierra Madre Road/Salisbury junction to the Rocky Ridge/Bull Ridge junction).

From the **Sierra Madre Road/Salisbury junction (4,920', 252756E 3855932N)**, follow the spur road down (northward) toward Salisbury Potrero. Continue straight at the **junction (0.5 mile, 4,740', 252454E 3856595N)** at the bottom; the road to your right (east) leads to the private inholding. While that route once led to the old Salisbury Canyon trail (26W03), it is currently off-limits. Please respect the private property and stay on the road.

Continue northward along the road, climbing out of the potrero to reach the **Salisbury Potrero campsite (1.3 miles, 4,805', 253509E 3857173N)**.

CAMP :: SALISBURY POTRERO

ELEVATION:	4,805'
MAPS:	USGS *Salisbury Potrero*; Conant's *San Rafael Wilderness*
UTM:	253509E 3857173N

This barren and largely shadeless site features excellent views of both Salisbury Potrero to the north and the numerous drainages above the Cuyama Valley but little else. There is no water here.

From the camp's spur trail, continue along the increasingly thin but still viable double-track along the ridge dividing the Newsome and Salisbury watersheds. The road begins to fade to singletrack at a **gap (3.3 miles, 3,875', 254352E 3858936N)** just as you begin a rather steep northwest descent into Newsome Canyon. This stretch can be a bit brushed-in during spring, but overall has remained in fairly good shape despite its general lack of use (cattle traffic may contribute to this).

After a mile of toe-pounding descent into Newsome Canyon, the **road (4.4 miles, 2,950', 252949E 3860424N)** picks up again across the often-dry but usually green and overgrown creek bed just upstream from **Lower Newsome Spring (4.5 miles, 2,900', 253012E 3860589N)**.

Follow the road another 2 miles (crossing the creek a few times) to reach the **junction (6.6 miles, 2,620', 252400E 3862317N)** with the Rocky Ridge Trail (26W01) at the Newsome/Lion confluence.

Route 38

SANTA BARBARA POTRERO and SIERRA MADRE ROAD

LENGTH AND TYPE:	5.6-mile one-way from Alamo Canyon gate to Santa Barbara Potrero Camp (11.2-mile out-and-back)
RATING:	Moderate to strenuous (climb)
TRAIL CONDITION:	Well maintained (service roads)
MAP(S):	USGS *Fox Mountain* and *Salisbury Potrero*; Conant's *San Rafael Wilderness*
CAMP(S):	Santa Barbara Potrero (site doesn't appear on most maps)
HIGHLIGHTS:	Fantastic views along the climb and from along the Sierra Madre Ridge

TO REACH THE TRAILHEAD(S): Use the Alamo Canyon Trailhead for this route.

TRIP SUMMARY: From Alamo Canyon, this route rises rather steeply along the Buckhorn and Sierra Madre Roads to Santa Barbara Potrero. Options for longer routes along the Sierra Madre Ridge all the way to McPherson are also available (see sidebar on the following pages).

Trip Description

From the **Alamo Canyon Trailhead (3,478', 263324E 3851071N)**, pass through the gate and follow the dirt Big Pine–Buckhorn Road (Forest Road 9N11) west along the Alamo drainage. Piñons, oaks, and scrub dominate along the lower portion. And while cattle are supposed to

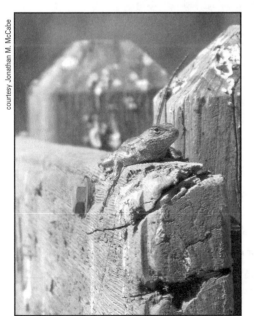

courtesy Jonathan M. McCabe

be restricted to the stretch east of the gate, the grazing bovines do occasionally get onto the road beyond. Keep an eye out.

The canyon narrows and the road leaves the main Alamo drainage after 0.75 mile, after which you'll soon endeavor along a steady climb comprised of a pair of switchbacks and a long straight section of climbing. Rather quickly, views of Santa Barbara and Dry Canyons, Cuyama Peak, and—farther in the distance—the Caliente Range and the San Emigdio Mountains come into view. There is seldom much shade along this route, so pace yourself accordingly.

Your progress follows not only the edge of the Dick Smith Wilderness boundary here but also the perimeter of the 2007 Zaca Fire. Reaching the junction with the **Sierra Madre Road (Forest Road 32S13) (4.5 miles, 5,230', 258661E 3851024N)** marks the end of the strenuous climbing; head straight (west) here along the Sierra Madre. The road leads you easily up to the **gap (4.8 miles, 5,260', 258324E 3850832N)** along the southern flank of a low knoll, where you'll gain your first good views of the grassy expanse that is Santa Barbara Potrero.

From the gap, it's an easy descent to the junction with the **signed spur road (5.3 miles, 5,100', 258020E 3851488N)**. Follow this less-traveled doubletrack down (south) a winding 0.33 mile to the fenced-in flat where sits **Santa Barbara Potrero campsite (5.6 miles, 4,950', 257693E 3851207N)** and from where the Judell Trail (26W05) heads down the drainage toward the Sisquoc River.

CAMP :: SANTA BARBARA POTRERO

ELEVATION:	4,950'
MAPS:	USGS *Salisbury Potrero;* Conant's *San Rafael Wilderness* (not shown on maps)
UTM:	257693E 3851207N

Once the site of the Sierra Madre Guard Station, what remains of the Santa Barbara Potrero site is limited (as of this writing) to a single table on a fenced-in flat. There is no fire ring or stove here; given the nature of the area it should remain so.

A County of Santa Barbara rain gauge and US Forest Service trail register sit just outside the northwest corner of the fencing; farther down are some old Pratt & Whitney aircraft engine–shipping containers used as water tanks. Water can be pulled from Oak Spring, a short walk along a cattle-rutted trail down the drainage.

TREASURES OF THE SIERRA MADRE ▨ ▨ ▨ ▨ ▨ ▨ ▨ ▨ ▨ ▨

Farther west along the ridge road, there are a handful of features worth consideration. First are trailheads to five other routes (three of which are detailed in this guide), as well as the McPherson Trailhead at the other end of this closed stretch of forest road.

Second—and by far more important—is the Chumash rock art along the Sierra Madre. Because the art of the ridge is well documented and there are signs along the road and some camp areas where the rock art is especially accessible, the Chumash art in this area is one of the few locations this guide discusses. Please show the ancient pictographs the respect they deserve.

From the Santa Barbara Potrero spur road/Sierra Madre Road junction, here are the points of note as one heads west along the road.

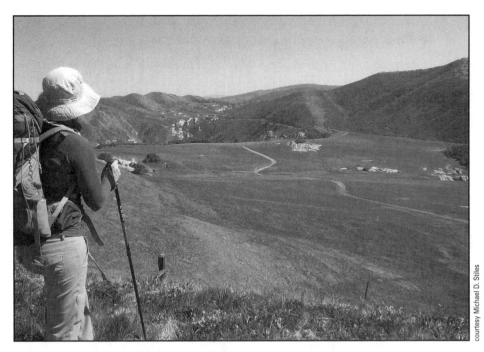

Montgomery Potrero

Salisbury Potrero Junction (4,920', 252756E 3855932N)

This dirt road, 5.3 miles from the Santa Barbara Potrero spur road/Sierra Madre Road junction, leads north down into the Salisbury Potrero (site of a large inholding). This is also the upper trailhead for the Bull Ridge Trail (26W01); see *Route 37.*

Sweetwater Trailhead (4,870', 252067E 3856162N)

The Sweetwater Trailhead, 5.8 miles from the junction, marks the upper stretch of the Sweetwater Trail (27W06), which drops 7 miles southward to the Sisquoc River.

Pine Corral (4,550', 250206E 3856988N)

Pine Corral, 7.5 miles from the junction, is a wide potrero punctuated by towering rock formations. Because of the numerous springs nearby, cattle tend to gravitate toward this area. The namesake spring is not to be relied upon during the summer, and water should be treated year-round.

Montgomery Potrero, Painted Rock, and the Rocky Ridge Trailhead (4,580', 248134E 3858204N)

The short spur road here, 9 miles from the junction, heads north to the Painted Rock campsite and its famous pictographs. Just short of the campsite is the trailhead for the Rocky Ridge Trail (27W04); see *Route 36* for both the trail description as well as the Montgomery Potrero/Painted Rock area.

Jackson Trailhead (4,640', 247622E 3858322N)

The Jackson Trailhead, 9.5 miles from the junction, marks the upper stretch of the Jackson Trail (27W05), which leads 4.5 miles south to the Sisquoc River and Sycamore Camp.

McPherson/Aliso Trailhead (4,960', 243762E 3862602N)

This is the upper trailhead, 14.9 miles from the junction, for the McPherson Trail (27W01), which drops 4.7 miles northward to Aliso Park Campground (see *Route 35*).

McPherson Corral (5,050', 243499E 3863195N)

The corral here, 15.4 miles from the junction, marks the extent of allowed vehicle traffic coming from the west (CA 166, Miranda Pines Campground, etc.) and serves as the western trailhead/parking area for those exploring the Sierra Madre ridge.

■　　■　　■　　■　　■　　■　　■　　■　　■　　■　　■　　■　　■

Dick Smith Wilderness

*This chapter details routes through
and near the Dick Smith Wilderness.*

NAMED FOR THE FAMED SANTA BARBARA newspaperman who championed the
establishment of the San Rafael Wilderness and the welfare of the California condor, the
Dick Smith Wilderness was established in 1984. Bordered on its western edge by the San
Rafael Wilderness and by CA 33 on its east, some lament it is the "forgotten wilderness" of
the southern Los Padres, as it receives very little maintenance and is lightly traveled. It's an
ideal swath of backcountry for those seeking solitude (and willing to work for it).

Well over 90% of the Dick Smith burned in the 2007 Zaca Fire. While the forest has
been quick to begin its recovery, the system of trails has not fared well. Many of the routes
described herein rely heavily (some exclusively) on the efforts of volunteers to keep the routes
clear, or at least viable. Think about getting involved yourself, and contact the Santa Barbara
or Mt. Pinos Ranger Districts about joining any of the numerous volunteer projects. Or, just
carry a good set of loppers while you explore the trails.

Dick Smith Wilderness Trailheads

Deal Trailhead (Bear Canyon) (3,680', 283285E 3839918N)

From the junction of CA 33 and CA 150 in Ojai, drive north along CA 33 (beyond the Pine
Mountain summit) approximately 37.7 miles to an easy-to-miss roadside parking area on the
left (north) side of the highway. There are no facilities here.

Deal Connector Trailhead (4,280', 282639E 3838666N)

From the junction of CA 33 and CA 150 in Ojai, drive north along CA 33 (beyond the Pine
Mountain summit) approximately 34 miles to a small and easy-to-miss dirt turnoff on the
left (west) side of the road just past mile marker 45.27—exercise caution crossing the road
to access the turnoff. The dirt road drops into an old parking area, now the trailhead for the
Deal Connector Trail (24W10). There are no facilities here.

Don Victor (5,190', 276179E 3834880N)

From Pine Mountain summit along CA 33, follow the dirt Potrero Seco Road (Forest Road 6N03; permit required) eastward, passing Potrero Seco Campground and the private inholdings after 3.5 miles, and reaching the split with the Don Victor Fire Trail (6N11) at 5 miles from CA 33. Phone (805) 646-4348 or visit the Ojai Ranger District in Ojai for permit specifics. In addition to the special-use permit, a US Forest Service Adventure Pass, federal Interagency Pass, or equivalent is required to use the road or park anywhere along it. There are no facilities here.

Santa Barbara Canyon
(3,350', 264440E 3851106N)

From CA 33 in the Cuyama Valley, head west along Foothill Road just south of the Santa Barbara/San Luis Obispo County line for 2.1 miles—crossing the Cuyama River en route—to Santa Barbara Canyon Road. Turn left (south) here and follow Santa Barbara Canyon Road/Forest Route 9N11 (which turns to dirt near the ranches) approximately 11.6 miles (keep right at the split with Dry Canyon Road), passing through Cox Flat to reach a small parking area on your right (west) marked by an old juniper. (If you find yourself in Alamo Canyon at the gated start of the Big Pine service road and all its fetid cattle mess, you've gone too far.) There are no facilities here.

If coming from Santa Maria or points north—or if the Cuyama presents too great an obstacle for your vehicle (either due to your vehicle's clearance or capabilities or due to the river's level)—you can also access Santa Barbara Canyon through a series of surface roads from the town of Cuyama along CA 166 (thereby utilizing the state highway to cross the river). From CA 166 just east of Cuyama, follow Kirschenmann Road southward approximately 2.4 miles to Foothill Road. Turn left (east) onto Foothill Road and follow it 3 miles to Santa Barbara Canyon Road, turning right (south) here. It's then 12.5 miles along Santa Barbara Canyon Road/Forest Route 9N11 to the destination described above.

Rancho Nuevo Trailhead
(3,520', 280357E 3841870N)

Four-wheel drive is recommended. From the junction of CA 33 and CA 150 in Ojai, drive north along CA 33 (beyond the Pine Mountain summit) approximately 40.7 miles to Forest Route 7N04A. Turn left (west) and proceed along the dirt road across the Cuyama River (impassable during and immediately after rains) and along the Rancho Nuevo watershed for 0.8 mile. Bear left (southwest) at the junction with Tinta Creek Road and continue another 0.7 mile (crossing the creek twice) to Rancho Nuevo Campground (which is effectively a turnaround with two campfire rings). There are no facilities here.

Tinta Trailhead (3,630', 278775E 3844169N)

Four-wheel drive is recommended. From the junction of CA 33 and CA 150 in Ojai, drive north along CA 33 (beyond the Pine Mountain summit) approximately 40.7 miles to Forest Route 7N04A. Turn left (west) and proceed along the dirt road across the Cuyama River (impassable during and immediately after rains) and along the Rancho Nuevo watershed for 0.8 mile. Stay straight (west) at the split with the Rancho Nuevo Road and continue another 2 miles to the camp. There are three sites and a pit toilet here. This route serves as the lower trailhead of the Tinta Trail (24W02), which skirts the northern edge of the Dick Smith and is a popular but challenging motorcycle route (Trail 101).

Dry Canyon Trailhead (4,630', 271372E 3848074N)

Located 5.8 miles along Dry Canyon Road (8N19) from Santa Barbara Canyon Road, this trailhead is the upper trailhead of the Tinta Trail. It's a rather steep 2.2 miles up the dirt road to Cuyama Peak. There are no facilities here.

■ ■ ■ ■ ■ ■ ■ ■ ■ ■ ■ ■ ■ ■ ■ ■ **DICK SMITH**

Born in 1920 in Minnesota, Dick Smith was an artist and newspaperman by profession whose contributions to the environment (and subsequent legacy) have far outshone his journalistic pursuits. A gifted photographer and artist, Smith was also an avid backpacker, naturalist, and environmentalist—in an era before it had become socially popular. His coverage of the 1969 Santa Barbara oil spill helped spark what is generally regarded as the modern environmental movement in the US.

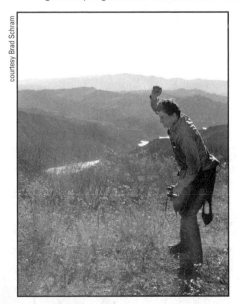

courtesy Brad Schram

Smith moved to Santa Barbara in 1948, after working for *Minneapolis Star-Tribune* and serving in the US Navy in World War II. He secured work with the *Santa Barbara News-Press* and, upon taking his first hike to nearby Figueroa Mountain, saw his life transformed. Already savvy as a wildlife artist and naturalist, Smith found in his new stomping ground great inspiration and worked toward its protection.

Smith joined with local lawmakers to help found the San Rafael Wilderness, the first recognized under the 1964 Wilderness Act. He was especially fond of the Madulce region adjacent to the San Rafael Wilderness, and after his passing in 1977, friends, peers, and supporters lobbied for Madulce and nearby lands to be preserved as wilderness. In 1984 the targeted area—65,000 acres—was made the Dick Smith Wilderness, commemorating Smith's huge contributions to the Santa Barbara backcountry. (As an idle point of trivia, Smith is one of only three people after whom a California wilderness has been named. The others are John Muir and Ansel Adams.)

■ ■ ■ ■ ■ ■ ■ ■ ■ ■ ■ ■ ■ ■ ■ ■ ■ ■

CUYAMA PEAK (5,878', 273346E 3848558N) ■ ■ ■ ■ ■

Follow the directions for Santa Barbara Canyon. Once on the dirt stretch of road past Santa Barbara Canyon Ranch, head south 7.6 miles until you reach the junction with Forest Route 8N19. Make the sharp left (east) here and follow 8N19 for 9 miles to the peak. The last 2.5 miles can be rather rough and are not recommended for passenger cars.

See page 13 for information about the lookout here and elsewhere in the southern Los Padres.

■ ■ ■ ■ ■ ■ ■ ■ ■ ■ ■ ■ ■ ■ ■ ■ ■ ■ ■

Cuyama Peak Lookout; courtesy D. S. Carey

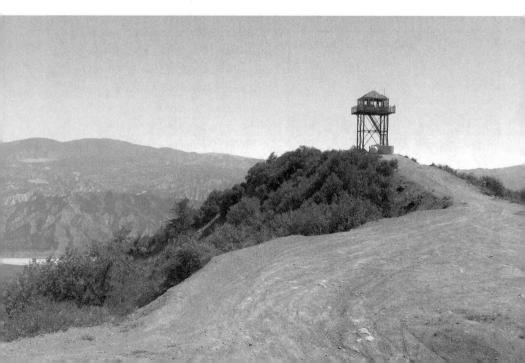

■ ■ ■ ■ ■ ■ ■ ■ ■ ■ ■ ■ ■ ■ ■ ■ ■

A ROAD RUNS THROUGH IT: THE BIG PINE–BUCKHORN ROAD

In the 1930s, the National Industrial Recovery Act (NIRA) contributed a great deal of labor and construction to the national forests. One of the best (and most useful) examples in the southern Los Padres are the Camuesa and Big Pine–Buckhorn Roads.

In his 1984 historical overview of the Los Padres, noted historian E. R. "Jim" Blakley gives a brief rundown of the roads' development and impact:

On the Santa Barbara Ranger District the construction of the Camuesa and Buckhorn Roads was probably the CCC project that had the most lasting influence on this portion of the Forest. The Buckhorn Road connected the southern part of the Forest with the Cuyama Valley. It put an end to the use of the Mono-Alamar pack trail, which previously had been the main trail crossing the Forest. The Madulce and Mono-Pendola Ranger Stations were no longer on the main trail and soon fell into disuse. New stations were built at Little Pine, Bluff Camp and Alamar Saddle. Today, both the Little Pine and Alamar Stations are gone. Bears destroyed the Alamar Station and human vandalism caused so much damage to the Little Pine "Happy Hollow" Station that the Forest Service finally crushed and burned it. The site of Bluff Camp Station was one of the temporary spike camps used by the CCC while they were constructing the road and the trails in that portion of the Forest. Now, in 1984, the station is used by trail crews, study programs, and the interagency Condor Recovery Team when they are working in this part of the Forest.

Because the Buckhorn Road (also known as the Big Pine Road) effectively connects the southern Los Padres (at Upper Oso) with the Cuyama Valley (at Santa Barbara Canyon), it makes for a great corridor when planning longer treks through either the San Rafael or Dick Smith Wildernesses.

■ ■ ■ ■ ■ ■ ■ ■ ■ ■ ■ ■ ■ ■ ■ ■

Route 39

ALAMAR TRAIL (20W06)

LENGTH AND TYPE:	6.4-mile one-way from Loma Pelona/Don Victor Fire Road to Alamar Camp
RATING:	Moderate
TRAIL CONDITION:	Passable to difficult (seasonal deadfall; little maintenance)
MAP(S):	USGS *Big Pine Mountain* and *Madulce Peak*; Conant's *Matilija & Dick Smith Wilderness*
CAMP(S):	Dutch Oven, Bill Faris, and Alamar
HIGHLIGHTS:	Remote and riparian trekking; great views of Madulce Peak

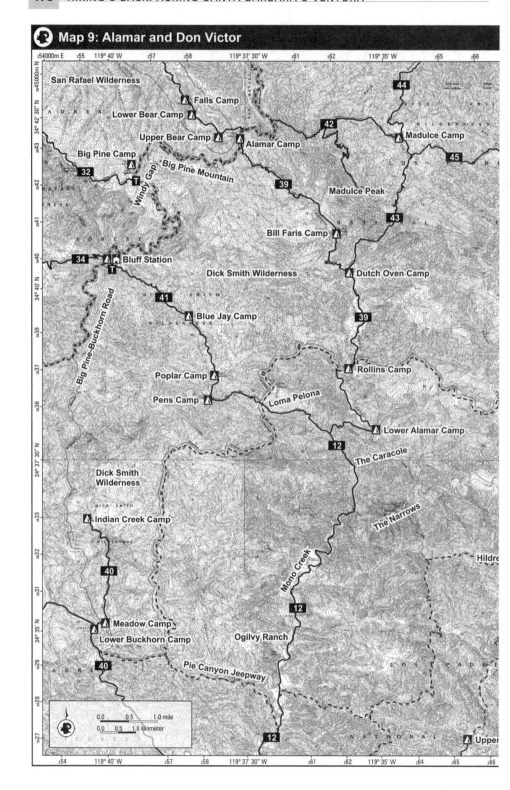

Map 9: Alamar and Don Victor

San Rafael Wilderness

Falls Camp

Lower Bear Camp

44

42

Madulce Camp

Upper Bear Camp

Alamar Camp

45

Big Pine Camp

Big Pine Mountain

32

39

Madulce Peak

Windy Gap

43

Bill Faris Camp

34

Bluff Station

Dick Smith Wilderness

Dutch Oven Camp

Big Pine-Buckhorn Road

41

39

Blue Jay Camp

Poplar Camp

Rollins Camp

Pens Camp

Loma Pelona

Lower Alamar Camp

12

The Caracole

Dick Smith Wilderness

The Narrows

Indian Creek Camp

40

Mono Creek

Meadow Camp

12

Lower Buckhorn Camp

Ogilvy Ranch

40

Pie Canyon Jeepway

12

Hildre

Upper

0.0   0.5   1.0 mile
0.0   0.5   1.0 kilometer

MAP 9 Alamar and Don Victor 179

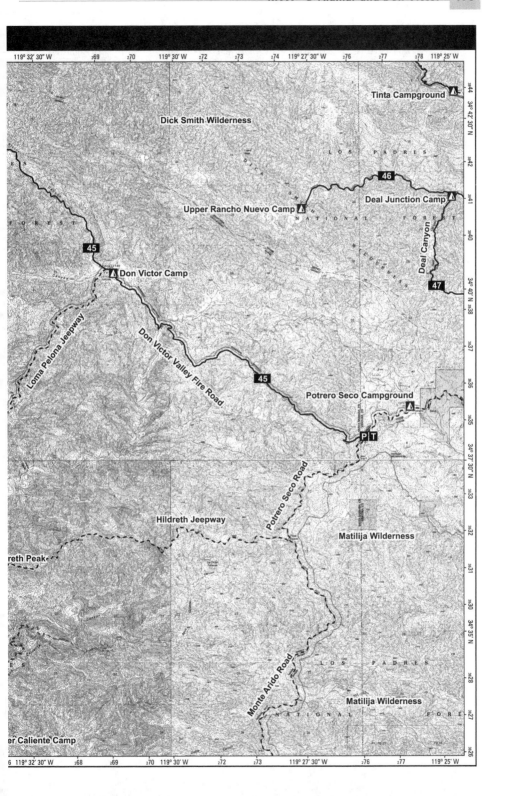

TO REACH THE TRAILHEAD(S): Along a desolate stretch of the Dick Smith, the Alamar Trail is most often approached either via the Mono-Alamar Trail (see *Route 12*) or from Alamar Camp along the Big Pine–Buckhorn Road. See Conant's *Matilija & Dick Smith Wilderness* and Map 9 to plot your approach.

TRIP SUMMARY: This route is described south to north and leads from the Loma Pelona/ Don Victor Fire Road along Alamar Canyon to the Alamar Camp along Big Pine– Buckhorn Road.

Trip Description

From the **Alamar Trailhead (3,125', 262351E 3837123N)** along Loma Pelona/Don Victor Fire Road (just east of Rollins campsite), follow the singletrack northward along Alamar Creek, crossing the creek numerous times along a 2-mile stretch that can be a bit thick along the creek but is generally easygoing on the chaparral slopes. **Dutch Oven campsite (1.9 miles, 3,680', 262325E 3839608N)** is situated among a cluster of fire-scarred oaks on your right (east).

CAMP :: DUTCH OVEN

ELEVATION:	3,680'
MAP:	USGS *Madulce Peak*
UTM:	262325E 3839608N

Dutch Oven—said to be named for cast-iron cookware left at this camp decades ago— is a small site set in a grass clearing near the confluence of Alamar Creek and the Puerto Suelo drainage. There are a few oaks on the edge of camp, and water can be retrieved from the creek. There are still several ice can stoves and a rock fire ring.

Immediately upstream from camp you'll reach the junction with the **Puerto Suelo Trail (1.9 miles, 3,680', 262294E 3839618N**; see *Route 43*). Take the left (west) fork here and continue along the Alamar drainage, crossing the creek and keeping to the north side of the drainage and leaving the oaks. The trail here can be hard to find post–Zaca Fire, both due to growth and fire damage, but keep an eye out for signs of the trail bed to follow the cut upstream. Views of Madulce Peak are especially good from this vantage point.

The cover here turns to low chaparral, especially heavy with yerba santa, as you climb on a gentle grade progressing clockwise around a knoll to reach **Bill Faris Camp (3.2 miles, 4,200', 261877E 3840714N).**

CAMP :: BILL FARIS

ELEVATION:	4,200'
MAP:	USGS *Madulce Peak*
UTM:	261877E 3840714N

Often misspelled "Bill Farris," this site was established in 1962 in memory of William L. Faris (1932–1960), a Santa Barbara– and Pomona-area Scouter, teacher, and U.S. Army officer. It was severely burned in the Zaca Fire; the oaks around camp bear the scars of their ordeal, but overall the site is clearer than in years past, when it was choked with growth and received little attention. The kitchen still retains its fire ring and several old ice can stoves. Water can be retrieved from the creek, and there is a nice grassy meadow behind camp.

From Bill Faris, the trail follows the increasingly narrow Alamar drainage, crossing the creek a handful of times early on before climbing somewhat steeply along the western drainage through charred forests of Coulter pines. This stretch, though often worked by volunteer crews, often features a fair amount of downfall (especially after winter or windstorms). Be prepared to scramble across fallen trees. The steady ascent finally deposits you on the **side road** (**6.4 miles, 5,685', 259310E 3843353N**) connecting Alamar Camp with the Big Pine–Buckhorn Road; it's about 200 feet to the right (east) to **Alamar Camp** (**6.4 miles, 5,675', 259390E 3843335N**).

CAMP :: ALAMAR

ELEVATION:	5,675'
MAP:	USGS *Big Pine Mountain*
UTM:	259390E 3843335N

In 1937 a US Forest Service guard station was built on this site, situated just off the Big Pine–Buckhorn Road built during the Depression. Over the years a group of pines matured to provide ample shade. The station was razed in the mid-1960s, and the camp placed there afterward. The site was very badly burned in the 2007 Zaca Fire and is now a barren and far more open incarnation of its former self. Seats have been fashioned from rounds cut from the numerous felled trees. There is no water available here, but the site has a modern fire ring, grate stove, and table.

Route 40

INDIAN CREEK TRAIL (Lower 27W12 and Lower 26W08)

LENGTH AND TYPE:	12.4-mile out-and-back to Indian Creek Camp; 4.8-mile one-way to Meadow Camp
RATING:	Moderate
TRAIL CONDITION:	Clear to passable
MAP(S):	USGS *Little Pine Mountain*; Conant's *Matilija & Wilderness*
CAMP(S):	Lower Buckhorn, Meadow, and Indian Creek
HIGHLIGHTS:	Fascinating geology; riparian trekking; cascades; swimming holes

TO REACH THE TRAILHEAD(S): Use the Mono Creek Gate Trailhead along Romero-Camuesa Road as described in Chapter 4 to access this route.

TRIP SUMMARY: This entry details the lower half of noncontiguous sections of trail 26W8, from Romero-Camuesa Road near the Mono/Indian confluence to Indian Creek Camp.

Trip Description

From the **gate (1,520', 258686E 3824656N)** at Romero-Camuesa Road (5N15), head west 0.9 mile along the dirt road to reach the **Indian Canyon Trailhead (1,520', 257760E 3825399N)**. This stretch entails a number of crossings of both Mono and Indian Creeks; be prepared for wet feet in the spring and after storms.

From the Indian Canyon Trailhead, follow the singletrack easily through open yucca-dotted terrain, crossing the creek adjacent to a low weir and following the Indian Creek drainage rather easily through talus and scree. This length of trail is technically the lower portion of the Buckhorn (27W12) route.

Stocky junipers mix with the chaparral before you enter a straight section, along which you'll traverse an exposed cross section of the fault here. Beyond, the route slowly gains in vegetation, and you'll enjoy numerous stretches of willow- and oak-shaded terrain as you cross the creek again and again before reaching the signed junction with the old **Pie Canyon Jeepway (3.5 miles, 1,820', 255000E 3828785N)**. Continue along the trail here, quickly reaching the **Pie Canyon Trail junction (4 miles, 1,875', 255020E 3829495N)**, situated at the confluence of Buckhorn and Indian Creeks. Here, follow the trail upstream along Buckhorn Creek a short way to the junction with the spur trail leading to **Lower Buckhorn Camp (4.4 miles, 1,950', 254886E 3830083N)**.

CAMP :: **LOWER BUCKHORN**

ELEVATION:	1,950'
MAP:	USGS *Little Pine Mountain*
UTM:	254886E 3830083N

Lower Buckhorn is an old site that has seen better days. Set at the edge of a small meadow beneath a cluster of mature live oaks, the site contains a fire ring, stove, and a table quite literally on its last legs. The site is said to be near a legendary Chumash hunting camp.

Just up the hill from the turnoff to Lower Buckhorn is the junction with the Buckhorn Trail. Follow the right (east) option to stay on the Indian Trail (now 26W08); it's the wider and typically better maintained of the two and is a former roadbed, so it is fairly easy to navigate. This route climbs easily for a few hundred yards to another junction with an old firebreak, this one leading around the northern edge of the knoll below which Buckhorn and Indian Creeks met just earlier in your hike. Crest the saddle to your right (east) and drop into the meadow below, regaining the Indian Creek drainage. At the southeast corner of the large meadow into which you descend you'll find **Meadow Camp (4.8 miles, 1,955', 255269E 3830179N)**.

CAMP :: **MEADOW**

ELEVATION:	1,955'
MAP:	USGS *Little Pine Mountain*
UTM:	255269E 3830179N

Formerly known as Indian Meadow, this camp is situated just outside the wilderness boundary, so while uncommon, mountain bikers shouldn't cause alarm. The site features a dilapidated table and fire ring. Water can be retrieved from the creek but shouldn't be relied upon in summer. There is virtually no shade here. *Note:* This site does not appear on current USFS or USGS maps.

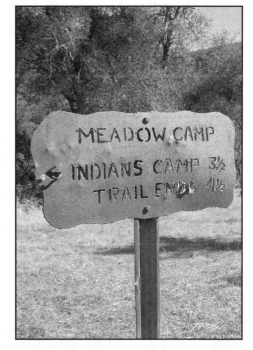

From Meadow Camp, Indian Trail continues northward through the meadow and into the hedge of chamises and manzanitas along Indian Creek's western banks. Follow the trail—again, there are many creek crossings along this stretch—into the southern reach of the Zaca Fire. The route here is a combination of arroyo willow, alder- and sycamore-lined riparian creek bed, and oak woodland. As the canyon narrows, you'll spot a few clusters of mature oaks that escaped the fire unscathed and a series of unique cobble-laden rock formations at the creek crossings. Once through a narrow stretch up the canyon, the walls ease and on a long meadow dotted with oaks you'll find **Indian Creek Camp (6.2 miles, 2,260', 254758E 3833170N**).

CAMP :: INDIAN CREEK

ELEVATION:	2,260'
MAP:	USGS *Little Pine Mountain*
UTM:	254758E 3833170N

Originally known as Indian Canyon Camp, this site represents the upper extent of the lower Indian Creek Trail. The main kitchen area is situated beneath a massive mature live oak, and in 2010 local district rangers and volunteers delivered and assembled a new table here. A second and almost forgotten kitchen is located just upstream in the meadow near a fallen oak. Water is available from the creek in all but the driest months.

The trail beyond camp is rarely (officially never) maintained, but there is some semblance of a route, which leads about another mile to an impressive two-tier waterfall deep within Indian Canyon. The going isn't easy and entails a heavy amount of rock-hopping, but it makes a fine day sojourn for those spending the night at Indian Creek Camp.

Route 41

INDIAN-POPLAR TRAIL (Upper 26W08)

LENGTH AND TYPE:	6.4-mile out-and-back from Bluff to Poplar; 3.7-mile one-way to Pens Camp and junction with Alamar Hill Trail
RATING:	Moderate
TRAIL CONDITION:	Clear to passable
MAP(S):	USGS *Big Pine Mountain*; Conant's *Matilija & Dick Smith Wilderness*
CAMP(S):	Bluff, Blue Jay, Poplar, and Pens
HIGHLIGHTS:	Fascinating geology; historic Bluff station; riparian trekking

TO REACH THE TRAILHEAD(S): This route begins at Bluff Station along the Big Pine–Buckhorn Road, some 25 miles from the nearest public road. See the prescribed maps and Map 9 for planning your approach.

TRIP SUMMARY: From Bluff Guard Station along the Big Pine–Buckhorn Road, this upper portion of trail 26W08 descends along Indian Creek to Pens Camp.

Trip Description

CAMP :: BLUFF

ELEVATION:	4,485'
MAP:	USGS *Big Pine Mountain*
UTM:	255708E 3840085N

Set just behind the Bluff Guard Station, this pleasant and well-groomed site—spared the ravages of recent fires due to its proximity to the station—features two tables, a fire ring, and a stove. It is surrounded by a cluster of mature live oaks. Water is

Namesake bluffs loom over the Big Pine–Buckhorn Road and Bluff Station.

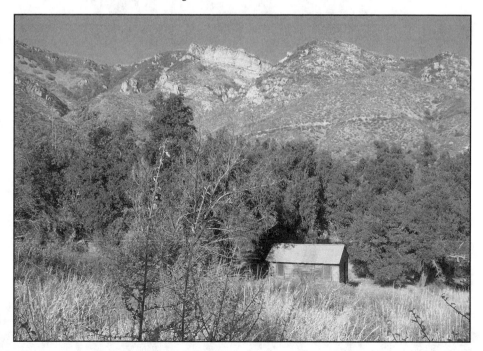

available along the headwaters of Indian Creek just down from camp (purify), and the station's latrine just to the northwest is available to campers.

From Bluff, the Indian-Poplar Trail enters the Dick Smith Wilderness from the south end of the vehicle turnaround in front of the guard station (near the old horse corral). Follow the long-retired road grade easily for about a mile—weaving in and out of intermittent tributary channels and a few perennial springs—before dropping down a series of switchbacks to regain the floor of the canyon. Willows, cottonwoods, and oaks mingle with chaparral here as you stay on the south side of the creek until the first of three **crossings (2 miles, 257593E 3838609N)** in fairly quick succession. Just after the third crossing, you'll find Blue Jay Camp on the right (southwest) side of the trail.

CAMP :: **BLUE JAY**

ELEVATION:	3,740'
MAP:	USGS *Big Pine Mountain*
UTM:	257827E 3838474N

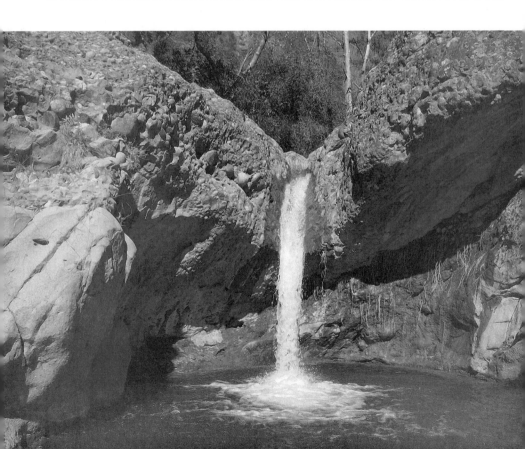

This nearly forgotten site is situated just off the trail on a small, grassy flat above the creek. There is one stove and little else; fire-scarred goldcup oaks mark the southern edge of camp. Some of the pools in the creek near camp are ideal for relaxing, and the bluffs east and west of camp seem to attract red-tailed hawks. Resident ornithologists will likely note proper blue jays (*Cyanocitta cristata*) do not actually reside this side of the Rocky Mountains; conventional wisdom is that the site is named after its cousin the Steller's jay (*Cyanocitta stelleri*), a bird common in this stretch of wilderness. *Note:* This site does not appear on current USFS or USGS maps.

From Blue Jay Camp, the trail crisscrosses Indian Creek numerous times, descending into a narrower stretch of the canyon with a healthy bigcone Douglas-fir population (many of which survived the Zaca Fire). After 0.5 mile of this narrower stretch, the canyon widens again and your route continues southward along some easy arroyo willow stretches. As the trees begin to thin and you follow a stretch along the west side of the creek, you'll reach an easy-to-miss spur leading to **Poplar Camp (3.2 miles, 3,350', 258476E 3836876N)** just before the trail crosses back to the east side of the creek.

CAMP :: POPLAR

ELEVATION:	3,350'
MAP:	USGS *Big Pine Mountain*
UTM:	258476E 3836876N

Situated on an oak-shaded flat but named for the poplar (cottonwood) trees in the drainage below, Poplar is a pleasant spot with greater space than its more compact neighbor 0.5 mile down the trail (Pens). A table and stove are here, and water can be retrieved from the creek.

From Poplar, continue 0.5 mile downstream to reach the junction of the Indian-Poplar and Alamar Hill (26W16) trails and **Pens Camp (3.7 miles, 3,300', 258285E 3836285N)**. See *Route 39* for the climb leading eastward out of Indian Canyon (via the Alamar Trail) to Loma Pelona.

CAMP :: PENS

ELEVATION:	3,300'
MAP:	USGS *Big Pine Mountain*
UTM:	258285E 3836285N

Also known as Lower Poplar (and further incorrectly labeled "Indian Can" on some late-1970s and early-1980s USFS maps), this small but tidy site has an ice

Map 10: Santa Barbara Canyon and Madulce Peak

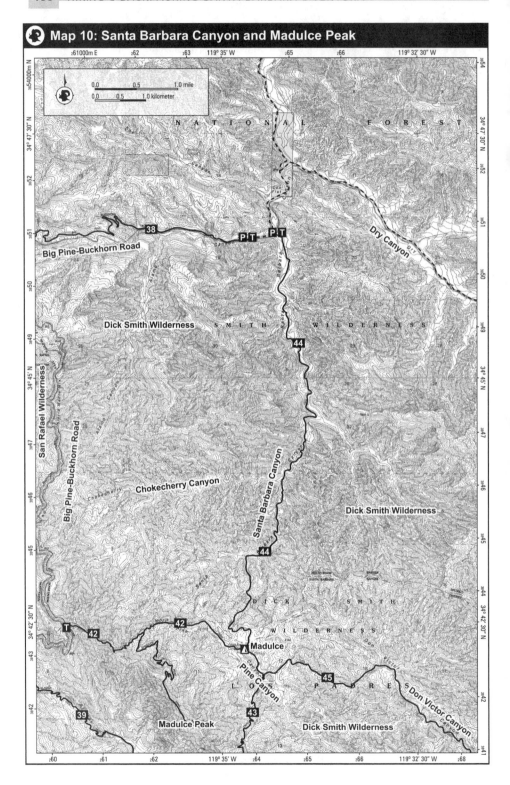

can stove and grill. Evidence of the camp's origins (stock pens) can still be found along the perimeter; old rolls of barbed wire and other accoutrements are scattered throughout.

Route 42

MADULCE (26W20) and MADULCE PEAK (25W13) TRAILS

LENGTH AND TYPE:	3.2-mile one-way from lower Madulce Camp to Big Pine–Buckhorn Road; 9-mile out-and-back from lower Madulce Camp to Madulce Peak
RATING:	Moderate east to west (climb); easy west to east
TRAIL CONDITION:	Clear (well-traveled singletrack) to passable (tree fall after storms and in winter)
MAP(S):	USGS *Madulce Peak*; Conant's *Matilija & Dick Smith Wilderness*
CAMP(S):	Madulce (see *Route 44*)
HIGHLIGHTS:	Conifer forest; peak ascent

TO REACH THE TRAILHEAD(S): Use the Santa Barbara Canyon Trailhead for this route.

TRIP SUMMARY: This short route connects the Madulce camps with the Madulce Peak Trail and is described as coming from the old Madulce Cabin site near the junction with the Santa Barbara Canyon Trail (25W02; see *Route 44*). The other direction (east), the trail follows Pine Creek 0.5 mile to the Don Victor/Puerto Suelo **junction (4,730', 264047E 3842746N)**.

Trip Description

From the old cabin site, follow the route westward up the Pine Creek drainage, crossing the creek once and entering into a thick grove of incense cedars, interior oaks, and ponderosa pines. You'll pass the **upper Madulce trail camp (0.1 mile, 4,850', 263616E 3843242N)** as the trail clambers into a dark boulder-strewn stretch. Cross the creek a handful of times. Much of this stretch is well shaded by incense cedars and Douglas-firs. You'll follow the drainage along a fairly easy ascent for about a mile until the trail leads out along the northern banks of the creek and to a ridge from where you will have increasingly impressive views of not only Santa Barbara Canyon and the Cuyama to the north but also—beyond the smog-hazed Central Valley—the snowcapped Sierra Nevada.

Continue climbing (now through groves of massive fire-ruined ponderosa and sugar pines and some pleasant sandstone boulder formations) along the northern flank of Madulce Peak along an increasingly steep series of switchbacks to the junction with the **Madulce Peak Trail (2.2 miles, 6,070', 261386E 3843264N)**. An old steel sign is posted here.

To gain Madulce Peak, follow the peak trail up the left (south) fork, which leads above the headwaters of Pine Creek's various tributaries. Soon you'll endeavor upon a series of switchbacks set beneath the towering survivors of the fire.

After a second series of switchbacks, you'll follow a fairly straightforward—and not overly aggressive—track heading southeast to **Madulce Peak (4.5 miles, 6,536', 262637E 3841833N)**. Views here are some of the best to be had in the Dick Smith, from Alamar Canyon directly below (to your south) out to the Channel Islands and the Pacific. The concrete footings you see here are remnants of the old Madulce Peak fire lookout, erected in 1934 and burned by the US Forest Service in the late 1970s.

From the junction with the peak trail, it's another mile up some additional switchbacks and then along an easily navigated and exposed, chaparral-dotted ridgeline (still with the Pacific in view) to reach the trailhead at **Buckhorn–Big Pine Road (3.2 miles, 6,170', 260225E 3843738N)**. A trail register is just short of the road.

Route 43

PUERTO SUELO (25W20)

LENGTH AND TYPE:	3-mile one-way from Pine Creek junction to junction with Alamar Trail
RATING:	Moderate (damaged and lightly traveled)
TRAIL CONDITION:	Passable
MAP(S):	USGS *Madulce Peak*; Conant's *Matilija & Dick Smith Wilderness*
CAMP(S):	—
HIGHLIGHTS:	Excellent views

TO REACH THE TRAILHEAD(S): This remote stretch of trail within the Dick Smith Wilderness can be approached by a number of routes; see Map 9 and Conant's *Matilija & Dick Smith Wilderness* to plan your route.

TRIP SUMMARY: This 3-mile route leads from the Don Victor–Madulce junction on the banks of Pine Creek to a small gap (the route's namesake) and then follows a drainage to Alamar Canyon to join the Alamar Trail. *Note:* There are numerous permutations of this route's name found on US Forest Service, USGS, and other maps; other spellings have included (but are not limited to) Puerto Suello, Puerta Suelo, and Puerto Suela.

Trip Description

Not to be confused with the Puerto Suello Trail (3E08) in the Monterey Ranger District, this route has suffered from lack of use and lack of maintenance over the past few years in the wake of the damage done by the Zaca Fire.

From the **Don Victor–Madulce junction (4,730', 264047E 3842746N)**, follow the single-track southward (sometimes steeply) a mile up to the namesake **Puerto Suelo (0.9 mile, 5,220', 263671E 3841457N)**. This gap between the Pine and Alamar drainages marks your high point here; to the south the views are extensive.

From the gap, drop rather steeply along the erosion-chewed route toward the southwest; some navigation will be necessary here. Doing this stretch in reverse can prove fairly strenuous, especially with the route difficult to find.

Small pockets of the canyon were spared complete destruction by the Zaca Fire, and as a result stands of bigcone Douglas-firs, oaks, and big-leaf maples lend welcome shade along fern-clad stretches during warmer days. But there are also numerous trees that were subjected to the fire and have since fallen, making for several points at which you'll find yourself crawling over or scrambling around blowdowns.

As the draw begins to open, you'll reach the junction with the **Alamar Trail (3 miles, 3,680', 262294E 3839618N)**. Dutch Oven Camp is mere yards to the south from here; see *Route 39*.

Route 44

SANTA BARBARA CANYON (25W02)

LENGTH AND TYPE:	7-mile one-way to Madulce Camp
RATING:	Moderate (elevation and distance)
TRAIL CONDITION:	Clear to passable
MAP(S):	USGS *Fox Mountain* and *Madulce Peak*; Conant's *Matilija & Dick Smith Wilderness* and *San Rafael Wilderness*
CAMP(S):	Madulce
HIGHLIGHTS:	Arroyo willow and oak woodland trekking along Santa Barbara Canyon; expansive views and conifer forests along Pine Canyon

TO REACH THE TRAILHEAD(S): Use the Santa Barbara Canyon Trailhead to access this route.

TRIP SUMMARY: This pleasant route follows a retired service road easily for a few miles and then through the slightly more choked and steeper route up Santa Barbara Canyon and one of its tributaries to Madulce Camp along the northeast flank of Madulce Peak.

Trip Description

The **trailhead (3,350', 264476E 3851108N)** is across and back a bit along the road from the parking area. Follow the trail eastward through the site of the old Willow car campground, crossing the creek after only about 250 feet. You will also see a trail register just as you come to the wilderness boundary. The route here follows a long-retired service road along the banks of lower Santa Barbara Canyon. Cattle often roam this stretch of the canyon, so mind your step. The creek crossings are in the dozens (especially later), so this trail description eschews marking each one.

As you progress southward, the canyon narrows some and many of the geologic features of the area present themselves more plainly. After some easy hiking and numerous creek crossings through willow- and cottonwood-shaded canyons, your route will follow a left (west) fork of the creek; it feels like the lesser of the two but is indeed the main fork. Soon you'll pass beneath a dark coppice of mature live **oaks**

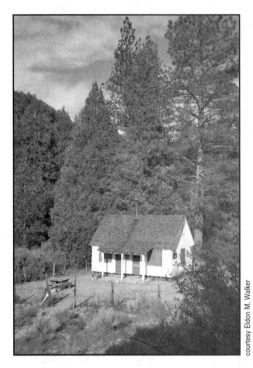

Madulce Cabin, 1983

courtesy Eldon M. Walker

(**3 miles, 3,730', 265017E 3847421N**) lined with a smattering of bigcone Douglas-firs that survived the fires. After another 0.5 mile Chokecherry Creek comes into the canyon from your right (west). From here, the going can be slow—wild roses, willow saplings, coffeeberries, and a multitude of lighter chaparral often encroach upon the trail. Though none of it prevents your progress, it certainly tempers any attempts at a land-speed record.

Soon you'll come into a quite lovely potrero, with views of upper Santa Barbara Canyon to your west. It's here you'll come to the **turn** (**5.3 miles, 4,140', 263835E 3844977N**) left (south) leading you up a tributary to Santa Barbara Canyon. Through this canyon the bands of different ecosystems become very thin, overlapping frequently (arroyo willow shaded by thick conifer spreads, with ferns on either side) and interspersed with weatherworn sandstone outcrops. Follow the easy trail 0.5 mile to the **fork** (**5.8 miles, 4,300', 263832E 3844250N**) of two rocky creek beds; follow the left (eastern) fork up a ways to the base of a fire-scarred and erosion-chewed hill. This next stretch—infamous among local hikers and dubbed Heartbreak Hill for its relatively unforgiving and straightforward approach—is a steep affair, often deeply rutted and choked with wild roses (especially post-Zaca). Labor up this 0.5-mile portion to reach a crest and then follow a lazy descent eastward another 0.5 mile into Pine

Canyon, where you'll find the junction with the Madulce Trail at **Madulce Camp** (**7 miles, 4,850', 263734E 3843191N**).

CAMP :: MADULCE CABIN SITE

ELEVATION:	4,850'
MAP:	USGS *Madulce Peak*
UTM:	263734E 3843191N

Nestled in a shallow area of tree-shaded Pine Canyon, Madulce consists of two sites near the old cabin grounds. The first site, heavily used and in plain sight as one approaches, is based around the foundation of the old cabin. This site—frequented by horse packers as well as backpackers—often has high lines strung between the massive creekside cedars. The kitchen features a large fire ring with a non-USFS grill, and often has implements (kettles, pans, etc.) stored in the remains of the cabin's old woodburning stove, which sits rusting in the elements beside the kitchen. This site is ideal for large groups.

CAMP :: MADULCE

ELEVATION:	4,850'
MAP:	USGS *Madulce Peak*
UTM:	263616E 3843242N

The actual trail camp, a few hundred yards up-trail from the old cabin site and generally considered the nicer of the two, enjoys far greater tree coverage, well shaded by firs, oaks, pines, and cedars (all still showing damage from the Zaca Fire). There is a fire ring and a cluster of old ice can stoves in the kitchen, and water is usually available in the creek beside the camp. *Note:* The 1995 *Madulce Peak* map shows the camp on the north side of Pine Creek; it is actually south of the creek, reached after crossing the creek one time past the old cabin site.

■ ■ ■ ■ ■ ■ ■ ■ ■ ■ ■ ■ ■ ■ MADULCE CABIN

The foundation remnants visible in the lower camp are those of Madulce Cabin, which burned in 1999. Originally the site of a hunting cabin from the 1880s, the best-known incarnation of the cabin was built in 1929. Its position here beside Pine Creek—nearly the junction of four major backcountry routes—gave it an ideal location, and the station was used by the US Forest Service (USFS) as a guard station. With the construction of the Buckhorn and Camuesa Roads by the Civilian Conservation Corps in the

1930s, the Mono-Alamar Trail was no longer a main route for traversing the forest, and Madulce Guard Station (along with Mono-Pendola Guard Station) eventually fell into disuse in the 1940s.

In the 1970s efforts by the USFS and local volunteers led to the revival of the station, and in 1978 it was awarded a place on the National Register of Historic Places. Subsequent upkeep by volunteers made it a popular place for backpackers, and the single-story wood structure—complete with an old wood stove, some furniture, and a small kitchen—was also often used by USFS personnel and work crews. Some of its contents (most notably the stove) can still be found around the lower camp.

Route 45

DON VICTOR VALLEY FIRE ROAD (6N11) and DON VICTOR TRAIL (25W03)

LENGTH AND TYPE:	13.2-mile out-and-back from Potrero Seco Road to Don Victor Camp; 13-mile one-way from Potrero Seco Road to Madulce Camp
RATING:	Moderate (damaged and lightly traveled) to difficult (miles of potential bushwacking)
TRAIL CONDITION:	Passable (old fire road) to challenging (nearly abandoned route)
MAP(S):	USGS *Madulce Peak* and *Rancho Nuevo Creek*; Conant's *Matilija & Dick Smith Wilderness*
CAMP(S):	Don Victor
HIGHLIGHTS:	Fantastic views of Dick Smith Wilderness

TO REACH THE TRAILHEAD(S): Use the Don Victor Trailhead to access this route.

TRIP SUMMARY: From Potrero Seco Road, this route follows the old Don Victor Valley Fire Road to Don Victor Camp, and then the Don Victor singletrack to Madulce Camp. The route is described east to west.

Trip Description

From the **split (5,190′, 276179E 3834880N)** at Don Victor Valley Fire Road (6N11) and Potrero Seco Road (6N03), head westward along the old fire road, passing through a gate and following the doubletrack easily up a short climb and then along a steady descent toward Mono Creek. Views along this entire route are fantastic: as you slowly gain on Madulce Peak some 13 miles distant, the Don Victor Valley and much of the Dick Smith Wilderness are laid out to your right (north); to your left (south), the upper Mono drainage is directly below you, and immediately beyond is Hildreth Peak. In the wake of the Zaca Fire, this route can prove brushy, but there is no mistaking the route. Numerous routes—including the Roblar (25W16) and Potrero Seco/East Fork Mono (25W04) Trails—that have either been officially or de facto abandoned over the years once used this stretch of road as a launching point: as a general rule don't follow any of the sometime tempting singletracks and instead stick to the road (unless you've done your homework).

It's a 5-mile trek to reach the first crossing of **Mono Creek** (**5.2 miles, 3,380',** **270503E 3837947N**). Here the road follows the meandering willow-clad Mono Creek—crossing several times—another 1.5 miles into Don Victor Valley and to **Don Victor Camp** (**6.6 miles, 3,475', 269285E 3839279N**). Wildflower displays are impressive here in the spring.

CAMP :: DON VICTOR

ELEVATION:	3,475'
MAP:	USGS *Madulce Peak*
UTM:	269285E 3839279N

Nearly all of what once existed of this site has been lost to history, but with space enough to bed down and nearby water, the flats near the junction with the Loma Pelona Jeepway mark the old site environs. Remains of the homestead's chimney were visible here as late as the 1960s but are now barely discernible. The US Forest Service does not maintain this site any longer, but it is still shown on forest maps.

From camp, continue eastward—crossing Mono Creek once more—to the junction with the singletrack Don Victor Trail. An old steel sign here indicates the direction; this stretch is often grassy and seeing the tread often proves difficult. (If you find yourself continuing southward along the road, you've missed it.)

Now your route becomes more difficult and is far less easy to discern. After the damage wrought by the Zaca Fire, all the maintenance in this area has been performed by a very small crew of dedicated volunteers—there is no official maintenance as of this writing. Be prepared to navigate, bushwack, crawl, and generally make painfully slow progress for what seems a very long 6 miles through Don Victor Canyon and the headwaters of Mono Creek to reach the **Don Victor/Puerta Suelo junction** (**12.4 miles, 4,730', 264047E 3842746N**); see *Route 43* for the Puerta Suelo Trail heading south here.

From here, the final 0.5 mile to **Madulce camp** (**13 miles, 4,850', 263734E 3843191N**; see page 193)—while not leisurely—will feel very easy after your climb out of the Don Victor. From Madulce, you have the option to continue toward the peak and Big Pine–Buckhorn Road (*Route 42*) or drop into Santa Barbara Canyon toward Cox Flat (*Route 44*).

Map 11: Eastern Dick Smith Wilderness

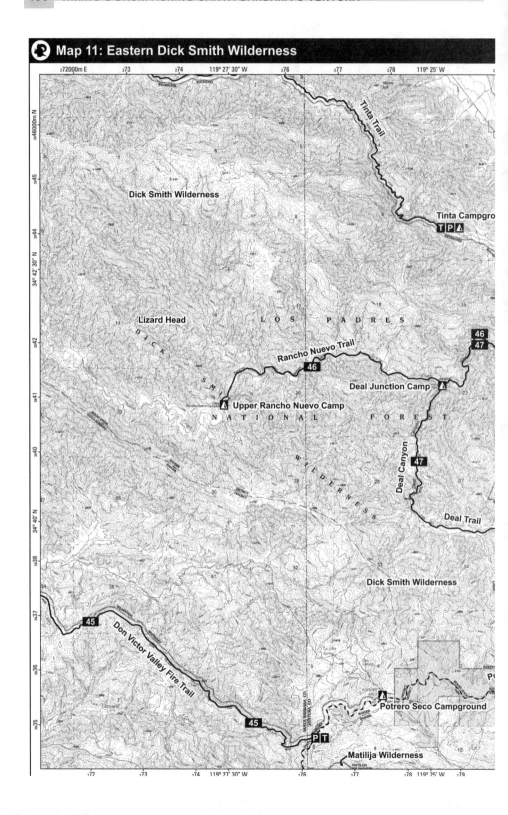

MAP 11 Eastern Dick Smith Wilderness **197**

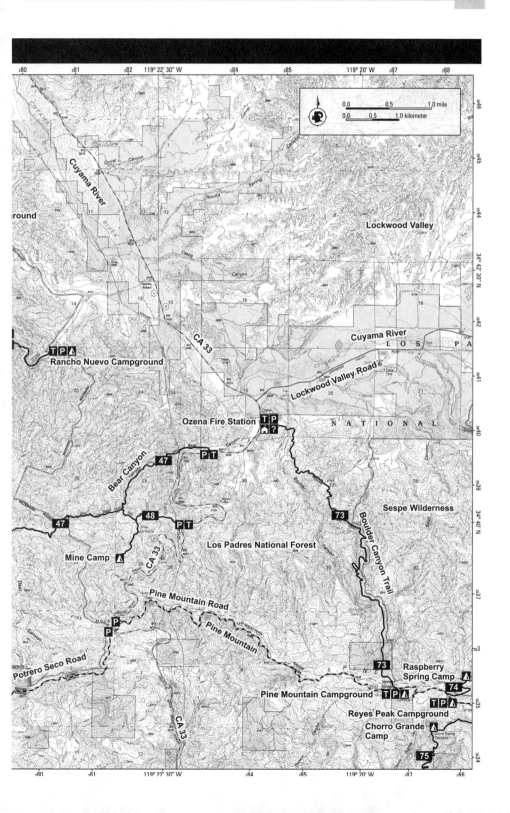

Lockwood Valley

Cuyama River

Rancho Nuevo Campground

CA 33

Ozena Fire Station

Bear Canyon

47

47

48

Mine Camp

CA 33

Pine Mountain Road

Pine Mountain

Potrero Seco Road

CA 33

Los Padres National Forest

73

Sespe Wilderness

Boulder Canyon Trail

73

Raspberry
Spring Camp

74

Pine Mountain Campground

Reyes Peak Campground

Chorro Grande
Camp

75

Route 46

UPPER RANCHO NUEVO CANYON (24W01)

LENGTH AND TYPE:	12-mile out-and-back
RATING:	Moderate (easy to Deal Junction)
TRAIL CONDITION:	Clear to passable
MAP(S):	USGS *Rancho Nuevo Creek*; Conant's *Matilija & Dick Smith Wilderness*
CAMP(S):	Deal Junction and Upper Rancho Nuevo
HIGHLIGHTS:	Sandstone cliffs of lower Rancho Nuevo Canyon

TO REACH THE TRAILHEAD(S): Use the Rancho Nuevo Trailhead to access this route.

TRIP SUMMARY: From the Rancho Nuevo car campground, this route follows Rancho Nuevo Creek 6 miles westward through the lower gorge and to Deal Junction, and then along the narrow ravines to Upper Rancho Nuevo trail camp.

Trip Description

From the **Rancho Nuevo Campground (3,520', 280357E 3841870N)**, follow the trail westward along the creek's southern bank. Almost immediately you'll pass an old stock **gate (0.1 mile, 3,550', 280050E 3841623N)** and then your route passes comfortably upstream through oak- and fir-lined trail, crossing the creek and then working the long stretch on the north slopes above the impressive sandstone formations of the lower canyon. This portion of the trail remains in good tread even after the Zaca Fire and makes for easy hiking until you reach **Deal Junction (2.4 miles, 3,750', 278747E 3841257N)**. Here the Deal Canyon trail heads south toward the slopes of Pine Mountain (see *Route 47*). A camp is just to your left (south) past the junction, along the grassy flat.

CAMP :: DEAL JUNCTION

ELEVATION:	3,750'
MAP:	USGS *Rancho Nuevo Creek*
UTM:	278740E 3841251N

A former cowboy camp made official USFS trail camp in the 1960s, Deal Junction Camp is a simple site set among the grasses and brush of a creekside flat with a single stove (one has gone missing in recent decades) and little else. Water is available from Rancho Nuevo Creek (except during summer), but Deal Creek is usually a more reliable source.

From Deal Junction, continue westward up the creek bed along the increasingly narrow canyon. Rains post–Zaca Fire have washed considerable portions of the trail away, and postfire regrowth (the most painfully apparent being wide swaths of California wild roses) can make the going slow in spots.

When the roses are high and thick, pants, gaiters, and patience are necessary to keep your trek from becoming one of lacerations and general discomfort, so enter this stretch prepared. Your route climbs easily (most effort is spent in any cross-country or rock-hopping, not in elevation gain) for just over 3.5 miles until you reach **Upper Rancho Nuevo Camp (6 miles, 4,150', 274580E 3841000N)**, set along the south side of the creek upon a small flat and surrounded by watersheds on three sides.

CAMP :: UPPER RANCHO NUEVO

ELEVATION:	4,150'
MAP:	USGS *Rancho Nuevo Creek*
UTM:	274580E 3841000N

A remote and cramped site, Upper Rancho Nuevo is a shadow of its former self, harassed by floods and fires and receiving little care or maintenance over the years. In the 1970s it possessed a pair of tables and four stoves, but amenities are now reduced to a single stove (grill) and an old New Deal–era ice can stove, the latter being more useful for most as a seat than for meal preparation. Water is available in wetter seasons from the creek.

From Upper Rancho Nuevo Camp, you may wish to consider trekking to the Lizard Head formation above the creek's northern drainage another 2 miles of cross-country to the northwest. Otherwise, once rested and ready to begin your return trip, retrace your steps back toward Deal Junction.

¿QUIÉN FUE LA FAMILIA REYES?

In the early 1800s, a several-year dry spell prompted the Reyes family—prominent ranchers from the northern San Fernando Valley outside Los Angeles—to head north literally in search of greener pastures. Traveling over the Tejon Pass and into the Cuyama, the family pioneered along the Cuyama watershed and immediate environs, gaining prominence throughout Ventura and Santa Barbara Counties. Many of the local features are named after the family (especially Jacinto D. Reyes, perhaps the most famous of the early Los Padres rangers) or their endeavors, among them

Reyes Creek, Reyes Peak, Beartrap Creek (after the men's hunting activities), and Rancho Nuevo ("new ranch").

■ ■

Route 47

BEAR, DEAL, and LOWER RANCHO NUEVO CANYONS (24W04 and 24W01)

LENGTH AND TYPE:	8.8 miles (shuttle)
RATING:	Moderate (for some trail-finding and occasional cross-country)
TRAIL CONDITION:	Clear to passable
MAP(S):	USGS *Reyes Peak* and *Rancho Nuevo Creek*; Conant's *Matilija & Dick Smith Wilderness*
CAMP(S):	Deal Junction
HIGHLIGHTS:	Sandstone formations and canyons; lower Rancho Nuevo Canyon

TO REACH THE TRAILHEAD(S): Use the Rancho Nuevo and Bear Canyon Trailheads for this shuttle.

TRIP SUMMARY: From the old Bear Canyon Trailhead, this near-loop trek follows Bear Canyon upstream to the ridgeline of the Zaca Fire–scarred Dick Smith Wilderness, dropping into the Deal Creek drainage and making a long northwesterly arc through the sandstone formations of lower Deal Canyon to the confluence with Rancho Nuevo Creek, and then east to the Rancho Nuevo car campground.

Trip Description

From the **Bear Canyon Trailhead (3,680', 283319E 3839929N)**, drop into the Bear Creek drainage and follow the trail westward for an easy ascent through the fire-scarred landscape. The canyon narrows and exhibits some fascinating sandstone features before opening back up just as you approach the Deal Connector Trail **junction (1.6 miles, 4,060', 281609E 3838894N)**; see *Route 48*. Your route steepens slightly as it begins to turn toward the west, gaining nearly 600 vertical feet in just under a mile. At the **crest (2.7 miles, 4,643', 280410E 3838684N)** you'll gain a fine view of Deal Canyon and the eastern edge of the Dick Smith Wilderness framed by charred piñons and scrub oaks. You can also take solace in the knowledge you've completed your elevation gain for the trip: it's (quite literally) all downhill from here.

Follow the switchbacks down into the Deal watershed, cutting right (west) just before the wash. Isolated stands of burnt Coulter pines mix among the more common piñons, manzanitas, and scrub. Your route follows the watershed—with the main fork and additional tributaries of Deal Creek coming in on your left (south) as you progress—and curves northward as sandstone formations rise above the creek bed and the canyon narrows. Much of the trail has been washed away post–Zaca Fire: depending on repair efforts, you may find yourself simply following the drainage for easy stretches rather than hiking along a trail proper. Signs of black bear (scat, prints, and raked tree trunks) are common along this portion of the hike.

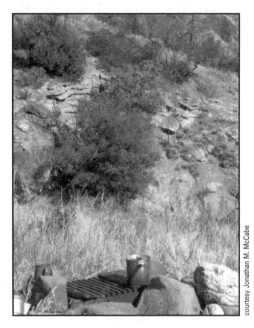

courtesy Jonathan M. McCabe

Deal Junction

■ ■ ■ ■ ■ ■ ■ ■ ■ **SMOKE ON THE MOUNTAIN**

In the summer of 2004—before the 2007 Zaca Fire decimated the Dick Smith and San Rafael Wildernesses—a US Forest Service (USFS) firefighting crew was flown into Deal Canyon to extinguish a 3-acre fire along a slide high above the creek bed. The fire wasn't in a location consistent with a neglected campfire or careless campers.

What the firefighters and investigators determined—and geologists and researchers from the USFS, USGS, and the University of California also soon confirmed—was that the fire had been caused by superheated fumaroles, some registering well over 500°F (far beyond the burn point of grass, wood, and other such combustibles). Geothermal and volcanic vents typically register around 200°F (near water's boiling point).

The immediate region has no significant coal or oil deposits, Geiger counter readings indicated no abnormal radioactivity, and there appears to be no evidence of volcanic or geothermal activity.

Theories abound as to the cause of these rather unprecedented hot spots, but the most likely explanation—according to the scientists still researching the phenomenon—is that the tertiary marine shale of which most of this region is composed contributed to a chemical reaction, and that the reaction is burning the shale's organic material—those bathymetric flora and fauna trapped on the seafloor some 45 millions year ago.

■ ■ ■ ■ ■ ■ ■ ■ ■ ■ ■ ■ ■ ■ ■ ■ ■ ■

Follow the narrow creek canyon through swaths of bigcone Douglas-firs and live oaks spared by the Zaca Fire (mostly along the trail, though with several creek crossings and an occasional rock-hopping episode, depending on trail condition) another 2 miles downstream

Deal Canyon

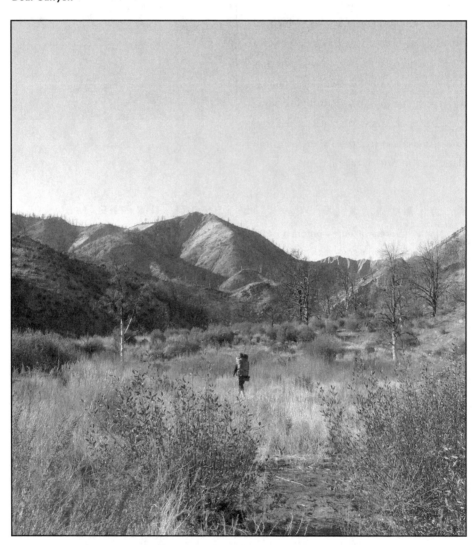

until the convergence with the **Rancho Nuevo Creek Trail (6.4 miles, 3,750', 278747E 3841257N)**. The **Deal Junction campsite** is to your immediate left (west), at the base of the slope along Rancho Nuevo Creek's southern banks.

CAMP :: DEAL JUNCTION

ELEVATION:	3,750'
MAP:	USGS *Rancho Nuevo Creek*
UTM:	278740E 3841251N

A former cowboy camp, Deal Junction is a simple site set among the grasses and brush of a creekside flat with a single stove and little else. Water is available from Rancho Nuevo Creek (except during summer), but Deal Creek is usually the more reliable source.

From Deal Junction, you can access the upper stretches of Rancho Nuevo Creek; see *Route 46* for the route west of the junction. To continue your route, join the Rancho Nuevo Creek Trail and head right (east). Here the trail remains in good tread, and you'll make quick time as you follow the creek through thick stands of oaks and firs and hike opposite the soaring and quite impressive sandstone cliffs of the lower canyon. Shortly after passing an old stock **gate (8.7 miles, 3,550', 280050E 3841623N)**, the trail opens to the **Rancho Nuevo Campground,** where your first vehicle is parked (**8.8 miles, 3,520', 280357E 3841870N**).

Route 48

MINE CAMP via Deal Connector (24W10)

LENGTH AND TYPE:	2.6-mile out-and-back
RATING:	Easy
TRAIL CONDITION:	Clear
MAP(S):	USGS *Reyes Peak* and *Rancho Nuevo Creek*; Conant's *Matilija & Dick Smith Wilderness*
CAMP(S):	Mine
HIGHLIGHTS:	Cool, quiet canyon; nice picnic spot

TO REACH THE TRAILHEAD(S): Use the Deal Connector Trailhead to access this route.

TRIP SUMMARY: From the parking area, the Deal Connector Trail (24W10) tracks west 0.75 mile along an easy grade to the junction with the Mine Spur Trail, and then heads south to a former prospectors' (and US Forest Service [USFS]) camp.

Trip Description

This very easy hike just outside the Dick Smith Wilderness boundary begins at the parking area and follows an old jeep trail into a shallow, grassy valley. Follow the thin strip of trail through the recovering grasses (burned in the 2007 Zaca Fire) along a shallow drainage and then toward the confluence of another small creek coming from the south. The trail ascends a knoll and cuts right (south), where it converges with the **Mine Spur Trail (0.6 mile, 4,170', 281871E 3838688N)**. Heavily burned during the 2007 Zaca Fire, the lower portion of the canyon still shows signs of the conflagration, with heavy stands of bigberry manzanitas standing bleached and bare.

From the junction, stay left (south) and continue along this easy grade. (To reach the Deal Trail, see "Making the Connection," opposite.) The upper stretches of this short canyon were largely spared from the recent fire; conifers and some canyon and interior live oaks here show minimal damage. The trail can be thin at points, but you'll still find it to be a simple walk up the canyon.

Cross the stream (usually barely a trickle) a few times, and after 0.5 mile there is a lovely stretch of the old jeep trail that hugs the west bank of the creek—but for the rock debris and fallen trees, the grade is still wide and pleasant, set in the narrowing canyon under increasing cover of the larger trees.

After the short stretch of road, follow the trail left (southeast) once more across the creek and up a short but steep few yards to the flat where **Mine Camp** stands (**1.3 miles, 4,300'**,

Mine Camp

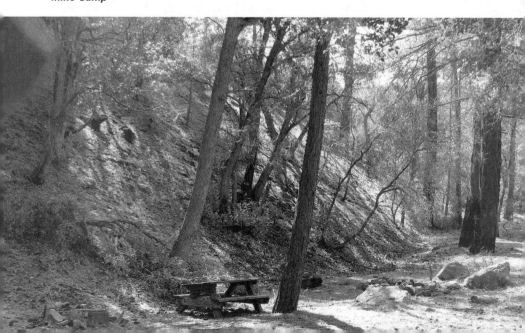

281558E 3837991N). The site makes for an ideal lunch spot, still in possession of an old wooden table and surrounded by mature bigcone Douglas-firs. When ready, retrace your steps to your vehicle or venture farther along the Deal Connector once back at the junction.

CAMP :: MINE

ELEVATION:	4,300'
MAP:	USGS *Rancho Nuevo Creek*
UTM:	281558E 3837991N

When the Atomic Energy Commission was encouraging uranium prospecting and mining throughout the area in the 1940s, Mine Camp was established by prospectors, and it later became a drive-in campground managed and maintained by the USFS (the remaining stove is one of the large concrete and cast-iron varieties and still bears the USFS stamp).

Mine Camp appears on the 1995 USGS *Rancho Nuevo Creek* topographic map but is shown quite north of its actual location (and was wholly absent from previous editions). It also appeared on older USFS recreation maps from the mid-1950s into the 1980s. The 4WD road was retired to trail use in the 1970s, and the trail and camp were both abandoned in the 1980s. But the site still features one of the old wooden picnic tables, and the charred remains of the latrine vault are still located just upstream.

MAKING THE CONNECTION

To reach the Deal Trail, continue along the right (westward) fork from the Mine Spur **junction (0.6 mile, 4,170', 281871E 3838688N)** and along the banks of the larger drainage to the junction with the Deal Trail (24W04) in **Bear Canyon (0.9 mile, 4,100', 281609E 3838894N)**—see *Route 47.* In the spring several species of wildflowers dot the creek banks, including monkeyflowers, larkspurs, and Matilija poppies. The landscape is classic chaparral, with recovering stands of manzanitas and mountain mahoganies throughout. Larger trees surround the higher points.

The Deal Connector is a popular alternate route for those hiking out of Bear Canyon and into Deal Canyon Camp, as this connector cuts 0.5 mile and nearly 500 feet of elevation gain from the starting length of the route.

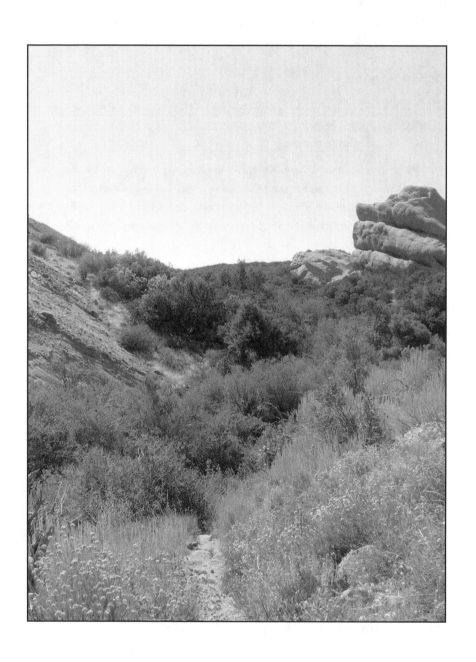

PART TWO

■　■　■　■　■　■　■　■　■　■　■　■

Eastern Mt. Pinos and
Ojai Ranger Districts

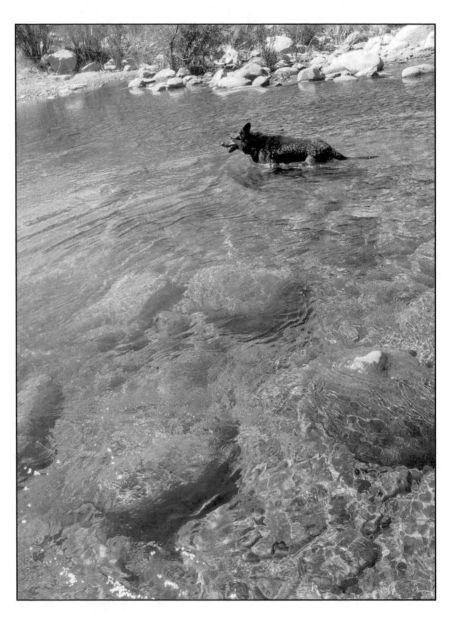

Cooling off in Matilija Canyon

Matilija Creek and Matilija Wilderness

This chapter details the routes of the Matilija Wilderness and upper Matilija watershed.

WEIGHING IN AT A (RELATIVELY SPEAKING) LIGHT 29,600 ACRES, the Matilija Wilderness is one of the smallest such-designated areas in the southern Los Padres, and it was part of the 1992 expansion of the Los Padres wilderness areas.

Historically, the Matilija drainage was an important route for accessing the backcountry from Ojai and Ventura (and vice versa). An old mail route followed in part what is now the only trail in the Matilija Wilderness, the Upper North Fork Trail (*Route 51*), and for years this route was also the primary (often only) means of communication between what is now northern Ventura County and the coastal communities. Louis L'Amour fans will recognize the Upper North Fork as part of the route followed by Sean Mulkerin in *The Californios*.

South of the Middle Fork, Murietta Canyon is the terminus (or beginning) of an important corridor into the Santa Ynez drainage via the Murietta Divide. Forest Road 5N13—pushed through to completion by the Civilian Conservation Corps during the Depression—connects the Matilija drainage with the Upper Santa Ynez Recreation Area (see Chapter 4). Most of the road is closed to private vehicles, but it does enable horse packers, hikers, mountain bikers, and emergency vehicles a through-route.

Matilija Trailheads

Cherry Creek Turnoff (4,110', 283883E 3831907N)

From the junction of CA 33 and CA 150 (the "Y") in Ojai, drive 27 miles north along CA 33 to the turnoff for Cherry Creek Road. During the winter or after heavy rains, the gate will be closed, and you will need to park beside the highway.

Cannon Creek Trailhead (2,240', 290358E 3821594N)

From the junction of CA 33 and CA 150 (the "Y") in Ojai, follow CA 33 approximately 9.5 miles (passing Wheeler Gorge Campground and the visitor center) to a group of turnouts just past Holiday Group Campground. The trailhead here is just across from mile marker 20.80.

Matilija Canyon Trailhead (1,560', 281995E 3820713N)

From the junction of CA 33 and CA 150 (the "Y") in Ojai, drive 5 miles north along CA 33 to Matilija Canyon Road on the left (west). The road passes through a community of small cabins and houses, and while suitable for passenger cars, it's narrow at places and often has rockfall and other debris. Drive 4.8 miles west along Matilija Canyon Road to the dirt parking area on the left (south) side of the road.

Ortega Hill (4,980', 283579E 3828090N)

From the junction of CA 33 and CA 150 (the "Y") in Ojai, drive 27 miles north along CA 33 to the turnoff for Cherry Creek Road. Turn left (south) onto the dirt road and follow it 2.75 miles to Ortega Hill. It's closed in winter.

Route 49

MURIETTA TRAIL (24W07)

LENGTH AND TYPE:	3.2-mile out-and-back or 5-mile loop
RATING:	Easy
TRAIL CONDITION:	Clear
MAP(S):	USGS *Old Man Mountain* and *White Ledge Peak*; Conant's *Matilija & Dick Smith Wilderness*
CAMP(S):	Murietta
HIGHLIGHTS:	Great for kids or first-timers; rock-hopping opportunities

TO REACH THE TRAILHEAD(S): Use the Matilija Canyon Trailhead to access this route.

TRIP SUMMARY: Named for the infamous 19th-century Mexican bandit who is believed to have used the canyon as one of his many hideouts, this hike makes for an easy (and child-friendly) day trip. From the south side of Forest Road 5N13, this very easy hike ascends the lower reaches of Murietta Creek to Murietta Camp. Total elevation gain is less than 250 vertical feet over 1.5 miles. The route can also be done as a slightly more challenging 5-mile loop via the Murietta service road.

Map 12: Murietta Divide and Divide Peak

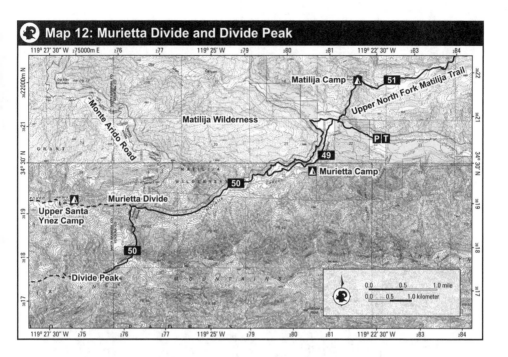

Trip Description

From the **parking area** (**1,560', 281995E 3820713N**), hike westward along the road beyond the gate and through the public access granted by the privately owned **Matilija Sanctuary**. You'll cross a branch of Matilija Creek twice. Shortly after the rise past the second crossing is the **Upper North Fork Trailhead** (**0.6 mile, 1,620', 281096E 3821130N**) on the right (north) side (see *Route 51*); continue a short stretch to the **Murietta Trailhead** (**0.7 mile, 1,625', 280939E 3821186N**).

Head south along the trail through high scrub and chaparral until the canyon narrows and live oaks and sycamores come into the mix, and you begin to follow an often-dry tributary to Murietta Creek. Ferns dot the shadier stretches of trail, as do blackberries and poison oak. Cottonwoods and alders begin to appear, and after 0.5 mile, you'll begin a very short ascent shaded by a massive live oak and its compatriots—this shade-dappled portion is often choked with poison oak.

Your route curves to meet **Murietta Creek** (**1.3 miles, 1,700', 280642E 3820459N**); the creek bed here is a lovely and broad swath of boulders and cobbles set beneath a long stretch of alders and a smattering of bays. The crossing is an ideal spot to allow younger hikers some time to perfect their rock-hopping skills, or to simply enjoy a short break.

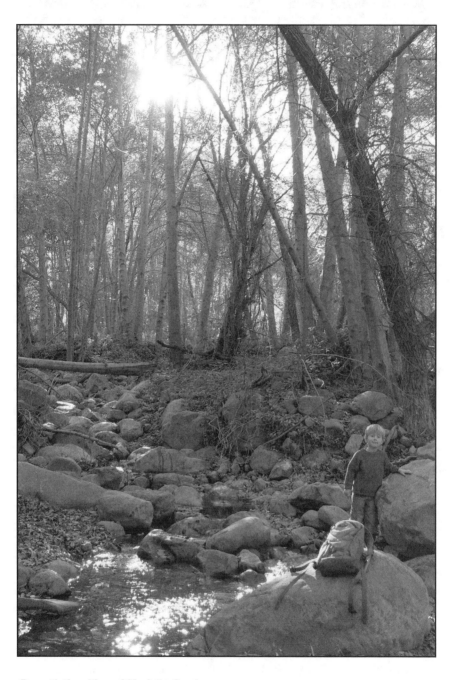

Beneath the alders of Murietta Creek

The trail cuts diagonally across to the other side of the cobble-strewn wash; follow the Forest Service markers to reconnect with the trail. *Note:* The USGS quads incorrectly mark the campground as being beside the creek here; you'll have to hike another 0.25 mile up-canyon to reach **Murietta Camp (1.6 miles, 1,800', 280354E 3820118N)**.

CAMP :: MURIETTA

ELEVATION:	1,800'
MAP:	USGS *White Ledge Peak*
UTM:	280354E 3820118N

A pleasant site tucked beneath a stand of mature live oaks, Murietta Camp is set along both sides of the trail, with one stove on the east and two along the west (creek) side. The old concrete form of the latrine that once stood in camp when it was accessible by 4WD sits in the southeast corner of camp. Be mindful of poison oak along the trail beyond camp.

From camp, you can either retrace your steps to return the way you came or continue beyond camp along what was once a spur route from Murietta Road for a slightly more challenging loop. From camp, the trail continues up-canyon through some lush sections, crossing the **creek (1.7 miles, 1,820', 280189E 3820182N)** just downstream from a narrower ravine and some inviting pools.

Follow the trail (a bit steeply, and—near one spring—a bit mucky at times) toward the **junction (2.4 miles, 2,170', 279419E 3820062N)** with the Murietta service road. It's then a simple matter of following the road about 2 miles down (east) and back to the **Murietta Trailhead (4.3 miles, 1,625', 280939E 3821186N)** where you first left the road. Retrace the final stretch back to your parked vehicle for a nice 5-mile loop.

Route 50

DIVIDE PEAK and THE MONTE ARIDO TRAIL (25W07)

LENGTH AND TYPE:	11.4-mile out-and-back
RATING:	Strenuous
TRAIL CONDITION:	Well maintained (service roads) to passable (unmaintained trail)
MAP(S):	USGS *Old Man Mountain* and *White Ledge Peak*; Conant's *Matilija & Dick Smith Wilderness*
CAMP(S):	—
HIGHLIGHTS:	Serious cardio workout; fantastic ocean and wilderness views

TO REACH THE TRAILHEAD(S): Use the Matilija Trailhead to access this route.

TRIP SUMMARY: This route follows the Murietta service road (5N13) steeply west to Murietta Divide, and then follows a largely abandoned singletrack southward to Divide Peak.

Trip Description

From Matilija Trailhead and **parking area (1,560', 281995E 3820713N)**, hike westward along the road beyond the gate and through the public access granted by the privately owned Matilija Sanctuary. You'll cross a branch of Matilija Creek twice; shortly after the rise past the second crossing is the **Upper North Fork Trailhead (0.6 mile, 1,620', 281096 3821130)** on the right (north) and the **Murietta Trailhead (0.7 mile, 1,625', 280939E 3821186N)** on the left (south). Continue following the road to a hairpin turn at the property line of the Blue Heron Ranch; make the left turn here and continue up the road, passing through the gate and beginning the long climb toward Murietta Divide.

A few springs and a few ravines over which the road crosses are dotted with sycamores and bays, but overall this route is largely bereft of shade, and bugs can be merciless in the summer. Despite that, the views of the bigcone Douglas-firs clinging to the hillsides to the west are outstanding and should help motivate you as the road becomes increasingly steep. After 2 miles you'll pass the upper junction with the **Murietta Trail (1.9 miles, 2,170', 279419E 3820062N)** described under the previous entry (*Route 49*).

Beyond the junction, follow the road up the steep and steady ascent, reaching **Murietta Divide (4.2 miles, 3,448', 276280E 3819286N)** after considerable elevation gain. Here, Potrero Seco/Monte Arido Road (6N03) comes in from the north, and to the south, the little-traveled Monte Arido Trail heads up toward the Santa Ynez ridge. The road along which you've been hiking continues now westward along the Santa Ynez River drainage; it's another mile to Upper Santa Ynez Camp, 4 miles to the east edge of Jameson Lake, and nearly 8 miles to Juncal. See Chapter 4 for hikes in that area.

To reach Divide Peak, follow now the Monte Arido (Spanish for "arid mountain") single-track southward for a very steep mile. Note here in place of the usual scrub and oaks, you are in the company of some of those majestic conifers you could view from far below. Views of the Channel Islands and Lake Casitas impress as you top out onto the eastern edge of the **Divide Peak OHV Route (5 miles, 4,570', 276052E 3818070N)**, part of what was once the epic Ocean View Trail (24W08). The boulders and landscape here are reminiscent of Pine Mountain and would perhaps beg to be climbed were the approach not already so strenuous.

Follow the OHV route a much easier 0.75 mile westward to **Divide Peak (5.7 miles, 4,707', 275506E 3817753N)**, actually a somewhat unimpressive pair of knolls. While the actual peak may not be impressive, the views couldn't be more so. A few hundred yards to the west near the water towers is where the old Rincon Trail (25W10)—the lower portion of which is shown on current US Forest Service maps but has been closed for years—once departed.

Unless you've sorted another exit or itinerary, return the way you came.

Route 51

UPPER NORTH FORK MATILIJA CREEK (23W07)

LENGTH AND TYPE:	2.6-mile out-and-back to Matilija Camp; 8.5-mile one-way to Ortega Junction (shuttle)
RATING:	Easy to Matilija; moderate to Upper Matilija; strenuous to Maple and Ortega Hill Trailhead
TRAIL CONDITION:	Clear to passable (seasonal)
MAP(S):	USGS *Old Man Mountain* and *Wheeler Springs*; Conant's *Matilija & Dick Smith Wilderness*; Harrison's *Sespe Wilderness*
CAMP(S):	Matilija, Middle Matilija, Upper Matilija, and Maple
HIGHLIGHTS:	Lush riparian hiking; wading pools; fractured geology

TO REACH THE TRAILHEAD(S): Use the Matilija Canyon Trailhead to access this route.

TRIP SUMMARY: From the north side of Forest Road 5N13, the North Fork Matilija Trail (23W07) ascends the Upper North Fork of Matilija Creek, passing through four trail camps—Matilija, Middle Matilija, Upper Matilija (officially abandoned but still in use), and Maple, as well as a handful of creekside guerrilla sites. The trail terminates at the junction of Cherry Creek Road (4WD and seasonal) and the Ortega Trail (23W08). The early portion of the trail makes an ideal day trip or first hike for youngsters.

Trip Description

From the **parking area (1,560', 281995E 3820713N)**, hike westward along the road beyond the gate and through the public access granted by the privately owned Matilija Sanctuary. You'll cross a branch of Matilija Creek twice; shortly after the rise past the second crossing, the **trail (0.6 mile, 1,620', 281096E 3821130N)** is on the right (north).

From the road, you'll drop slightly through a wired-off corridor into the Matilija Creek watershed. Cross the cobbled creek bottom (or rock-hop as necessary) to the sage-covered clearing directly across the creek bed. The trail angles across this small clearing toward the Upper North Fork of Matilija Creek, crossing the creek once more to the east bank (and entering the wilderness) and following the well-shaded and easy grade.

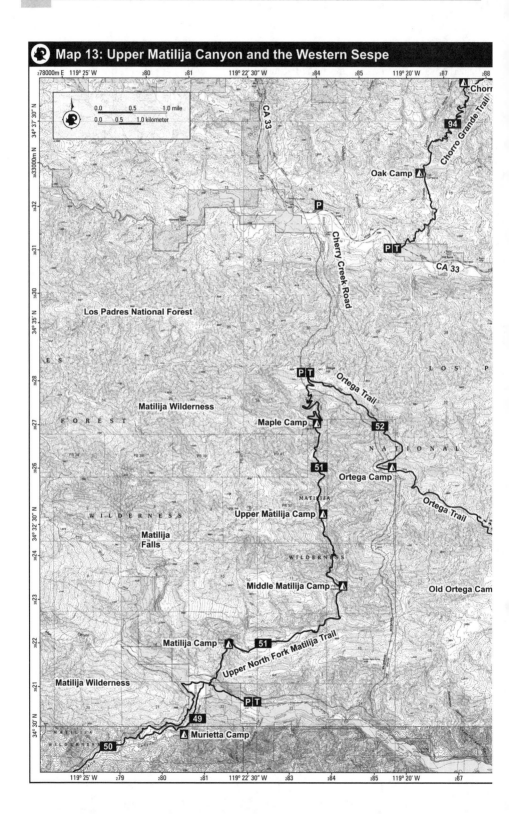

Map 13: Upper Matilija Canyon and the Western Sespe

Chorr
94
Oak Camp
P
Cherry Creek Road
Los Padres National Forest
P T
Ortega Trail
Matilija Wilderness
F O R E S T
Maple Camp
52
51
Ortega Camp
N A T I O N A L
Ortega Trail
MATILIJA
W I L D E R N E S S
Upper Matilija Camp
Matilija
Falls
W I L D E R N E S S
Middle Matilija Camp
Old Ortega Cam
Matilija Camp
51
Upper North Fork Matilija Trail
Matilija Wilderness
P T
49
M A T I L I J A
W I L D E R N E S S
50
Murietta Camp

CA 33
CA 33
Chorro Grande Trail

MAP 13 Upper Matilija Canyon and the Western Sespe 217

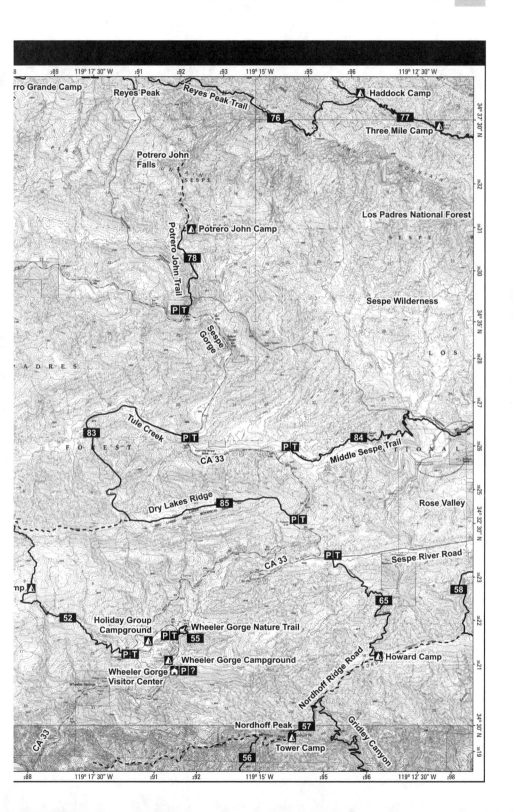

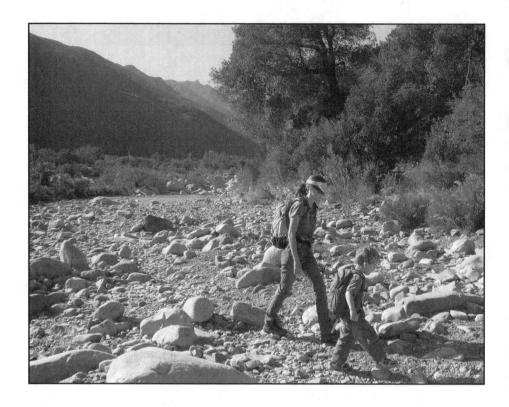

This area's geology is composed largely of marine sedimentary rocks from various geologic periods; the rock formations along the Upper North Fork are consistent with the southern extent of the Santa Ynez Mountains but also exhibit some dramatic uplift and fractured landscape along the route.

Shortly after a third stream crossing, **Matilija Camp (1.3 miles, 1,760', 281527E 3822042N)** will be on the right (east) side of the trail (though the 7.5-minute quad incorrectly marks it as west of the trail). The camp is situated between the trail and the creek in a wide, level area.

CAMP :: MATILIJA

ELEVATION:	1,760'
MAP:	USGS *Old Man Mountain*
UTM:	281527E 3822042N

Matilija is a well-shaded site with water available year-round from the Upper North Fork. Formerly the terminus of a jeep trail used as late as the 1960s, the camp has two main areas: the lower site is dominated by two massive live oaks (with California bay saplings along the creek bank) and contains one fire ring with grill;

the upper site is ringed by four oaks and several large boulders and contains three fire rings with grills.

The lower site is ideal for a solo or pair of backpackers; the upper site could accommodate a larger group. Both provide easy access to the creek and trail. The creek contains several nearby pools large enough for wading.

From Matilija Camp, continue north, crossing the creek once more a short distance from camp and setting out along the fairly level, well-worn trail. This stretch is clear and you can make good time as the trail departs the creek (if only briefly) and parallels it for nearly 0.5 mile before a series of eight creek crossings, a short set of switchbacks, and then another stretch of smooth travel.

The trail here affords especially good views of the creek and some ideal swimming holes as it tracks along the steep ravine wall. An old US Forest Service (USFS) sign leans against a moss- and lichen-encrusted boulder along the way, promising any tired boots they have only another 0.5 mile to Middle Matilija Camp.

The first of three crossings from the sign is a large tributary from the east; about 0.75 mile up this tributary is a waterfall worth investigating. Continuing along the trail, cross the main creek twice more and then come into a wide, grassy field dominated by a trio of large, gnarled oaks on the north end. Beneath the oaks sits **Middle Matilija Camp (3.9 miles, 2,360', 284218E 3823299N)**.

CAMP :: MIDDLE MATILIJA

ELEVATION:	2,360'
MAP:	USGS *Wheeler Springs*
UTM:	284218E 3823299N

Middle Matilija is another well-shaded site, located on the north end of a grassy shelf alongside the east bank of the Upper North Fork. There are two stoves, each situated beneath an oak on either side of the trail. Though damaged in the 1985 Wheeler Fire and by subsequent flooding the following winter, the camp has recovered well and is an ideal site for an easy weekend.

From Middle Matilija, ascend gradually into a short narrows, and after another half dozen crossings follow a series of switchbacks (exposed and quite warm in summer months but also exhibiting numerous plant specimens less-often encountered in the riparian areas below). Directly across from the switchbacks is a waterfall coming from one of the creek's western tributaries.

This exposed stretch of the trail parallels the ravine at the 2800' contour some 200 feet above the creek level for a distance of just over 0.25 mile. The trail's view here offers one a good perspective of the geology of the canyon as you hike away from the creek bed to rise high above the fractured landscape. The (literal) high point of the trail here crosses a unique rock "gate" at the Santa Ynez Fault, which you'll see on both sides of the canyon. From this point, descend gradually and return to the creek; after two more crossings is the abandoned **Upper Matilija Camp (5.5 miles, 2,900', 283836E 3824883N).**

CAMP :: UPPER MATILIJA

ELEVATION:	2,900'
MAP:	USGS *Wheeler Springs*
UTM:	283836E 3824883N

Upper Matilija, though officially abandoned in the 1970s as a cost-saving measure, is still in very good repair. The preceding switchbacks tend to discourage many day trekkers. A remote site, Upper Matilija is often mistaken for Maple Camp (another 1.5 miles upstream) because it isn't on the 7.5-minute *Wheeler Springs* map. The site possesses one large fire ring (no stove/grill) and—cast aside and almost an afterthought—a New Deal–era ice can stove.

From Upper Matilija, continue up-creek, crossing nearly a dozen times and gaining almost 1,000 feet of elevation in 1.5 miles between camps. In late winter and early spring this stretch can prove an exercise in bushwhacking at points. Midway through this bit between camps is another section of narrows.

As the chaparral and scrub begin to (if only briefly) give way to the larger conifers (bigcone Douglas-firs) and the canyon seems on the verge of submitting to Ortega Hill, a boulder jutting out from the soil on the right (east) side of the trail marks the spur to **Maple Camp (7 miles, 3,780', 283735E 3826997N).**

CAMP :: MAPLE

ELEVATION:	3,780'
MAP:	USGS *Wheeler Springs*
UTM:	283735E 3826997N

Maple is a spacious creekside camp encompassed by half a dozen big-leaf maples and a smattering of sycamores and bay laurel trees. The site features one large kitchen area and fire ring with a stove, as well as two ice can stoves. Though visited by the occasional day hiker from the Cherry Creek and Ortega Hill area upslope, it is seldom used for overnight camping.

Though named for the coppice of *Acer macrophyllum* found here, the camp (and much of this portion of the canyon) could have just as easily been called Bay, as the aromatic trees dominate the area.

Immediately north of camp are a few lazy switchbacks, followed by an ascent that snakes steeply up—making for an arduous though brief climb; in summer especially the rocky, south-facing slopes can become very warm. In 1.5 miles the trail gains over 1,200 feet in elevation to an open area just southwest of Ortega Hill and just outside the Matilija Wilderness boundary. It is here the Upper North Fork Trail and the Ortega Trail converge into **Cherry Creek Road (8.5 miles, 4,980', 283579E 3828090N)**.

Before the winter closures, this junction can be used as a parking area (USFS designates the road 4WD access only). During the off-season (and for those in passenger vehicles) it is another 2.75 miles to the **junction** of Cherry Creek Road and CA 33 (**11.25 miles, 4,110', 283883E 3831907N**). If you hike from this junction you'll pass the former Cherry Creek drive-in camp, an oak and mixed conifer area about 1 mile along the road. Until (temporarily) closed to recreational shooting by court order in the summer of 2011, this area was an extremely popular target-shooting area. It remains littered with spent shells and detritus from lax target shooters.

Route 52

ORTEGA TRAIL (23W08)

LENGTH AND TYPE:	8.9-mile one-way (shuttle)
RATING:	Moderate (distance; rocky terrain)
TRAIL CONDITION:	Well maintained (old 4WD and motorcycle route) to clear
MAP(S):	USGS *Wheeler Springs*; Conant's *Matilija & Dick Smith Wilderness*; Harrison's *Sespe Wilderness*
CAMP(S):	Ortega and Old Ortega (abandoned)
HIGHLIGHTS:	Excellent views of Tule and Matilija drainages, Channel Islands, and surrounding mountains

TO REACH THE TRAILHEAD(S): Use the Cannon Creek and Ortega Hill Trailheads for this shuttle.

TRIP SUMMARY: This slowly retiring OHV route descends from Ortega Hill along several easy ridgelines and then into the Cannon Creek drainage. At any given point, views of the

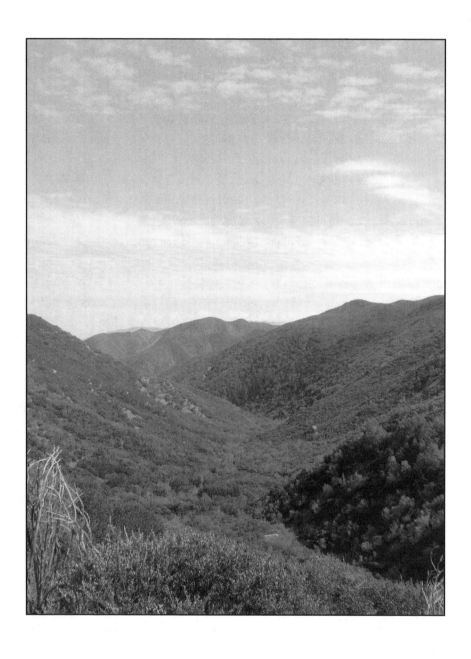

Channel Islands, Nordhoff Ridge, the Topatopa Mountains, and/or Pine Mountain can be had. This is a shuttle hike.

Trip Description

Note: Before the winter closures, this parking area just west of Ortega Hill can be used as a parking area (USFS designates the road 4WD access only). But if Cherry Creek Road is closed, factor in another 3 miles to your plans. From the junction of CA 33 and Cherry Creek Road/FS Route 6N01, follow the old 4WD road across Sespe Creek. Proceed up the canyon to the Ortega Hill shooting area and **junction (2.8 miles, 4,980', 283579E 3828090N)** with the Ortega (23W08) and Upper North Fork (23W07) Trails, passing the old Cherry Creek drive-in camps in an oak and mixed conifer area along the way.

Built by Ramón Ortega in the 1800s as a wintering route from the high country down into Nordhoff (now called Ojai), the Ortega Trail is now a very rough (and in places, extremely rocky) motorcycle trail best suited to experienced riders. Its use by motorcyclists seems to be diminishing over the years (storms in 2005 and subsequent erosion have made the trail quite difficult), and mountain bikers are even more infrequent. While OHV routes are not generally covered in this guide, this trail can make for a fine destination during the off-season (especially after wet weather closes the route to motorcycles altogether).

This route is not recommended in the summer when motorbike traffic *may* be more likely, and only the hardiest of dogs should be considered, even in cool weather, as the rocks alternate between abrasive sandstone and sharp talus. There is usually no water along this route, so plan accordingly.

From the Ortega Hill parking area, follow the road to the southeast and through the iron **barriers (~400 feet, 4,940', 283624E 3828014N)** intended to prevent larger vehicles from accessing this motorcycle trail. You'll gain great views of the Upper North Fork of Matilija Canyon and the trail descending toward Maple Camp to your right (west) as you follow the wide route steadily (descending the last 0.25 mile or so) to a **gap (1.4 miles, 5,150', 285189E 3826995N)** between that drainage and Tule Creek to your left (east). The cut that heads directly up the knoll follows the break created when the old Richfield Oil (later ARCO) natural gas pipeline was built along these hills in the late 1940s; follow the road as it heads left and down the eastern flanks of the knoll.

Descend from the gap easily at first with a smattering of piñon pines, and then you'll begin to curve clockwise down around the knoll rather steeply. This stretch is often the first of what local hikers term the "ankle-breaker" sections—rocky and requiring some diligence. Follow the road down about 0.5 mile with nearly 500 feet of elevation loss before climbing back up to a barren, rock-sheeted stretch of road and the new incarnation of **Ortega Camp (2.8 miles, 4,900', 285495E 3825986N)**.

CAMP :: ORTEGA

ELEVATION:	4,900'
MAP:	USGS *Wheeler Springs*
UTM:	285495E 3825986N

A site built by industrious OHV enthusiasts near the end of the old service road, the "new" Ortega campsite is a spacious site set atop a plateau and commanding excellent views of the nearby mountains and Tule Creek drainage. Two tables—one an old wooden affair and one a hardier and more recent metal specimen—complement five widely spaced fire pits (some with grills). There is no shade here (the highest vegetation is shoulder-height manzanita along the site's perimeter), but it does make for a good lunch spot for those hiking through.

From camp, you'll note the route again heading high atop the knoll directly to your south. This route follows a long-abandoned (though documented as recently at the 1995 *Wheeler Springs* 7.5-minute quad) route (the former pipeline service road) several miles southward that roughly follows the course of the pipeline (paralleling the Matilija Wilderness boundary) before reaching a tributary of Matilija's Upper North Fork just short of North Fork Point. From the creek, the route rock-hops to some very secluded falls before following the drainage out to the Upper North Fork route just downstream from the Middle Matilija Camp. This is a rewarding route to pursue, but one which entails a fairly long day, a great deal of uneven terrain, and a fair amount of bushwacking.

Instead, follow the road southeast from camp, where it quickly restricts quad-wheeled vehicles and constricts into classic singletrack. The going is quite rocky for a time, until stretches of far more manageable talus—hemmed in by scrub oaks and more manzanitas—lead you to a usually dry **crossing (3.4 miles, 4,680', 285947E 3825544N)** and then up an easy rise to a series of saddles and gaps that traverse and weave along the easy line of ridgetops separating the Matilija (later Ventura) and Tule (later Sespe) drainages.

This continues along a pleasantly easy grade—crossing an old firebreak constructed during the 1985 Wheeler Fire several times—with very little in the way of elevation change to the upper **junction (4.5 miles, 4,700', 287435E 3824914N)** with the Dry Lakes fuelbreak. Your route continues south toward the Cannon Creek drainage.

Here your route begins to descend noticeably, and your views are restricted to primarily points south. In short time you'll find yourself in a gap over which old sandstone formations loom (the trail here becomes quite rocky again); some use trails wander about these rocks. Just beyond (after crossing the headwaters of Cannon Creek) you'll come to the **original Ortega campsite (5.9 miles, 4,240', 288149E 3823488N)**.

CAMP :: OLD ORTEGA

ELEVATION:	4,240'
MAP:	USGS *Wheeler Springs*
UTM:	288149E 3823488N

This tiny and largely forgotten site is situated alongside the usually dry cobble-strewn wash that is upper Cannon Creek. While it contains two New Deal–era ice can stoves and a fire ring, the camp barely has enough room for more than two or three campers' bedrolls and has little shade. The nearby rock formations do make for a pleasant view, but the sparse site (these days) is likely best suited for day use and as a lunch spot.

Note: This site, built in the 1930s by the CCC, is no longer shown on USGS quads (last seen on the 1991 edition) or the recent editions of the USFS Los Padres visitor maps. It is, however, shown on the Conant map (labeled "Ortega Vieja").

From the Old Ortega site, the trail leads you down through the Cannon Creek drainage, eschewing the harder chapparal and rocky route for easier going along a packed shale and talus trail; for a stretch you'll follow another old fuelbreak before a sharp **drop** (**7 miles, 3,650', 288469E 3822505N**) to your left (east). From here your descent is dotted by ferns along some north-facing slopes, and while sections remain fairly rutted from a combination of erosion and motorcycles, the going is easy for most of the way down. About a mile down you may notice a large east-facing sandstone **boulder** (**8 miles, 2,940', 289594E 3821936N**) with the inscription JB KING 1908 JAN 30—nobody's quite certain about the identity of the author, though a 1995 article that appeared in the *Los Angeles Times* theorized the carving may have been the work of Ojai-area Reverend John B. King of the long-shuttered Holiness Church.

Toward the end, several long switchbacks ease the drop until finally you'll hear the vehicles on the highway below and reach the **junction** (**8.7 miles, 2,320', 290155E 3821641N**) with another old break that actually does lead to a roadwork staging area farther down along CA 33 across from Holiday Group Campground. Older incarnations of this side trail also provided options for dropping into the Wheeler Gorge Campground and the now-shuttered Wheeler Hot Springs.

Stay on the trail you've been following—now a wide and easy path under cover of sycamores—and head toward the cluster of sycamores due east, where the trail meets **CA 33** (**8.9 miles, 2,240', 290358E 3821594N**) directly across from mile marker 20.80.

Ojai Frontcountry, Nordhoff Ridge, and Rose Valley

This chapter details the trails of the Ojai and Santa Paula frontcountry (including those leading to Nordhoff Ridge) and Rose Valley.

THE CITY OF OJAI—HOME TO FEWER THAN 10,000 SOULS—is an artisan community situated at the foot of the Topatopa Mountains and Nordhoff Ridge. It is effectively the gateway town to most of the Ojai Ranger District's frontcountry. Originally named Nordhoff, after the Prussian-American writer Charles Nordhoff, during the Great War the town adopted its old Chumash place-name as a concession to anti-German sentiment of the time.

Aside from those in Rose Valley (see "Campgrounds" on page 230), the other two car campgrounds are Wheeler Gorge (70 sites) and Holiday Group Campgrounds (8 sites; reservations required). Both are managed by the Rocky Mountain Recreation Company (**rockymountainrec.com**). The Wheeler Gorge Visitor Center—open weekends 9 a.m.– 3 p.m.—provides interpretive and educational activities and programs and is located across the highway from Wheeler Gorge Campground, about 8 miles north of Ojai along CA 33.

Trailheads of the Ojai Frontcountry, Nordhoff Ridge, and Rose Valley

Cozy Dell Trailhead (880', 289605E 3817584N)

From the junction of CA 33 and CA 150 (the "Y") in Ojai, drive north along CA 33 approximately 3.3 miles to a parking area on the west side of the road. There are no facilities here. The trail is across the road.

Gridley Trailhead (1,160', 295798E 3816421N)

From the junction of CA 33 and CA 150 (the "Y") in Ojai, drive east along CA 150 (Ojai

Avenue) through Ojai for 2 miles to Gridley Road. Turn left (north) on Gridley Road and continue 1.5 miles to what is effectively the end of the road. Park your vehicle in this cul-de-sac.

Horn Canyon (Thacher School) Trailhead (1,450', 299919E 3815677N)

From the junction of CA 33 and CA 150 (the "Y") in Ojai, drive east along CA 150 (Ojai Avenue) through Ojai for 3.4 miles and make a slight left (east by northeast) onto Reeves Road (at Boccali's restaurant, at the base of Dennison Grade). Follow Reeves Road 1.1 miles and turn left (north) at McAndrew Road. Continue north along McAndrew Road another 1.1 miles until you reach the entrance to the private Thacher School on your right (if you make a 90-degree turn to the left and begin heading downhill, you've missed it—this entrance can be easy to miss). Turn right into the Thacher School grounds—you are now on private property. Bear right at the first junction just inside the property and continue eastward through the parking areas for 0.2 mile. Stay right at this next junction as well, heading eastward onto a dirt road and crossing Horn Creek. (A vehicle with higher-than-average clearance is recommended if you're making this trip after any measurable rains.) The road passes through an avocado orchard beside an athletics field for approximately 250 feet. The parking area is in front of the gate. There are no facilities here.

Howard Creek Trailhead (3,480', 295234E 3823677N)

From the junction of CA 33 and CA 150 (the "Y") in Ojai, drive north along CA 33 approximately 14.5 miles to Forest Road 6N31 (Rose Valley Road). Turn right (south) onto this road and continue east for 0.5 mile to the turnoff for a gated service road on your right (south); park on either side of the service road here. A Forest Service Adventure Pass, federal Interagency Pass, or equivalent permit is required to park a vehicle anywhere in the Rose Valley Recreation Area. There are no facilities here, but restrooms are available farther down the road at Rose Valley Campground, Middle Lion Campground, and the Piedra Blanca Trailhead.

Oso Trailhead (735', 289601E 3815388N)

From the intersection of Fairview Road and CA 33 in Ojai, follow Fairview Road westward approximately 0.3 mile to a dogleg at Rice Road. Proceed straight/right (north) here for 0.2 mile to the intersection with Meyer Road. Turn left (west) at Meyer and proceed another 0.3 mile (staying straight and passing through the gate at the Oso Road intersection) to the dirt parking area. This parking area is managed by the Ojai Valley Land Conservancy.

Note: As of this writing the gate leading to the Oso Trailhead (at the Meyer/Oso intersection) is open 8 a.m.–7:30 p.m. during summer (April–October) and 8 a.m.–5 p.m. during the off-season (November–March). Plan accordingly.

Rose Valley Campground (3,420', 299648E 3823278N)

From the junction of CA 33 and CA 150 (the "Y") in Ojai, drive north along CA 33 approximately 14.5 miles to Forest Road 6N31 (Rose Valley Road). Turn right (south) onto this road and continue east for 3.1 miles to the intersection with Rose Valley Lake Road. Turn right (north) here and continue 0.6 mile northward to Rose Valley car camp. A small parking space is located between sites 3 and 4 for day hikers, but a Forest Service Adventure Pass, federal Interagency Pass, or equivalent grants rights to one of the campgrounds if you're inclined. There is no water here, but there are restrooms.

Santa Paula Canyon (Thomas Aquinas College/Ferndale) (975', 307824E 3811547N)

From Ojai, take CA 150 (North Ojai Road) eastward 11.9 miles (over Dennison Grade) to the parking area just west of the Thomas Aquinas College entrance. From CA 126 in Santa Paula, take Exit 12 (10th Street/CA 150) and follow CA 150 approximately 5.9 miles to the trailhead.

The Ventura County Sheriff's Department has posted signs warning hikers against leaving any valuables in their vehicles here, as break-ins have been on the rise in recent years.

Sisar Canyon (1,800', 303945E 3814064N)

From the junction of CA 33 and CA 150 (the "Y") in Ojai, drive east along CA 150 (Ojai Avenue) 8.9 miles (over Dennison Grade) to the turnoff for Sisar Road on your left (north). Alternately, from CA 126 in Santa Paula, take Exit 12 (10th Street/CA 150) and follow CA 150 approximately 8.9 miles to the turnoff for Sisar Road on your right (north).

Sisar Road is a residential area; drive slowly and watch for pets and children. Drive north on Sisar Road approximately 0.5 mile to where the road splits to the right onto the dirt Forest Service road (now called Sisar *Canyon* Road). Here you'll note private vehicles parked; there is about 400 feet of road between the turnoff and a pair of water towers along which you'll find a few spots for parking if you're in a low-clearance passenger vehicle. If you have better-than-average clearance, continue along the road another (sometimes rough) 0.5 mile to a parking area just before the Forest Service gate. There are no facilities here.

Stewart Canyon Debris Basin (960', 293338E 3815506N)

From the junction of CA 33 and CA 150 (the "Y") in Ojai, drive east along CA 150 (Ojai Avenue) through Ojai for 1 mile to North Signal Street. Turn left (north) onto Signal Street and continue 0.9 mile (making a left turn to stay on Signal at the dogleg with Grand Avenue at 0.4 mile) to the Spelway Dam/Stewart Canyon Debris Basin road on your left (a USFS sign here indicates the way). Turn left (west) and continue 0.2 mile to the turnoff on your left for the Pratt Trailhead and parking area.

Topatopa Bluff Trailhead (5,300', 305818E 3819629N)

Note: Access to this trailhead requires a permit from the Ojai Ranger District; visit the office or call (805) 646-4348 for details.

From Rose Valley Campground (see description on page 230), pass through the locked gate and follow the 4WD road 1.3 miles up to its junction with Nordhoff Ridge Road. Turn left (east) here and continue 8.1 miles along the ridge road (passing Elder Camp) to a small parking area just down from the road gate and wilderness boundary.

Wheeler Gorge Nature Trail Turnoff (1,940', 291538E 3821970N)

From the junction of CA 33 and CA 150 (the "Y") in Ojai, drive north along CA 33 8.5 miles to a small parking area north of the USFS fire station and just before the North Fork Matilija Creek bridge (there is also space to park just up the road, on the other side of the bridge). The parking space is on the left (west) side of the highway; exercise caution crossing the highway and please be sure not to block the gate. There are no facilities here, but restrooms are located at the Wheeler Gorge Campground just down the road on the west side of the highway.

Nordhoff Ridge Road

Nordhoff Ridge Road is a key route for Ojai-area hikes. The road cuts across the top of the Nordhoff ridgeline from above Wheeler Canyon to the Sespe Wilderness boundary in the east, where the old road tread continues a few miles into the wilderness toward Hines Peak and Red Reef Canyon. Several trails lead to the road from Rose Valley or Ojai.

The main vehicle access to the road is via the steep Chief Peak Road (also known as Seabee Road), built in the 1950s by the Naval Construction Battalion's heavy equipment operators when the Navy maintained the base in Rose Valley. Sisar Road is gated and not open to public vehicles coming from Nordhoff Ridge.

Access to both Nordhoff and Chief Peak Roads are by permit only; the Ojai Ranger District office issues a maximum of 20 permits a day. During hunting season, permits are usually difficult to obtain, but other times you will seldom see others atop the ridge. Call (805) 646-4348 to arrange for a permit—they are good for three days. A Forest Service Adventure Pass, federal Interagency Pass, or equivalent is also required to drive the road.

Three dry camps are along the ridge: Howard, at the upper terminus of the Howard Creek Trail (not to be confused with the old Howard Creek Campground at the Howard/Sespe confluence); Tower, set beneath the remains of the old Nordhoff Peak lookout tower;

and Elder, just east of the lower Red Reef section that drops into Sisar Canyon. All of these sites provide a table and fire pit but lack water and facilities.

Rose Valley

Rose Valley, said to be named for the wild roses growing along the surrounding hillsides, has had a long and storied history in the annals of both the Los Padres wilderness and Ventura County.

In the 1960s—when the Sespe Road was a prime destination for off-roaders, target shooters, and tailgating outdoor enthusiasts—those passing through Rose Valley were witness to the might of the U.S. Naval Construction Battalion (the Seabees) at its height. Established as a training area by the Seabees in the early 1950s, the Rose Valley facility was a bustling scene of Quonset huts, a landing strip, several outbuildings, and heavy equipment of all descriptions. It was those Seabees who bulldozed numerous roads—notable among them Chief Peak Road—into the nearby hillsides; half a century later their works remain the routes used by countless hikers and mountain bikers. The two artificial lakes—popular with local anglers—were also the Navy's handiwork.

When the Navy scaled back to their base of operations in Port Hueneme farther south, the facilities were used as a base for large-scale firefighting operations by the USFS until 1986, when arrangements were made for the Ventura County Sheriff's Department to use the facility as a work camp for low-security inmates. That use, however, only lasted until 1992, about the time the additional wilderness legislation and endangered species protections were signed into law.

A part of the area was—in the '70s and '80s—colloquially known as Sparkle Mountain for the volume of blasted glass, bottles, and other detritus left by target shooters. (The trail directly behind the shooting area heading up the Howard Creek drainage toward Nordhoff Ridge was subsequently abandoned.) Shooting is no longer allowed in the area (with the exception of that under the auspices of The Ojai Valley Gun Club, which was founded in 1960 and maintains a range in Rose Valley under an agreement with the USFS).

Campgrounds

Two camps are located in Rose Valley: the eponymous Rose Valley Campground (9 sites; access to Rose Valley Falls and Chief Peak) and Middle Lion Campground (7 sites; access to Lion Canyon). Both only require a Forest Service Adventure Pass, federal Interagency Pass, or equivalent for use, and they are first come, first served. There are restrooms but no water. These camps can be a bit rambunctious on weekends, so weekday trips are recommended.

Route 53

KENNEDY RIDGE

LENGTH AND TYPE:	3.5-mile out-and-back
RATING:	Moderate
TRAIL CONDITION:	Clear to passable
MAP(S):	USGS *Matilija*
CAMP(S):	—
HIGHLIGHTS:	Panoramic views of Lake Casitas, the Ojai Valley, and the Pacific

TO REACH THE TRAILHEAD(S): Use the Oso Trailhead to access this route.

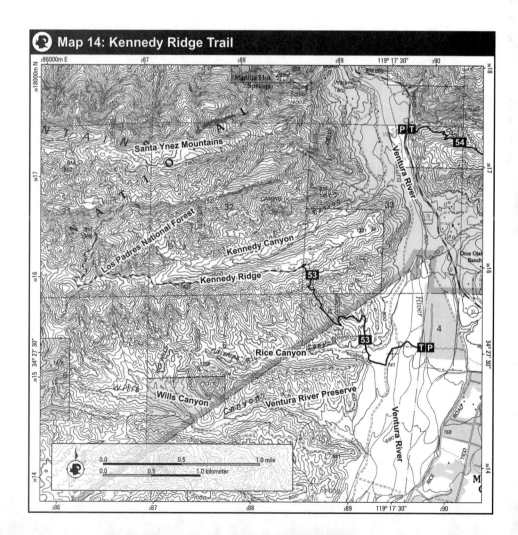

Map 14: Kennedy Ridge Trail

TRIP SUMMARY: This new and still-in-progress route begins along the Rice Canyon Trail in the Ojai Valley Land Conservancy's beautiful Ventura River Preserve, and then climbs into forestlands toward an old ridgeline trail. This trail is a joint effort of the OVLC and the US Forest Service's Ojai Ranger District.

Trip Description

The first mile of this route is a matter of connecting the proverbial dots along various bits of other trails, retired roads, and rights-of-way.

From the **Oso Trailhead (735', 289601E 3815388N)**, follow the singletrack westward to the Rice/Wills junction a few yards distant. Head right (north) here and follow the trail through shrub and willows to the banks of the **Ventura River (150 yards, 725', 289505E 3815451N)**. This crossing is often a dry, cobble-strewn affair, but during the winter and after rains it can result in wet feet.

After crossing the river, follow the trail up to a retired service road and head southward above the riverbank. Here you'll pass a long-abandoned orange grove (this route has been labeled the Orange Grove Trail, but the signage may not reflect that), where old and gnarled trees (many of which still bear fruit) are intertwined with laurel sumacs, some nonnative volunteers, and even the occasional manzanita.

At the **upper junction (0.25 mile, 750', 289339E 3815270N)** with the Wills Canyon Trail, where Rice Creek crosses beneath the road, take the right (westbound) fork that cuts between the orchard and follow the creek toward the **Los Robles Diversion Canal (0.45 mile, 774', 289143E 3815424N)**. Cross the bridge here; just up ahead is the **junction (0.5 mile, 790', 289100E 3815441N)** where the Kennedy Ridge route splits from the Rice Canyon route. Head up the draw, connecting with a service road at 0.65 mile (head left here), and then follow this road. The route treads across Sespe sandstone and its red, silty soils and is lined periodically with black walnuts. Views of the Ventura River watershed are quite nice on clear days. You'll turn off the road once again and return to **singletrack (0.85 mile, 880', 288869E 3815759N)** in a shallow draw. Now the hike truly begins!

Follow the singletrack through the classic chaparral and sandstone-punctuated terrain of the eastern Santa Ynez Mountains for an at-times steep mile. *Note:* GPS data sets and some old maps show an old dozer line ascending this ridge; your route does not follow that line, so don't rely overly on a GPS receiver to navigate. The trail is clear and easy enough to follow. After some effort you'll reach the **junction (1.7 miles, 1,470', 288534E 3816242N)** with an old legacy trail. Just yards to the right (east) is a picnic table set in a clearing beneath a formation of Coldwater sandstone boulders.

The picnic table represents the end of this entry's narrative (the trail heading left [west] from the junction eventually fades into the brush), but with any luck the route's ultimate goal of reaching the East Camino Cielo and eventually the historic Ocean View Trail will someday be a reality. To help with the ongoing efforts to maintain and extend this route, visit **ovlc.org**.

Route 54

COZY DELL TRAIL (23W26)

LENGTH AND TYPE:	4-mile out-and-back to Cozy Dell service road (Forest Route 5N34); 2.1-mile one-way to Foothill Trail junction; 3.2-mile one-way to Pratt Trail junction
RATING:	Moderate (easy after the initial climb)
TRAIL CONDITION:	Clear
MAP(S):	USGS *Matilija*; Conant's *Matilija & Dick Smith Wilderness*; Harrison's *Sespe Wilderness*
CAMP(S):	—
HIGHLIGHTS:	Views of Ojai Valley and Ventura River watershed

TO REACH THE TRAILHEAD(S): Use the Cozy Dell Trailhead to access this route as described, or the Stewart Debris Basin if coming via the Pratt Trail.

TRIP SUMMARY: From CA 33, the Cozy Dell Trail climbs out of the Sheldon Canyon drainage into Cozy Dell Canyon to Cozy Dell Creek and Forest Route 5N34. Numerous spur trails, many of which follow fuelbreaks and dozer lines of varied ages, crisscross the area

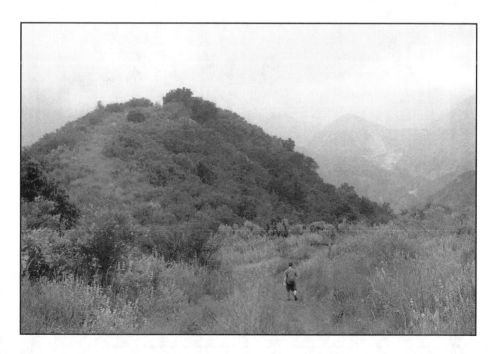

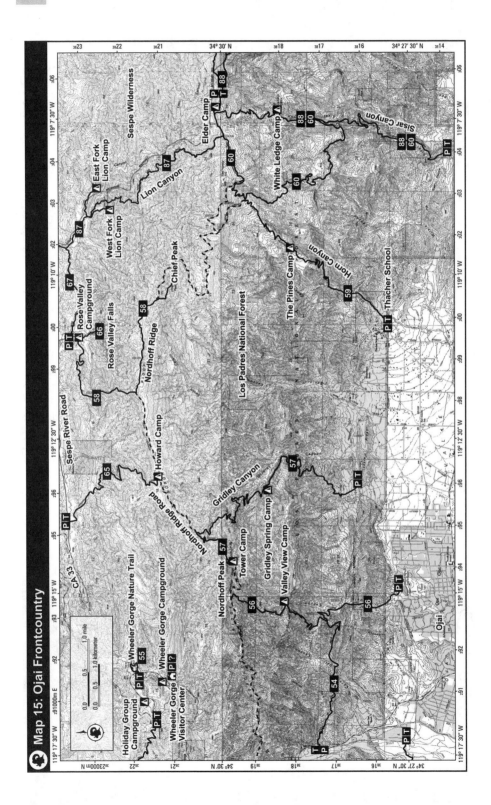

Map 15: Ojai Frontcountry

and intersect with your route. The lower portion of the trail is heavy with poison oak, and bugs can be troublesome in hot weather.

Trip Description

From CA 33, cross the road to the **trailhead (880', 289620E 3817616N)** just south of the guardrail across Sheldon Creek. Follow this route into the canyon, crossing the intermittent creek twice in fairly rapid succession and then climbing along its southern slope through dense oak- and scrub-shaded trail. Poison oak is heavy along the early stretches. Less-irritating flora you'll encounter along the at-times steep switchbacks include chamises, scarlet buglers, miner's lettuce, various ferns and grasses, and the invasive fennel. Orange, spaghetti-like dodders can be seen clinging to spots on the slopes opposite, and *Dudleya* (canyon liveforevers) cling to rock faces as you make your way to the grassy **saddle (1.1 miles, 1,580', 290493E 3817258N)** between the Sheldon and Cozy Dell drainages.

Here, views from the rocks just to your right (south) offer a great perspective of the Ojai Valley and the Ventura River watershed, and monkeyflowers, purple sage, and lupines dot the grassy slopes. Stay to the trail that continues eastward here; a thread of a trail heads left (north) up the knoll popular with geocachers and those exploring some of the old fire cuts toward Nordhoff Ridge to the north. Here your route follows an old US Forest Service road down into the Cozy Dell drainage; the tread here is much easier than some of the rockier and steep sections from which you've just emerged. Mustard, grasses, and thistles are ambitious and encroach on the old road in the spring. Hollyleaf cherries and laurel sumacs form a thick blanket across the hillsides.

The road drops into a shallow drainage and then climbs easily back again to another **gap (1.5 miles, 1,580', 290917E 3817146N)**, where more fire cuts and spur trails head north and south. Stay on the main route and drop again easily along the pleasant route, crossing two intermittent tributaries lined with live oaks and sycamores before coming to the willow- and sycamore-lined **Cozy Dell Creek (2 miles, 1,390', 291552E 3817135N)** and moments thereafter the **junction (2 miles, 1,410', 291551E 3817101N)** with the Cozy Dell service road (Forest Route 5N34).

The meeting of the road and trail is technically the end of the Cozy Dell Trail, but you have numerous options from here if you wish to make a longer trip of it. From the junction, it's an easy 0.1 mile north along the service road to the western trailhead of the **Foothill Trail (2.1 miles, 1,440', 291623E 3817103N)**. To connect with the trails in Stewart Canyon, continue along the road another mile under the shade of massive mature live oaks to a **junction (2.9 miles, 1,850', 292659E 3816987N)** with Forest Route 5N34 and a second service road. The lower portion of Stewart Canyon is laid out before you to the east.

Bear left (north) here and climb around a prominent knoll to the junction with the **Pratt/Stewart Canyon Trail (3.2 miles, 2,050', 292668E 3817300N)**; see *Route 56.*

Route 55

WHEELER GORGE NATURE TRAIL

LENGTH AND TYPE:	0.75-mile loop
RATING:	Easy
TRAIL CONDITION:	Clear
MAP(S):	USGS *Wheeler Springs*; Conant's *Matilija & Dick Smith Wilderness*; Harrison's *Sespe Wilderness*
CAMP(S):	—
HIGHLIGHTS:	Pleasant and very easy riparian and chaparral hike; excellent for children

TO REACH THE TRAILHEAD(S): Use the Wheeler Gorge Nature Trail turnoff to access this route.

TRIP SUMMARY: Built by the Youth Conservation Corps in 1979 and refurbished after the 1985 Wheeler Fire, this easy loop trail follows the alder-shaded North Fork of Matilija Creek for its first leg and then wraps around through scrub and chaparral on its return. This is a great hike for youngsters, and interpretive brochures for a self-guided hike are available for a small donation at the Ojai Ranger District office (weekdays) and the Wheeler Gorge Visitor Center (weekends). The brochures and signposts were redesigned and updated by a local Eagle Scout candidate in the summer of 2011.

Trip Description

From the **trailhead (1,920', 291538E 3821970N)** follow the trail down into the North Fork of Matilija Creek (the tributary on the left side of the highway is Cannon Creek). Almost immediately you'll be faced with poison oak along the base of a large oak and elsewhere along the trail, so do exercise caution. After passing beneath CA 33, you'll find the alders provide ample shade as you follow the path toward the single creek crossing. From this spot—popular with picnickers, rock-hopping children, and (unfortunately) careless litterers—cross the creek and follow the track to the right, joining the counterclockwise circuit (a spur comes in from your left from the overflow parking). This early stretch follows the North Fork of Matilija Creek (there is good access to a nice stretch of creek across from signpost No. 5).

Soon you'll begin to climb easily along the oak- and manzanita-shaded trail, eventually climbing to the **high point (0.4 mile, 2,060', 291749E 3822222N)** of the hike. Dry Lakes Ridge (see *Route 85*) is visible to the northeast. Turn left (westward) and descend easily through the arid, rocky trail through the chamises and woolly bluecurls. Your route leads back toward CA 33, turning left (south) just above the highway.

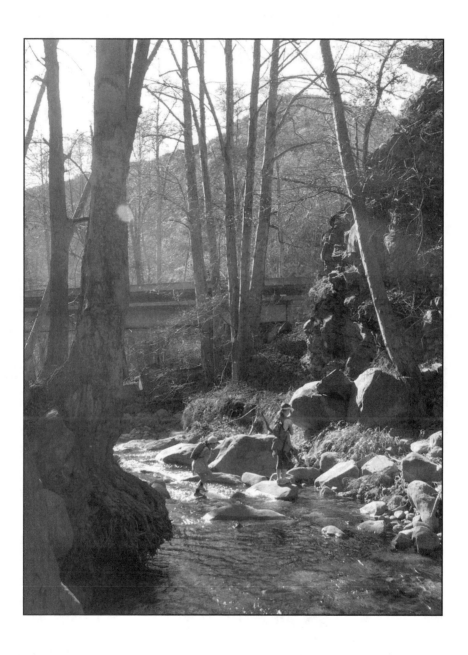

Continuing above the road, note the large live oak on your right. The hollowed trunk is especially popular with young hikers. Another hundred yards and you'll again make a left to return to the creek crossing (or cut right to the overflow parking area).

WHEELER GORGE NATURE TRAIL MARKERS ▪ ▪ ▪ ▪ ▪

1 *BEWARE OF POISON OAK!*

2 WHITE ALDER

3 LAUREL SUMAC

4 YERBA SANTA

5 COAST LIVE OAK

6 HOLLYLEAF CHERRY AND WILD CUCUMBER

7 ARROYO WILLOW

8 SYCAMORE AND BLACKBERRY

9 TRANSITIONAL OAK WOODLAND

10 BLACK SAGE

11 CHAMISE

12 TOYON

13 WESTERN MOUNTAIN MAHOGANY

14 SCRUB OAK

15 FLOWERING ASH

See the self-guided tour brochure for additional details.

▪ ▪ ▪ ▪ ▪ ▪ ▪ ▪ ▪ ▪ ▪ ▪ ▪ ▪ ▪ ▪ ▪ ▪ ▪

Route 56

STEWART CANYON via Pratt Trail (23W09)

LENGTH AND TYPE:	7-mile out-and-back to Valley View Camp; 9.6-mile out-and-back to Nordhoff Ridge Road; 11.6-mile out-and-back to Nordhoff tower
RATING:	Strenuous
TRAIL CONDITION:	Clear
MAP(S):	USGS *Matilija* and *Ojai*; Conant's *Matilija & Dick Smith Wilderness*; Harrison's *Sespe Wilderness*
CAMP(S):	Valley View
HIGHLIGHTS:	Excellent views of the Ojai Valley and beyond; lush Valley View Campground

TO REACH THE TRAILHEAD(S): Use the Stewart Canyon Debris Basin Trailhead to access this route.

TRIP SUMMARY: From the Stewart Canyon Debris Basin, this steep route climbs 3,000 feet along Stewart Canyon through chaparral and scrub forest to Nordhoff Ridge Road (with the

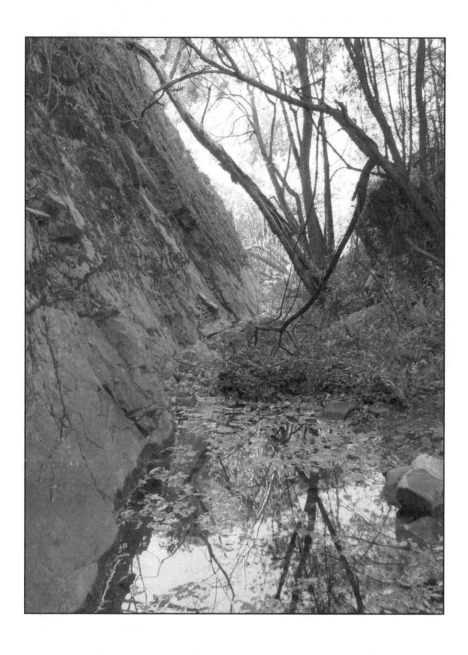

option to continue to the Nordhoff Peak). Spectacular 360-degree views and several other route options can be had from the ridgeline.

SIDE TRIP: VALLEY VIEW SPUR ▪ ▪ ▪ ▪ ▪ ▪ ▪ ▪ ▪ ▪

The easy 0.2-mile drop into Valley View makes for an ideal lunch or picnic spot; water is easily accessible here beneath the cool shade of bays and big-leaf maples. The creek runs along the base of the slab you admired from the junction before dropping precipitously toward your starting point.

▪ ▪

Trip Description

From the Pratt Trail **parking area** (**960', 293338E 3815506N**), the trail begins outside of the forest boundary in the southwest corner of the parking area, near some US Forest Service signage and information panels.

Follow the well-marked trail along several stretches of public access through private property along the lower stretches of Stewart Creek; please respect the property owners and stay to the trail. Several nonnative trees (Peruvian pepper, crape myrtle, and various eucalypti) line your route. Twice the route crosses residential portions of Foothill Road before reaching an **information sign and gate** just inside the forest boundary (**1 mile, 1,130', 293088E 3816522N**). Continue past the gate and follow the dirt road up the canyon, passing a water tank and signage indicating the Foothill Trail. Mature sycamores and live oaks border the road much of the way. Stay left when your route joins **Fuel Break Road** (**1.3 miles, 1,625', 293060E 3816977N**) and continue up the road as it winds higher along the canyon and then cuts westward away from Stewart Canyon, finally reaching a saddle and **turnoff** onto the singletrack (**2 miles, 2,050', 292668E 3817300N**).

The singletrack will lead you steadily up along a well-worn trail dominated by ceanothus and scrub oak, rounding a knoll and continuing to drift westward away from the canyon. Upon reaching the ridge dividing Stewart Canyon and Cozy Dell Canyon to the west, the trail realigns northward and you'll continue climbing by way of numerous switchbacks; much of the ascent here is lined with bigberry manzanitas, and the trail is quite rocky in spots. Enjoy the vistas of the Ojai Valley, which come into view quickly as the trail begins to bend back toward the east. After a gain of 1,000 vertical feet in just over a mile, your route rejoins the main Stewart Creek drainage, and after a quick realignment northward you'll find yourself at the junction with the **spur trail** leading down to Valley View Camp (**3.3 miles, 3,000', 293092E 3818311N**). The dramatic uplift caused by the Santa

Ynez Fault in this area is especially apparent standing at this junction and looking eastward across the chasm. The massive slab of sandstone from which Stewart Creek begins its steep descent sits at a 70-degree angle, so steep it's largely bare of the heavy chaparral of its neighboring hillsides.

CAMP :: VALLEY VIEW

ELEVATION:	2,820'
MAP:	USGS *Matilija*
UTM:	293209E 3818336N

A secluded camp set beneath a single live oak and numerous bay trees, Valley View is a relatively recent addition to the Los Padres, installed after the Wheeler Fire. Valley View is actually a bit of a misnomer, as little is visible through the thick canopy of bays, oaks, and big-leaf maples, and the massive sandstone slab that constitutes the southern edge of the creek here blocks any view. The creek beside camp is a lovely water-carved affair of large boulders and stone creek bottom.

You can enjoy the namesake view of the Ojai Valley from either the trail junction along the Pratt Trail or at a clear spot of trail a hundred yards before camp (just as rows of aromatic bay trees form a tunnel along the final approach to the site).

There is one stove here and one ideal flat for a tent just north of the kitchen. But poison oak is also present—between the kitchen and the lower creek access—so it's best to access the creek along the trail just upstream.

From the junction with the Valley View spur trail, the Pratt Trail continues to lead you up-canyon, eschewing switchbacks altogether for much of the climb and steadily gaining another 1,000 feet in another 1.5 miles along varied ridgelines until reaching the junction with **Nordhoff Ridge Road** (**4.7 miles, 3,980', 293147E 3819636N**).

Views from atop the road are excellent; you have the option to continue right (east) and hike the road another 0.9 mile to the junction with the **turnoff** to the fire lookout (**5.6 miles, 4,400', 294139E 3819598N**).

Continue to your left (northward) and follow the approach road as it wraps around the base of **Nordhoff Peak** (**5.8 miles, 4,850', 294144 3819683**) to deposit you at a beautiful vista, directly beneath the fire lookout. Ascend the lookout's narrow and steep concrete-and-steel staircase for fantastic surrounding views. Stretched out before you southward are the Channel Islands (on a clear day one can easily identify a minimum of six of the eight islands, including all those that comprise Channel Islands National Park), Lake Casitas, and many other features. To the north are views of Pine Mountain, Dry Lakes Ridge, and the western expanse of the Sespe Wilderness. Several of the prominent Ventura County peaks can be identified from this vantage point as well, most notably Chief Peak (the highest point along Nordhoff Ridge) to the east.

While neither facilities nor water are available here, a sturdy picnic table and fire ring are set beneath the tower.

You have several options for descending from here; the most practical (unless you've arranged a shuttle) is to return the way you came. With some planning, a descent along Gridley Canyon is viable, the trailhead being only a mile east along the road (see *Route 57*).

Route 57

GRIDLEY CANYON (22W05) and NORDHOFF PEAK (5N08)

LENGTH AND TYPE:	5.4-mile out-and-back to Gridley Spring; 14.2-mile out-and-back to Nordhoff Peak
RATING:	Moderate to Gridley Spring; strenuous to Nordhoff Peak
TRAIL CONDITION:	Clear (popular trail) and well maintained (service road)
MAP(S):	USGS *Ojai* and *Lion Canyon*; Conant's *Matilija & Dick Smith Wilderness*; Harrison's *Sespe Wilderness*
CAMP(S):	Gridley Spring
HIGHLIGHTS:	360-degree views, including Ojai Valley, Oxnard Plain, Rose Valley, Pine Mountain, Lake Casitas, and Channel Islands

TO REACH THE TRAILHEAD(S): Use the Gridley Road Trailhead to access this route.

TRIP SUMMARY: From the end of Gridley Road, this steady but pleasant climb—considered the most popular route for accessing Nordhoff Ridge—bisects a privately held avocado orchard via a public-access trail and service road and then climbs along the western slopes of Gridley Canyon to the old Gridley Spring Camp. Mountain bikes are common along this route.

Trip Description

From the signed **trailhead (1,160', 295756E 3816407N)**, walk along the ravine northward for approximately 0.5 mile until you reach the **junction (0.4 mile, 1,420', 295786E 3816965N)** with a dirt road. Note this portion of the hike passes through private property; do be respectful of the owners and stay to the trail. (The US Forest Service [USFS] has placed numerous trail markers to ensure you can keep your way.) Your route will continue northeast along a branch of the road, passing through the ranch until a **five-way intersection (1 mile, 1,640', 296189E 3817313N)** of dirt roads and trails; take the marked route at your 10 o'clock and continue past the upper stretches of the avocado orchard.

Soon your route departs from the agricultural endeavors and cuts northeast through high chaparral along what was years ago the old Gridley Canyon service road; your ascent is punctuated by the surprisingly audible sounds of Gridley Creek rushing far below. The trail here winds along steep slopes made easier due to being along the old road grade; cast a glance upward and through the chaparral and scrub downslope and you'll realize how steep the hillside truly is.

After climbing for nearly 2 miles, the trail turns west by northwest to provide an **expansive view** of Gridley Canyon and its tributaries below (**1.8 miles, 2,250', 296659E 3818352N**). Big-leaf maples begin to dot the hillside, and after a quick turn toward the southwest, the lush, north-facing slopes feature western brackens and other ferns and numerous big-leaf maples thriving in the moist and shaded shelter of the geologically jumbled hillsides.

At the crux of this canyon is your destination; you'll likely spot the horse trough fed by **Gridley Spring** (**2.7 miles, 2,480', 295858E 3818673N**) before you happen upon the spring itself. The old camp is just across the draw, along the hairpin of the trail.

CAMP :: GRIDLEY SPRING

ELEVATION:	2,480'
MAP:	USGS *Matilija*
UTM:	295858E 3818673N

Following the 1985 Wheeler Fire, rains washed out a once viable campsite (with a second stove and tables) and left behind what is now best used as a rest spot for the frequent hikers, mountain bikers, and equestrians. Though there is still an iron-pipe hitching rack and a stove, this camp's usable space is so limited that it prevents more than perhaps a pair of sleeping bags. That said, Gridley Spring (also labeled "Gridley" or most often "Gridley Springs" on earlier USFS and USGS maps) typically remains quite cool and comfortable and makes a good spot for lunch.

If Gridley Spring was your destination, return the way you came when you're ready. If you're pushing through to Nordhoff Peak, continue to follow the trail as it narrows and enters thick chaparral; in spots your route effectively tunnels through 12-foot-high scrub. The climb between the spring and Gridley Saddle ascends nearly 1,500 feet in 3 miles, and while you climb, occasional glimpses of the Nordhoff fire lookout can be had whenever the switchbacks lead in a northwesterly direction. Your route crosses a few spring-fed gullies (bay trees cluster along these points), which is often the last water along this stretch.

A last set of switchbacks cuts east around a final ridgeline to keep you in the Gridley watershed proper; along the ridge you'll spot the trail sign along Nordhoff Ridge Road. Only a hundred yards from the road, you'll cross a seasonal tributary over which stands a fire-blackened and windbeaten trio of bigcone Douglas-firs, hardy survivors of the 1985 Wheeler Fire. The **Gridley Saddle (5.8 miles, 3,800', 294921E 3820479N)** lies just beyond. Views down the north slope here are into Bear Creek, Rose Valley, and across CA 33 to the Dry Lakes Ridge.

From the saddle, proceed left (west) 1 mile along Nordhoff Ridge Road (FS Road 5N08) along the steep switchbacks to the **turnoff** to the fire lookout **(6.9 miles, 4,400', 294139E 3819598N)**. Continue to your right (northward) and follow the approach road as it wraps around the base of **Nordhoff Peak (7.1 miles, 4,850', 294144E 3819683N)** to deposit you at a beautiful vista directly beneath the fire lookout. The lookout's original wooden cab was destroyed in the 1948 Wheeler Fire. Its replacement burned in the 1970s; now only the steel frame remains.

Ascend the lookout's narrow and steep concrete-and-steel staircase for fantastic surrounding views. Stretched out before you southward are the Channel Islands (on a clear day one can easily identify a minimum of six of the eight islands, including all those that comprise Channel Islands National Park), Lake Casitas, and many other features. To the north are views of Pine Mountain, Dry Lakes Ridge, and the western expanse of the Sespe Wilderness. Several of the prominent Ventura County peaks can be identified from this vantage point as well, most notably Chief Peak (the highest point along Nordhoff Ridge) and Hines Peak, both to the east. A P-51 Mustang crashed into the mountain here in 1944, but most evidence of the crash has long since been recovered (or pilfered), and what remains is extremely difficult to reach.

While neither facilities nor water are available here, a sturdy picnic table and fire ring are set beneath the tower.

You have several options for descending from Nordhoff Ridge; the most practical (unless you've arranged a shuttle) is to return the way you came. But with some organization, a descent along Stewart Canyon via the Pratt Trail is viable (see *Route 56*); the trailhead is only a mile west along Nordhoff Ridge Road. The road can also be accessed by other routes, notably the Howard Creek Trail coming out of Rose Valley (see *Route 65*).

Route 58

CHIEF PEAK

LENGTH AND TYPE:	8.6-mile out-and-back from Rose Valley Campground to peak
RATING:	Strenuous
TRAIL CONDITION:	Well maintained (service road) to passable (unofficial route)
MAP(S):	USGS *Lion Canyon*; Harrison's *Sespe Wilderness*
CAMP(S):	—
HIGHLIGHTS:	Great 360-degree views from Pine Mountain to the Pacific

TO REACH THE TRAILHEAD(S): Use Rose Valley Campground to access this route.

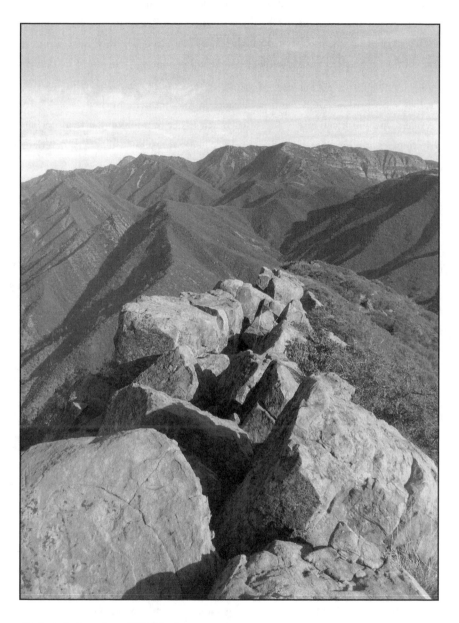

Eastward views from Chief Peak

TRIP SUMMARY: From Rose Valley Campground, this fairly strenuous ascent follows a dirt road through low chaparral for most of the route, but with some rock scrambling at the very end to one of the highest points in the Ojai frontcountry. Recreational 4WD vehicles and ATVs are allowed on this road, but through a fairly restrictive permit system administered by the US Forest Service. You're unlikely to encounter many—if any—off-roaders except on holiday weekends. The road is closed to vehicular use altogether during the rainy season (typically October–May). Bugs can be a nuisance in the summer months.

Note: Chief Peak can also be accessed much easier by obtaining a road permit and only hiking/scrambling the last 0.5 mile described below, but this entry describes the "traditional" route.

Trip Description

From the **road gate (3,420', 299610E 3823311N)** at the west end of the campground, follow Nordhoff Ridge Road. The road, now a dedicated 4WD and service route popular with mountain bikers, climbs steadily westward to a **bend (1.3 miles, 4,290', 298262E 3823102N)**, which affords you a view of Rancho Grande below and much of the surrounding environs. Here the road curves southward and gets steeper, and the soil composition—previously sandstone and graded rock—turns to marine sedimentary shale for a time. Bigcone Douglas-firs and an occasional white fir begin to mix with the scrub and oaks.

This, your steepest portion, soon joins with **Nordhoff Ridge Road (2.1 miles, 5,000', 298335E 3821925N)**; continue to your left (east) along the road. Views of the Ojai Valley and the Pacific are fantastic. The Nordhoff Fire Lookout can just be made out westward along the ridge (see *Route 57*), and Chief Peak and the Topatopa Mountains loom eastward. Follow the service road another 1.5 miles (passing a small spring-fed pond on your left) until you reach the **firebreak (3.7 miles, 5,140', 300529E 3821346N)**, which descends from the lower Chief Peak ridge to meet the road here along Chief Peak's northwestern flank.

Part from the road here and follow the firebreak up the slope, first southward and then curving eastward to the **lower ridge (4.1 miles, 5,450', 300767E 3821051N)**. From this point you'll drop into a saddle where the firebreak ends and then follow a thin but fairly clear trail through the rocky landscape. There are two approaches, both of which require a bit of scrambling, but the most practical skirts Chief Peak's western and southwestern exposure, climbing through the sparsely vegetated rock to the ridgeline and very small flat atop **Chief Peak (4.3 miles, 5,565', 300990E 3820901N)**. Enjoy impressive views of the eastern mountains; the east fork of Lion Canyon to the northeast; and Rose Valley, Pine Mountain, and all points west.

Once you've had time enough to soak up the 360-degree view, return the way you came.

Route 59

HORN CANYON (22W08)

LENGTH AND TYPE:	2.2-mile out-and-back to last and largest stream crossing; 5.2-mile out-and-back to The Pines; 9.8-mile out-and-back to Nordhoff Ridge Road
RATING:	Easy to last crossing; moderately strenuous to The Pines campground and Nordhoff Ridge Road
TRAIL CONDITION:	Clear
MAP(S):	USGS *Ojai*; Harrison's *Sespe Wilderness*
CAMP(S):	The Pines
HIGHLIGHTS:	Views of Ojai Valley; riparian trekking along lower stretch

TO REACH THE TRAILHEAD(S): Use the Horn Canyon Trailhead to access this route.

TRIP SUMMARY: From the Thacher School grounds, this popular hike follows the lush Horn Creek before leaving the watershed and climbing to The Pines, a campsite set beneath a grove of Coulter pines. Beyond camp, the route continues to Sisar and Nordhoff Ridge Roads. Due to its accessibility, the lower portion of the trail is very popular and can be almost crowded on weekends.

Trip Description

From the Thacher School **parking area (1,450', 299919E 3815677N)**, follow the wide service road northeast along the edge of the school grounds. After the first **stream crossing (0.4 mile, 1,640', 300389E 3816144N)**, alders begin to shade portions of the route. Springtime brings a bevy of wildflowers here, but all seasons bring poison oak along stretches of the lower canyon, so do exercise caution (especially when passing other hikers or stepping aside for any horses). Cross the creek twice more over the course of 0.75 mile until the **final crossing (1.1 miles, 2,000', 300758E 3817061N)**. This lush and spacious area beneath the alders is a popular turnaround spot for day hikers and ideal for a lunch or water break. This is also the last spot where water is easily accessible along the trail.

From this crossing, follow the trail eastward toward a fairly steep section of switchbacks that will lead you out of the drainage of Horn Creek's east fork and toward **The Pines (2.6 miles, 3,250', 301657E 3817920N)**.

CAMP :: THE PINES

ELEVATION:	3,250'
MAP:	USGS *Ojai*
UTM:	301657E 3817920N

A lovely and rather unexpected site, the camp is set on a flat high above the Horn Canyon drainage on Chief Peak's southern flanks on a stretch (geologically speaking) of sandstone and shale landslide debris. The Pines is a spacious site appointed with hitching rails, a trough, and ample space.

Legendary ranger Jacinto Reyes planted the namesake Coulter pines here as part of an experimental pine plantation at the turn of the century. The Pines was consumed by the 1932 Matilija Fire and damaged again during the 1948 Wheeler Fire. Since that time students of the nearby Thacher School have tended to and helped replant the site. It remains a popular day-trip destination, not only among Thacher students (or prospective students and their families) but also for many locals.

The site possesses two kitchens, one seldom used and more suitable for overflow; the main kitchen and stove is situated in the middle of the flat. In early 2011 a nice set of chainsaw-hewn benches were built here by firefighters removing a problem Coulter pine. Water is available about a hundred yards north of camp and down a fairly steep ravine if the troughed spring in the northwest corner of the camp is dry. The creek there is effectively the last water on the trail.

From The Pines, the trail continues climbing, now through "hard" chaparral in an area typically well maintained by the horse packers from Thacher School. This is the steepest part of the ascent, and switchbacks are for the most part mercilessly absent—you'll find yourself climbing some long, steep stretches of straight, rock-strewn trail. Be sure to enjoy the scenery and fantastic views of the Ojai Valley from this vantage point. When you come upon **Sisar Road (4.1 miles, 4,700', 303000E 3819056N)**, cross the road and continue to the trail connector to the right (east). Continue another 0.75 mile along a much less steep section of switchbacks to the junction with **Nordhoff Ridge Road (4.9 miles, 5,270', 303384E 3819108N)**.

Now along Nordhoff Ridge, the Lion Canyon Trail is 0.8 mile to your east (see *Route 87*), and the lower portion of the Red Reef/Sisar Trail is 1.3 miles to the east. Chief Peak and numerous features are accessible to the west.

Route 60

SISAR CANYON (Southern Red Reef Trail [21W08])

LENGTH AND TYPE:	16.8-mile loop (lollipop)
RATING:	Strenuous
TRAIL CONDITION:	Well maintained (service road) and clear
MAP(S):	USGS *Ojai*, *Santa Paula Peak*, and *Topatopa Mountains*; Harrison's *Sespe Wilderness*

CAMP(S):	White Ledge
HIGHLIGHTS:	Clear service-road hiking; fantastic views atop Nordhoff Ridge

TO REACH THE TRAILHEAD(S): Use the Sisar Canyon Trailhead to access this route.

TRIP SUMMARY: This strenuous but easily navigated loop (also extremely popular with mountain bikers) climbs nearly 10 miles along Sisar Canyon Road to the Topatopa/ Nordhoff Ridge service road (an ascent with an elevation gain of nearly 3,500 feet). It then climbs eastward before dropping back into Sisar Canyon proper along the lower stretch of the Red Reef Trail (21W08) to eventually reconnect with the lower portion of Sisar Canyon Road. Be mindful of the aforementioned mountain bikers—as well as horses— along this route.

Trip Description

From the **parking area (1,800', 303946E 3814072N)**, proceed north along the road, using the pedestrian/horse access on the right (creek) side of the gate. Oaks and white alders provide ample shade along the road, but poison oak is also present, so mind the roadsides and any young hikers. Your **first crossing (1,850', 303899E 3814193N)** of Sisar Creek is usually an easy affair but can result in wet feet after rains.

Sisar Road

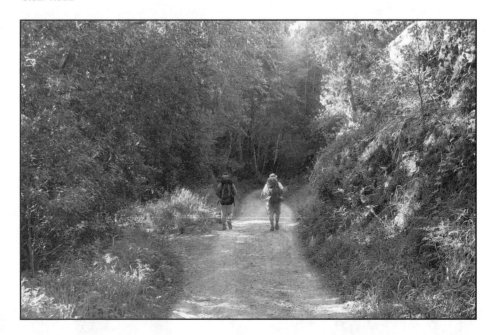

Continue climbing moderately now along the east banks of Sisar Creek; sycamores, California bays, and ferns sink their roots into the lush and moist cuts along the road and along the creek proper. Numerous cascades and pools make this stretch popular with waders and day-trippers; warm weekends especially can attract numerous visitors. Continue along this pleasant stretch another mile to the **second crossing (1.1 miles, 2,270', 304309E 3815478N)**, and your ascent begins to steepen slightly as you continue following the creek up-canyon. When you reach the **fork (1.5 miles, 2,540', 304681E 3815816N)**, stay left (the road to the right is a private easement).

Soon you'll reach a **hairpin turn (1.9 miles, 2,655', 304951E 3816254N)**, where the road leaves the creek and cuts left (west) away from the drainage. From here the route is much more exposed, as you'll be leaving the cover of the riparian habitat that makes Sisar Canyon so pleasant and find yourself hiking higher above the watershed. The road climbs in a generally northwest direction, zigzagging up the mountain. Many of the south-facing bends provide spectacular views of the Ojai Valley, Sulphur Mountain, and the Oxnard Plain and Channel Islands beyond. Views of the Topatopa Mountains to the northeast are consistently impressive.

Soon manzanitas join the rest of the exposed chaparral through which the road leads, and after 1.5 miles of climbing you'll reach a **gate (3.3 miles, 3,310', 304860E 3817310N)** at another hairpin in the road. This is where the trail from White Ledge joins the road (and where you'll be exiting the trail near the end of this loop).

Continue climbing along the road as it leaves the Sisar drainage for that of Wilsie Canyon to the west. Scattered **rock formations (5.6 miles, 4,125', 303462E 3817439N)** skirt the road near an old fire-road junction, and the road continues its snaking climb toward Nordhoff Ridge Road. Here the grade becomes slightly more forgiving, as by this point you've made a large portion of the elevation gain. The road passes beneath Wilsie Spring shortly afterward, and then you'll note the first intersection with the **Horn Canyon Trail (7.1 miles, 4,700', 303000E 3819056N;** see *Route 59*). Less than a mile up the road from here is the junction with **Nordhoff Ridge Road (7.9 miles, 4,900', 302158E 3819762N)**.

Turn right (east) onto Nordhoff Ridge Road and continue along the ridgetop, passing the **Horn Canyon Trailhead (9.1 miles, 5,270', 303384E 3819108N)** on your right (south), and then descend easily toward the **Lion Canyon Trailhead (9.9 miles, 5,140', 304517E 3819606N;** see *Route 87*) on your left (north) until you reach the junction for the lower portion of the **Red Reef Trail (10.4 miles, 5,230', 305145E 3815117N)** on your right (south).

Here the trail follows classic sunbaked chaparral along the descent into Sisar Canyon, popular with local mountain bikers, before dropping into the riparian environs of Sisar Creek and **White Ledge Camp (12.2 miles, 3,880', 304945E 3818139N)**.

CAMP :: WHITE LEDGE

ELEVATION:	3,880'
MAP:	USGS *Santa Paula Peak*
UTM:	304945E 3818139N

Not to be confused with the camp of the same name in the Santa Lucia Ranger District's portion of the San Rafael Wilderness (Santa Barbara County), White Ledge Camp is a very pleasant site shaded under heavy cover of primarily bay trees. White Ledge is situated at the crux between Sisar Creek and a spring that runs in all but the driest of months. There are three stoves at the site, and the main (center) kitchen has a spacious fire area and makes good use of the site's rocks. Sycamores and live oaks line this site's periphery. White Ledge is a frequent water or lunch spot for mountain bikers and hikers both.

From White Ledge Camp, the trail crosses the spring on the western edge of camp and then descends easily through lush chaparral and riparian terrain, meeting with the creek after a ways. Follow the singletrack southward until reaching the **road** (**13.6 miles, 3,300', 304862E 3817310N**) and the terminus of the Red Reef Trail. Continue now along the road you followed earlier, descending 3 miles to the **parking area** (**16.8 miles, 1,800', 303946E 3814072N**) at the start of Sisar Canyon Road.

Route 61

HINES PEAK

LENGTH AND TYPE:	0.9-mile out-and-back from Timber/Santa Paula Canyon Saddle; 6.7-mile out-and-back from end of Nordhoff Ridge Road via Red Reef; 20.7-mile out-and-back from Sisar Canyon Trailhead via Red Reef
RATING:	Strenuous (climb)
TRAIL CONDITION:	Passable (not a maintained route)
MAP(S):	USGS *Topatopa Mountains*; Harrison's *Sespe Wilderness* (final ascent not on map)
CAMP(S):	—
HIGHLIGHTS:	Relatively short Class 2 approach to the highest point of the Topatopa range with excellent 360-degree views from Mt Pinos to the Pacific; condor sightings possible

TO REACH THE TRAILHEAD(S): This route is accessed along the Red Reef Trail (21W08).

TRIP SUMMARY: From the saddle between the Timber Creek and Santa Paula drainages, this route follows a rough use trail to the summit of Hines Peak.

Trip Description

To start, follow the Red Reef Trail (*Route 88*) to the **saddle (6,020', 309046E 3820460N)** between Timber and Santa Paula Creeks. Approach the peak from the northwest.

From the saddle, climb along the thin use trail southeastward up the shale-and-talus edge, punctuated only by the occasional gnarled tree, until reaching the slightly more-stable rock of the peak's northern flank. The going here can be slow, with loose rock and scree. Keep your hands free, as numerous sections are steep enough to warrant scrambling on all fours.

Follow the route upward (it is often marked by cairns) to a **gap (0.35 mile from saddle, 6,565', 309327E 3820803N)** on the western edge of the peak. Head left (east) here for another 0.1 mile through the burn area to the benchmark and trail register atop **Hines Peak (0.45 mile, 6,704', 309466E 3820751N)**.

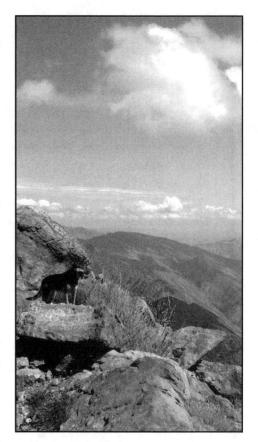

Farther eastward along the ridge, one can catch glimpses of the old Topatopa Peak Trail that skirted the southern flanks of the Hines long ago and led some 6 miles eastward to Topatopa Peak and the fire lookout tower that once stood there. The route fell into disuse when Topatopa Peak was included in the Sespe Condor Sanctuary as part of the sanctuary's 1954 expansion.

Route 62

LAST CHANCE TRAIL (21W09), SANTA PAULA CANYON, and TOPATOPA BLUFF

LENGTH AND TYPE:	7-mile out-and-back to Big Cone Camp; 3.6-mile one-way to East Fork junction; 7.4-mile out-and-back to Graffiti Falls; 11.8-mile out-and-back to Jackson Hole Camp; 6.1-mile one-way to Jackson Falls; 17-mile out-and-back to Last Chance Camp; 10.5-mile one-way to Last Chance Connector junction; 12.7-mile one-way to Topatopa Bluff; 13.5-mile one-way to Nordhoff Ridge Road

RATING:	Moderate to Big Cone; strenuous to Nordhoff Ridge Road
TRAIL CONDITION:	Well maintained (former service road) to passable (washed-out route requiring rock-hopping and scrambling)
MAP(S):	USGS *Santa Paula Peak* and *Topatopa Mountains*; Harrison's *Sespe Wilderness*
CAMP(S):	Big Cone, Cross, Jackson Hole, Last Chance, and Topatopa Lodge (abandoned)
HIGHLIGHTS:	Riparian trekking; some of the best swimming holes in Ventura County; conifer stands; unique geology

TO REACH THE TRAILHEAD(S): Use the Santa Paula Canyon (Thomas Aquinas/Ferndale) Trailhead to access this route as described south to north; use the Topatopa Bluff Trailhead for the upper terminus.

TRIP SUMMARY: This route ascends Santa Paula Canyon from the trailhead near Thomas Aquinas College, past the East Fork, and along the Last Chance (main) fork through riparian, oak woodland, and conifer-clad scenery and some extremely popular cliff-jumping and swimming spots. The lower stretch is by far the most heavily traveled in the Ojai Ranger District but is seldom followed all the way to its true northern terminus along the western edge of Topatopa Bluff. Litter and graffiti can be a problem along the lower trail, despite the efforts of local volunteers.

Trip Description

From the **parking area (975', 307824E 3811547N)**, walk east along the shoulder of CA 150 to the entrance of the Thomas Aquinas College grounds. Follow the well-marked road around the eastern edge of the college grounds for about a mile (respect the college's property and stay on the road) and through the Ferndale and Rancho Recuerdo properties, following signage throughout until the sealed road ends just before a pair of fenced-off **pump jacks (1.2 miles, 1,100', 308556E 3812697N)**. (Dogs must stay leashed through these stretches of privately held property.) Circumnavigate this fenced-off area on the creek side, and thereafter the old road (formerly 4N03) will lead you along the left (south) banks of Santa Paula Creek (the other side of the creek here is privately held).

Floods in 2005 scoured much of this stretch of the canyon, and portions of the trail were lost to the torrents. As a result, a bit of route-finding and rock-hopping is involved at points, but overall if you simply head up-canyon, you'll be fine. The US Forest Service has done a competent job of remarking the route as it currently stands, with a handful of Carsonite signs indicating the prescribed route.

You'll hike in both cobble-strewn creek bed and oak- and alder-shaded glens, where there is also a fair amount of poison oak (so be diligent in your route-finding, especially in

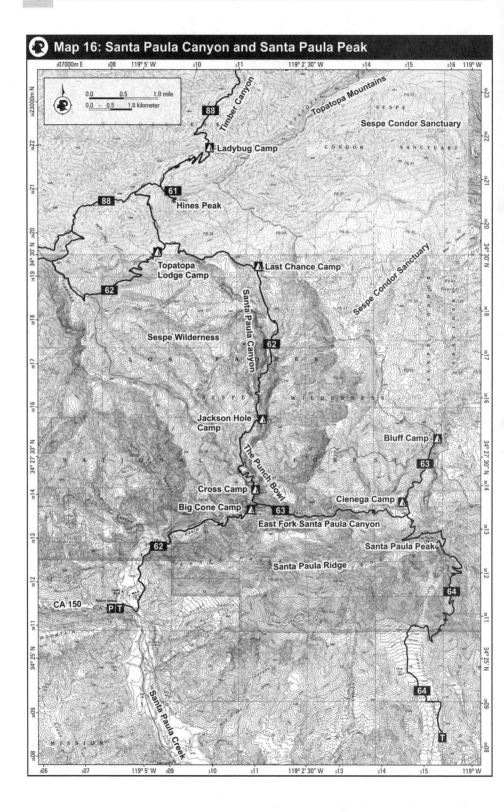

Map 16: Santa Paula Canyon and Santa Paula Peak

Timber Canyon

Topatopa Mountains

SESPE

Sespe Condor Sanctuary

88

Ladybug Camp

CONDOR   SANCTUARY

61

Hines Peak

88

Topatopa
Lodge Camp

Last Chance Camp

Sespe Condor Sanctuary

62

Sespe Wilderness

Santa Paula Canyon

LOS   PADRES

62

SESPE   WILDERNESS

Jackson Hole
Camp

Bluff Camp

The Punch Bowl

63

Cross Camp

NATIONAL   FOREST

Cienega Camp

Big Cone Camp

63

East Fork Santa Paula Canyon

62

Santa Paula Peak

Santa Paula Ridge

64

CA 150   P T

64

Santa Paula Creek

T

MISSION

the late fall and winter when much of the poison oak will be denuded and more difficult to identify). While you can make your own way of it, there are typically two main stream crossings (chosen at your discretion during the drier months, as numerous use trails will allow you progress upstream). The two waypoints most important are where the trail skirts the north bank of the creek to briefly follow a **spur trail (2.2 miles, 1,280', 309626E 3813226N)** to regain the old roadbed and—most important—where you gain the **roadbed** again (**2.7 miles, 1,390', 310298E 3813387N**) on the south side a short time after a second stream crossing. This is where many people lose their way and needlessly struggle up along the ravine.

Follow the roadbed steadily but not steeply up, gaining impressive views of the ravine below. Overall this stretch of the old road is in very good shape (with the exception of the washout that's rent a massive gouge in the route at one point along the high portion of the road) and will lead you along the east side of a knoll (Hill 1989). Just beyond is **Big Cone Camp (3.5 miles, 1,700', 311064E 3813717N)**.

CAMP :: BIG CONE

ELEVATION:	1,700'
MAP:	USGS *Santa Paula Peak*
UTM:	311064E 3813717N

Named for the *Pseudotsuga macrocarpa* (bigcone Douglas-fir) that join the oaks in shading this canyon, Big Cone is an old and well-worn site situated on a pleasant flat. Its beauty has been tarnished by graffiti on the large boulders strewn about camp. However, the general vandalism has diminished since the route became more difficult to access, but it still attracts its share of indifferent visitors, and litter can be a problem. A use trail toward the end of camp leads up to Hill 1989 and yields fantastic views of the canyon below; it's a popular spot for photographers to capture the best-known falls just north.

The site has space aplenty, four kitchens with varying combinations of fire pits and stoves, and water available in the creek below. Before the 2005 flood scoured much of lower Santa Paula Canyon and caused that massive cut along the upper portion of the old service road, this site was (physically) still accessible by 4WD.

From camp, follow the trail another few hundred yards down to the crossing of Santa Paula Creek's East Fork. This is another spot where many hikers seem to lose their way; be sure to cross the **East Fork (3.6 miles, 1,650', 311175E 3813787N)** here before following the trail back up and to the left (west) to the main canyon. Also just across the creek crossing is the fading junction with old East Fork Trail. This narrative describes the route continuing toward the waterfalls, the Punch Bowl, and other points along the main canyon; see *Route 63* for the route heading right (east).

Heading along the main fork again, you'll pass the best-known cascade (locally known as Graffiti Falls) along a fairly level route and then ascend a short series of switchbacks to reach **Cross Camp (4.1 miles, 1,800', 311111E 3814230N)**.

CAMP :: CROSS

ELEVATION:	1,800'
MAP:	USGS *Santa Paula Peak*
UTM:	311111E 3814230N

Named for the cross carved in a nearby rock, Cross Camp is a pleasant site with reliable water and shade, but its beauty is marred by graffiti (and often overrun by weekend revelers). It sees little overnight use by backpackers and is usually left to the party crowd. The famous slot swimming holes are nearby (often called the Punch Bowls, though the true Punch Bowls are up another ravine and less visited).

From Cross Camp, the **Punch Bowl formation (4.1 miles, 1,800')** is a few hundred yards across the flat upstream from camp and into the ravine where the creek and a tributary converge. This spot makes for fine photography when free of graffiti and becomes an eyesore when tagged by a rainbow of rattle cans. The more adventurous enjoy cliff-jumping from several nearby spots. Do exercise caution here—whether jumping or simply wading in—and treat the entire area as a fall zone.

From Cross Camp, the trail leads you northwest up a series of switchbacks. You'll gain some elevation on the Santa Paula Creek drainage and then level off with great views of the canyon below, following a fairly level cut for about a mile. Shortly you'll enter the riparian environs again just as you reach the junction with the spur trail leading to **Jackson Hole Camp (5.9 miles, 2,425', 311134E 3815400N)**. The camp is an easy walk down this spur trail.

CAMP :: JACKSON HOLE

ELEVATION:	2,425'
MAP:	USGS *Santa Paula Peak*
UTM:	311134E 3815400N

A shaded site beneath oak cover, Jackson Hole sees far less use than the canyon farther downstream. Another site—possibly the original forest camp—is east of the creek under a thick canopy of white alders. This upper camp is hemmed in by poison oak much of the year. *Note:* This camp is inexplicably shown along the steep canyon sides on the 1995 *Santa Paula Peak* quad; don't go looking for it there.

Another 0.25 mile up-trail from the Jackson Hole Camp junction, continue northward, soon coming upon lower Jackson Falls and then the namesake Jackson Hole. From the Jackson Hole formation, follow the trail easily alongside the creek for a stretch. The trail can be somewhat undefined for stretches here, but about 0.5 mile from camp the tread reappears quite clearly (though often overgrown) to begin the relentless ascent up a ridge rising above the creek's eastern banks. You'll lose sight of the creek rather quickly here but are still afforded excellent views of the bluffs and formations to your right (east). Hines Peak looms as you continue through open, rolling terrain to a **gap** (**8 miles, 4,325', 311536E 3818087N**) where you can enjoy a breather and then follow the trail along a more forgiving grade before it drops into the creek drainage and **Last Chance Camp** (**8.5 miles, 4,300', 311304E 3819182N**).

CAMP :: LAST CHANCE

ELEVATION:	4,300'
MAP:	USGS *Santa Paula Peak*
UTM:	311304E 3819182N

Set on a small flat between drainages and marked by boulders, Last Chance is a nearly forgotten site. Officially abandoned in the 1970s, it reappeared on maps and the collective forest radar in the late 1990s and early 2000s but still sees little use. An old ice can stove and rock fire ring are typically the only indicators of a kitchen. It can be a rather brushy site in late spring and summer.

Note: After the 2006 Day Fire, the trail bed along this section can feel nearly abandoned but remains fairly easily navigated. Without maintenance and/or regular use, it could disappear back into the growth within the next few years—or at least prove to be an exercise in bushwhacking.

From Last Chance Camp, the trail cuts west away from the creeks, up a draw, and then northward along the flank of Hines Peak to the **junction** (**10.5 miles, 5,175', 309077E 3819923N**) with the Last Chance Connector. The route heading up to your right (north) leads toward Hines Peak and the Sespe (via Timber Canyon). To exit the canyon here and gain the Red Reef Trail in just over a mile of fairly steep climbing, follow the old connector (see sidebar on page 259); otherwise, bear left (west) at this junction for the uppermost section of your route. This junction area—especially post–Day Fire—can be a bit tricky to navigate.

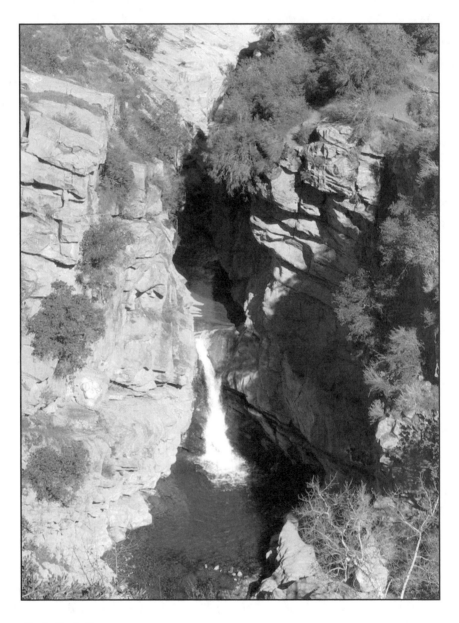

Santa Paula Canyon

LAST CHANCE CONNECTOR (21W20)

LENGTH AND TYPE:	1.2-mile one-way
RATING:	Easy southward; moderate northward (climb)
TRAIL CONDITION:	Passable
MAP(S):	USGS *Santa Paula Peak* and *Topatopa Mountains*; Harrison's *Sespe Wilderness*

This route—decades ago designated a connector to the Last Chance Trail but now considered by many to be the main approach from the north—drops southward between No-name and Hines Peaks to join the true upper 21W09. Further, note that the approach from Red Reef Trail differs from that depicted on the 1995 USGS *Topatopa Mountains* quad (primarily in the position of the trailhead coming off Red Reef and the curve of the route for the first 0.25 mile).

Now hiking the uppermost stretch of Last Chance Canyon, you'll quickly come into a willow-dotted **draw (10.7 miles, 5,100′, 308961E 3819868N)** that can typically be relied upon to have water even in the driest years (one of the main springs for this ravine is just up the canyon). From this crossing, continue through low, rolling alluvial hills and gullies laid bare by the Day Fire. In a rather incongruous spot of this open area stands the old **Topatopa Lodge Camp (10.8 miles, 5,035′, 308885E 3819611N)**.

CAMP :: TOPATOPA LODGE

ELEVATION:	5,035′
MAP:	USGS *Topatopa Mountains*
UTM:	308885E 3819611N

Officially abandoned in 1974, this largely forgotten site has been rediscovered by only a handful of backpackers and die-hard backcountry explorers after the 2006 Day Fire laid bare the brush that had consumed the site over the previous 30 years. Somewhat poorly positioned between the two main tributaries (it's not conveniently near either), it features a pair of large ice can stoves (but little else) and may have been chosen for its views both up- and down-canyon if used by hunters. There is room enough for really only one tent, but it still commands impressive views of Santa Paula Canyon and is a nice spot for a remote but relatively accessible camp.

Though the site only appeared intermittently on Los Padres visitor maps—that is, it wasn't on the 1967 or 1968 editions but did appear on the 1969 and 1972 editions, only to disappear again for later editions—it was a staple for Santa Paula– and Ojai-area trekkers for decades. The site was included in the USFS trail signage as early as the 1940s: U.S. Coast & Geodetic Survey records mention signage in their documenting of Hines Peak's monument indicating distances to "TOPA TOPA

LODGE" [sic] from both the junction ("2½ miles") and the junction with the Last Chance Trail just north of camp ("¼ mile").

It does not appear on any modern maps. And while not a magnificent site by any stretch, it's a fascinating and forgotten little corner of the Los Padres.

From the camp, continue westward through an often-dry draw and climb quickly out of this drainage and over another low rise to drop into the cool, often-overgrown crossing of **Santa Paula Creek (11.2 miles, 4,900', 308722E 3819389N)**. In years past, the trail followed a long series of well-cut switchbacks up the southern banks of the creek. As of this writing, however, the next section is still a bit of a pick-and-find, made a bit easier due to the flagging done by trail volunteers after the fire. This stretch of trail leading toward Topatopa Bluff is known locally as the Don Borad Memorial Trail, named for a tireless trail (and community) volunteer and mountaineer who passed away in 2008, but who had spent years clearing trail in the Ojai Ranger District.

After scrambling through ravines populated by the charred remnants of manzanitas and scrub, the tread slowly starts to reform, and eventually the old roadbed appears to lead you to the lower **Topatopa Bluff junction (12.6 miles, 6,270', 306418E 3819445N)**. Follow this track left (westward) to the **Topatopa Bluff vista (12.7 miles, 6,370', 305732E 3819582N)**. It's a somewhat steep but simple enough descent to **Nordhoff Ridge Road (13.5 miles, 5,460', 305739E 3819569N)** from here.

AT DAY'S END ▨ ▨ ▨ ▨ ▨ ▨ ▨ ▨ ▨ ▨ ▨ ▨ ▨ ▨

The Day Fire scorched huge sections of the southern Los Padres during its long march of destruction in September and October 2006. Roaring southward up the back side of the bluffs from the Sespe, the fire reached Topatopa Ridge, Tar Creek, and Bear Heaven on September 16—causing genuine concerns that the flames might reach the upper Ojai Valley—and stormed across Topatopa Peak, destroying the old fire lookout there. Though access had been prohibited for the general public for decades, as the peak was within the Sespe Condor Sanctuary, the site was still visited by some federal and state agencies and contained numerous historic records, now lost to the ages. The superstructure on which the cab sat is still visible from Sewart and Alamo Mountains, Tar Creek, Hines Peak, and other vantage points.

The Day Fire was finally extinguished almost a month later on October 13, 2006.

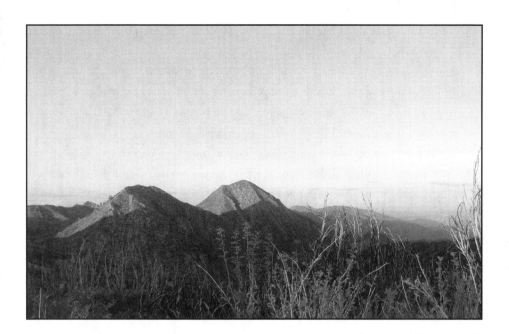

■ ■ ■ ■ ■ ■ ■ ■ ■ ■ SIDE TRIP: TOPATOPA BLUFF

LENGTH AND TYPE:	2.9-mile loop from Nordhoff Ridge Road
RATING:	Moderate plus strenuous climb (from Nordhoff Ridge Road); strenuous from Sisar Canyon
TRAIL CONDITION:	Clear from Nordhoff Ridge Road to the Bluffs lookout (trail receives regular use and care from volunteers); well maintained from lookout northeastward to junction with Red Reef and back (old service road)
MAP(S):	USGS *Topatopa Mountains* and *Santa Paula Peak*; Harrison's *Sespe Wilderness*
CAMP(S):	—
HIGHLIGHTS:	Panoramic views from vista point

TRIP SUMMARY: This route climbs from the end of Nordhoff Ridge Road to a fantastic vista above Topatopa Bluff, and then provides the option of an out-and-back or loop return.

Trip Description

This 2.9-mile loop begins at the very end of Nordhoff Ridge Road. *Note:* USGS topos show a different trail for the lower sections; in the years since the last updates and fires, the route has evolved considerably and the trailhead has relocated.

From the trailhead (**5,460', 305739E 3819569N**), follow the track up a series of increasingly steep switchbacks, first through chaparral and then rather directly following a zigzagging course of relaid trail along the dozer line cut during the 2006 Day Fire. Even from the start of your route, views along the ridge are excellent. Your progress becomes quite steep along the last section until you top out at the **vista** (**0.8 mile, 6,370', 305732E 3819582N**). A geocache/trail register is at the foot of the stone bench here, a fine place to rest your feet and enjoy a snack. Views of the Santa Barbara Channel, the Sespe, the very western edge of Topatopa Bluff, and nearly all points in a 360-degree arc are laid out before you (weather permitting).

If you have plans to hike the entire loop, note that the trail markers set southeast from the bench are those leading farther along the Bluff (first along an easy singletrack and then following an old service road) and not the loop as described here. If you explore the area above the Bluff, you will need to retrace your steps either the way you came or at least as far as the junction described below.

To make the loop, head northeast from the stone bench on an easy grade to meet the old **service road** (**1 mile, 6,325', 306604E 3819517N**). Follow the road to the left (northeast) with excellent views of No-name and Hines Peaks and the upper drainage of Santa Paula Canyon, switchbacking once until you reach the junction with the **Red Reef Trail** (**1.8 miles, 6,050', 306950E 3820198N**).

It's a fairly leisurely mile back to the trailhead (**2.9 miles, 5,460', 305739E 3819569N**).

Route 63

EAST FORK SANTA PAULA CANYON (21W11)

LENGTH AND TYPE:	7.2-mile out-and-back from East Fork junction to Cienega Camp; 9.6-mile out-and-back from East Fork junction to Bluff Camp
RATING:	Strenuous
TRAIL CONDITION:	Passable (abandoned trail) to challenging (some rock-hopping, Class 2 scrambling, and navigation necessary)
MAP(S):	USGS *Santa Paula Peak*
CAMP(S):	Cienega and Bluff
HIGHLIGHTS:	Route-finding and unique geology; dark forest; impressive sandstone formations

TO REACH THE TRAILHEAD(S): Use the Santa Paula Canyon (Thomas Aquinas/Ferndale) Trailhead to access this route.

TRIP SUMMARY: Trek through the fascinating geology and deep conifer forests of Santa Paula Canyon's upper east fork. Mileage begins at the route's departure from the main fork of Santa Paula Canyon, just beyond Big Cone Camp.

Trip Description

See *Route 62* for the first 3.6 miles of this route. *Note:* This route is not shown on Harrison's *Sespe Wilderness*. Further, what was in decades past a very nice route in this canyon had already fallen into a state of disuse when in 2005 a series of storms dropped enough rain in this canyon to cause massive flooding. Those storms redefined the canyon walls, obliterating much of the trail, and even rendering much of the topographic detail of the relevant maps inaccurate. This route should be approached as a cross-country rock-hop, as there is very little trail remaining. (And those portions that do remain often lead to sheer drop-offs where the floods have scoured portions of the canyon walls away, so it's often best to stick to the creek bed and resign oneself to relatively slow progress.)

From the crossing of the **East Fork** (**1,650', 311175E 3813787N**) just past Big Cone Camp, you can follow what's left of the old trail a short way, but progress will just as easily be made simply following the drainage eastward. At intervals you'll find pieces of old trail, but resist the temptation to follow one that loses sight of the creek, for you'll likely be forced to return the way you've come to regain the drainage. Bigcone Douglas-firs, big-leaf maples, ferns, oaks, and especially alders keep you company here, and it's those streamside alders through which you'll spend the most time clambering, pushing, and scrambling.

Sandstone formations above Bluff Camp

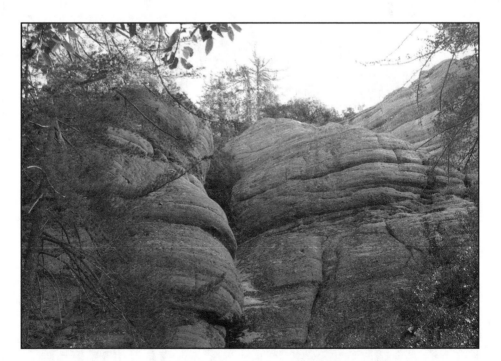

As you continue upstream (eastward), you'll note numerous channels down which debris (including boulders the size of delivery trucks) came crashing down during the 2005 storms. Many of those boulders you'll in turn be forced to navigate. After just more than 1.5 miles of progress the ravine will confine you to a short **narrows (1.7 miles from the junction upstream from Big Cone, 2,430', 313164E, 3813633N)** of upturned sedimentary layers. Here you can opt to navigate through or just around the first small cascade, but regardless you'll find yourself now in a unique stretch of white- and purple-striped siltstone, which when wet can be like walking through clay (or, as one hiker has likened it, plaster of Paris). Don't look to make overly fast progress through this section.

Atop this quagmire you'll find yourself in a rather pleasant **clearing (2.4 miles, 2,685', 313666E 3813593N)** shaded by mature trees. From here, you'll need to pick a line up the heavily wooded slope to your north, eschewing the rest of the drainage but also staying on the east bank of the drainage that has come in on your right (south). See Map 16 for additional edification. Upon the slope you'll eventually locate a portion of the old track where the **trail bed (2.6 miles, 2,850', 314036E 3813569N)** is still in fairly good repair, if a bit overgrown. Follow this route as it climbs out of the drainage eastward under heavy cover to the **junction (3.5 miles, 3,490', 314750E 3813499N)** with the Peak Trail (20W16). The terrain here—

Cienega Camp

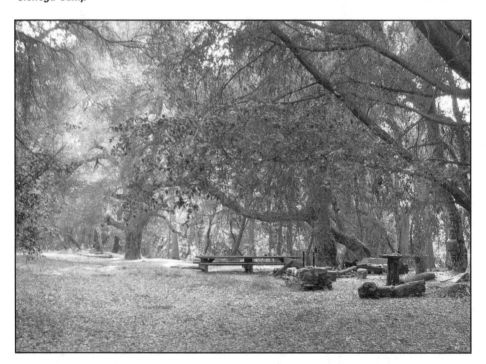

though covered well by decades of duff not singed since the Depression—is largely comprised of landslide deposits composed of broken and battered rock. Take the left (northeast) fork here and head north as you cross a number of small creeks through a lush, fern-lined stretch to reach **Cienega Camp (3.6 miles, 3,480', 314744E 3813710N)**. *Note:* The route from the junction and up to Bluff was once designated the Bluff Trail (21W10).

For the route to the right, which leads to Santa Paula Peak, see *Route 64*.

CAMP :: CIENEGA

ELEVATION:	3,480'
MAP:	USGS *Santa Paula Peak*
UTM:	314744E 3813710N

Spanish for "marsh," Cienega is named for the springy meadow nearby. This site is something of an unknown to many and doesn't tend to get the traffic such an attractive site might were it situated elsewhere. Dozens of mature oaks and a smattering of bays provide heavy shade along the flat here, and a bevy of camp accoutrements—a bona fide barbecue pit, large fire ring, 20-foot rough-hewn dining table, and other camp "furniture"—make this a very comfortable site, and one suitable for horse packers. A few springs and boulders nearby make for interesting side excursions.

You may note that unlike the terrain leading into camp, the soils in camp are a finer, often sandlike composition on the ground and with large boulders in the hills above. Most of this area is composed of the late-Eocene Cozy Dell shale and sandstone, which is what gives the soil its slightly red/purple hue. The sandstone higher up the canyon walls and toward Bluff Camp is composed of darker sandstone from the Sespe formation.

From Cienega, the trail continues briefly to the northwest under cover of trees, crossing the **stream (3.7 miles, 3,510', 314733E 3813815N)** on the other side of camp and through a gauntlet of massive boulders, but then quickly embarks on a steady climb to the northeast through chaparral and scrub. Views of the northern flank of Santa Paula Peak, Santa Paula's East Fork, and the Upper Ojai Valley are rather impressive from this route. Along this fairly steep affair you'll follow a series of long switchbacks for about a mile until reaching the first rock formations at the base of the namesake sandstone bluffs that have stood sentinel in the east during your ascent. This Sespe formation geology, easily identified for its red sandstone and cobble- and pebble-filled siltstone, extends for miles eastward into the condor sanctuary and the Sespe.

The trail levels and loses some altitude here, and then follows the shallow **drainage (4.7 miles, 4,560', 315360E 3814997N)** beneath massive erosion-sculpted sandstone monoliths to **Bluff Camp (4.8 miles, 4,600', 315417E 3815117N)**.

CAMP :: BLUFF

ELEVATION:	4,600'
MAP:	USGS *Santa Paula Peak*
UTM:	315417E 3815117N

This seldom-visited site is named for the red sandstone cliffs that dominate the eastern edge of this area; these bluffs form the edge of the Sespe Wilderness, and the eastern portion doubles as the boundary of the Sespe Condor Sanctuary. Views from the formations above camp are impressive, stretching across Bear Heaven, down the West Fork, east beyond the Sespe, and points southward (the bluffs are just higher than 4,957-foot Santa Paula Peak to the south). In addition to the bigcone Douglas-firs, which seem to heavily populate this corner of the forest, tall sugar pines join their company here. Water can be had from the spring-fed stream running through camp but cannot be relied upon year-round.

Though decades ago a trail did continue north of camp, Bluff is for all intents the end of this route. Beyond is the high point, which marks the southwestern border of the Sespe Condor Sanctuary, and just to your left (north) is the Sespe Wilderness boundary. The trail beyond seems to be a corridor for black bears into Santa Paula Canyon, as the route displays a disproportionate amount of scat and claw-raked trees.

Route 64

SANTA PAULA PEAK (20W16 and 21W16)

LENGTH AND TYPE:	10.3-mile out-and-back to Santa Paula Peak; 6.6-mile one-way to East Fork junction
RATING:	Strenuous
TRAIL CONDITION:	Well maintained to passable (ranch roads and well-defined trail; some scrambling to reach the peak)
MAP(S):	USGS *Santa Paula Peak*
CAMP(S):	—
HIGHLIGHTS:	Distant 360-degree views from atop Santa Paula Peak

TO REACH THE TRAILHEAD(S): From CA 126 in Santa Paula, follow Timber Canyon Road north approximately 1.8 miles to a **parking area (1,300', 315445E 3808437N)** on the shoulder of the road below a private residence (whichever side has space enough for your vehicle). As a courtesy to the owners—who thus far have been kind enough to allow hikers on their property—try to arrange a drop-off or pickup rather than leaving your vehicle parked on their property. There are no facilities here.

Note: Timber Canyon Road is gated, and you will need to contact the owners to gain access; their contact specifics are not provided here. Further, ownership could change without notice, and as there is no formal US Forest Service (USFS) easement here, access via Timber Canyon is not a permanent certainty.

See *Routes 62* and *63* if approaching via the East Fork of Santa Paula.

TRIP SUMMARY: From Timber Canyon, this fairly steep ascent heads easily through grazing pasture and then climbs the southern flanks of Santa Paula Peak to the summit. You also have the option to drop down the northern slope of Santa Paula Peak to the campgrounds at the East Fork headwaters. *Note:* There is almost never water in any of the tiny draws along the ascent toward Santa Paula Peak, so be sure you're carrying enough for your party to make the climb and return (10-plus miles round-trip).

Ascending Santa Paula Peak

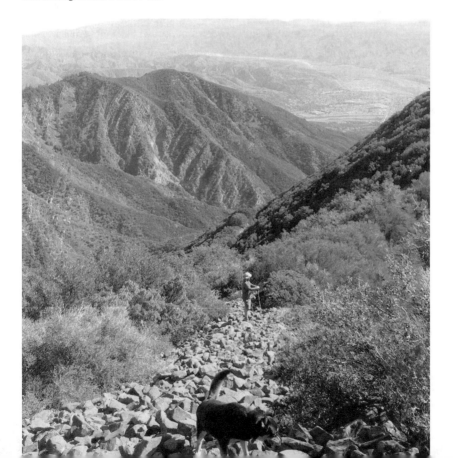

Trip Description

If approaching from the East Fork of Santa Paula Canyon, see *Routes 62* and *63* to reach the junction just south of Cienega Camp. From the junction, follow the Peak Trail southward and up the northern flanks of the peak 1.6 miles to the spur trail leading to the peak. *Note:* Neither approach to Santa Paula Peak is shown on Harrison's *Sespe Wilderness*.

From the **parking area (1,300', 315445E 3808437N)**, walk up the driveway to the dirt road on the right (east) side of the house. Follow this old road easily northward past rows of avocado trees, whereupon you'll come to a locked **gate (0.5 mile, 1,630', 315377E 3809198N)** and barbed-wire fence. There's no crawling under or slipping through: you will have to climb over this gate (or if you have a long enough inseam, carefully straddle the barbed wire). The fence is here to contain the ranch's cattle.

Once over the gate, continue following the doubletrack along the edge of a wide grove of live oaks. Mind your ankles in the hoof-carved ruts, and mind the cow pies (and while you're at it, mind the cattle—best not to spook them). Continue straight (north) when you reach a three-way **junction (1.5 miles, 2,200', 315019E 3810506N)**; the road is markedly less well traveled here. Continue northward until a switchback sends you up to your right (east) and then southward. In the spring, this is where the wildflowers become most apparent, and you'll enjoy the blankets of color laid across these lower hills. Another **junction (2 miles, 2,490', 315222E 3810580N)** on your left (east) is your desired turnoff; keep an eye out, as this can be easy to miss (even in the 1940s, the U.S. Coast & Geodetic Survey party described some of the junctions along this route as "dim"). If you come to another barbed-wire fence, you've gone about 50 feet too far; don't follow the deceptively well-worn trail along this fence.

From the junction, you're now on a USFS trail (20W16), which switchbacks slowly northward through chaparral and scrub, making this southern exposure a hot ascent in the summer. There is very little shade along this route, but it may be some consolation that your views of the Santa Clara River Valley and surrounding environs improve with every step. The geology of this higher area is dominated by sandstone of the Coldwater formation, a late-Eocene (and hard) rock you'll note in various spots off the sides of the trail.

After a few miles of steady climbing, you'll gain a ridgeline and then the **junction (5 miles, 4,720', 315529E 3812720N)** with the Santa Paula Peak spur trail. From the junction, follow the use trail up the eastern flank of Santa Paula Peak over the fairly well-maintained trail (one stretch clambers up a field of rockfall). A few stretches of this short trail edge some sheer drop-offs, so do exercise caution and mind any four-legged companions by staying well away from the edge (there's ample room to do so).

Climb this short route to the peak, where you'll first cross the burned-out footings of the old Santa Paula Peak lookout and onto the geographic top of **Santa Paula Peak (5.2 miles, 4,957', 315363E 3812816N)**.

■ ■ ■ ■ ■ ■ ■ ■ ■ **SANTA   PAULA   PEAK**

Stand here and you'll immediately understand why a fire lookout was placed atop this somewhat barren sandstone peak. On any reasonably clear day, the towers of downtown Los Angeles are visible to the south, as are the snowcapped San Gabriel Mountains, the Peninsular Ranges, and—if you're counting—seven of the eight Channel Islands (only San Clemente is typically indiscernible beyond—and nearly behind—Catalina Island). Also in view is the Santa Clara River Valley and nearby South Mountain, the Oxnard Plain, Lake Casitas, the ranges beyond the Matilija Wilderness, and—to the north—the Topatopa Mountains (including No-name, Hines, and Topatopa Peaks—look closely and you'll spy the tower upon which the Topatopa Peak lookout stood until destroyed in the 2006 Day Fire). San Cayetano Peak is the mountain to your east looming above the community of Fillmore.

■ ■ ■ ■ ■ ■ ■ ■ ■ ■ ■ ■ ■ ■ ■ ■ ■ ■ ■ ■

Beyond the junction, the trail drops around the northeast flank of the peak to a second **junction (5.3 miles from the Timber Canyon Trailhead excluding the Santa Paula Peak spur trail, 4,500', 315508E 3813117N)**. You'll have a good view of the East Fork of Santa Paula Canyon from this vantage point. The right (east) route is the old route (20W15) that once led to San Cayetano Mountain but has not been maintained for decades; the left (west) leads down the well-shaded northern flank of Santa Paula Peak through a long series of switchbacks of increasing steepness under cover of oaks, and then conifers and across moss-covered rock fields to the **junction (6.6 miles, 3,490', 314750E 3813499N)** with the East Fork Trail. Cienega Camp is only another 0.1 mile to the north; see *Route 63* for that route.

Route 65

HOWARD CREEK TRAIL (22W26)

LENGTH AND TYPE:	5.9-mile round-trip
RATING:	Moderate
TRAIL CONDITION:	Clear
MAP(S):	USGS *Lion Canyon*; Harrison's *Sespe Wilderness*
CAMP(S):	Howard
HIGHLIGHTS:	Excellent views

TO REACH THE TRAILHEAD(S): Use the Howard Creek Trailhead to access this route.

TRIP SUMMARY: From Rose Valley, this moderate climb follows the Howard Creek drainage from Rose Valley Road southward to Nordhoff Ridge. It's a great day trip.

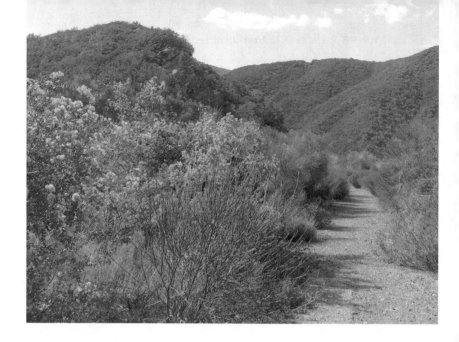

Trip Description

From the service road turnoff (**3,480', 295234E 3823677N**), hike past the gate and follow the road southward to the **singletrack junction (0.15 mile, 3,520', 295288E 3823468N)** on the left (east). Follow the track here eastward as it curves clockwise around a knoll; your route here is an old road lined by brooms and ceanothus, and while the remaining road base is coarse, it makes for easy hiking.

Once around the knoll, the trail straightens and heads south toward a **gap (0.4 mile, 3,650', 295730E 3823235N)** bordered by sandstone formations. Follow the trail down into one of Howard Creek's tributaries here, passing a small stand of Coulter and Digger pines, and stay left as you cross the drainage, taking a roughly southeast tack to begin weaving in and out of two additional tributaries to the main branch of Howard Creek. Here your route begins a steady but not overly taxing climb, and views of Pine Mountain, Piedra Blanca and the Sespe, Dry Lakes Ridge, and points in between quickly avail themselves. The facilities at Rancho Grande on your left (east) are also easily discerned.

A handful of seeps and small (often dry) fern-adorned drainages mark your progress until the second main **tributary (1.65 miles, 3,900', 296223E 3822338N)**, often dry during the summer. Here the trail cuts back left (east) sharply, working eastward along the southern flanks of the hill around which Howard Creek flows. The stretch just past this first tributary is well shaded by numerous interior live oaks and dotted with ferns and bays.

Continue the steady ascent southward, leaving the oaks and usually reliable shade for the more exposed scrub typical of Nordhoff Ridge until you reach a **gap (2.65 miles, 4,380', 296169E 3821616N)** with excellent panoramic views of points north, and then head right (south) along a newer cut of the trail to the **firebreak and junction** (**2.8 miles, 4,440', 296086E 3821430N**) with a spur trail. Following the right (southward) fork here will lead you down along the edge of a pleasant meadow to meet **Nordhoff Ridge Road** (5N08) (**2.9 miles, 4,400', 296064E 3821344N**). Gridley Saddle is a mile along the road from this junction, and beyond lay the Nordhoff lookout and the upper Pratt Trail access (see *Routes 57* and *56*, respectively).

Cutting left (east) at the junction will lead you up a short trail to **Howard Camp** (**4,500', 296209E 3821443N**), where a sturdy wooden table and heavy-duty fire ring installed in 1999 are available on a first-come, first-serve basis. (Don't confuse this with the old Howard Creek Campground at the Howard/Sespe confluence.) There are no facilities here. Coulter pines just south of the camp make for a pleasant rest spot, as there is no shade at the camp proper. Views of the Pacific, as well as the Ojai Valley and the Oxnard Plain, are especially good from this vantage point.

You can either return the way you came, or with some planning and a shuttle vehicle, you have numerous options to the east: Chief Peak, the upper Horn Canyon, Lion Canyon, Sisar Canyon accesses, the old Topatopa Lodge Trail, Santa Paula and Red Reef Canyons, and Hines Peak.

Route 66

ROSE VALLEY FALLS (22W15)

LENGTH AND TYPE:	0.8-mile out-and-back
RATING:	Easy
TRAIL CONDITION:	Clear
MAP(S):	USGS *Lion Canyon;* Harrison's *Sespe Wilderness*
CAMP(S):	—
HIGHLIGHTS:	Easy and pleasant hike; waterfall

TO REACH THE TRAILHEAD(S): Use Rose Valley Campground to access this route.

TRIP SUMMARY: This very easy and popular hike leads to the lower Rose Valley Falls. It's ideal for children and first-timers.

Trip Description

From the Rose Valley Campground **parking space** (**3,420', 299648E 3823278N**), walk to the southern edge of camp and proceed down the clearly marked trail, crossing the creek a few times before climbing slightly to parallel the drainage along the western banks. Your route is lined with some scrub along the very early portion but soon is dominated by alders, bays, and the occasional live oak.

The route here, though uphill, is wide, very easily navigated, and composed largely of well-compacted shale. Numerous side trails drop into the creek, mostly at opportune wading pools and swimming holes. In very little time you'll reach the pleasant **lower Rose Valley Falls** (**0.4 mile, 3,600', 299853E 3822788N**), which cascade over a formation of arkosic (feldspar-heavy) sandstone that has withstood erosion over the ages better than the softer surrounding sandstone and shale. The upper falls, which are equally impressive, are accessible by a tenuous scrambling route over loose shale; exercise extreme caution if you attempt this approach—every local area hiker knows someone or a friend of someone killed attempting to access the upper falls from this canyon. For a technical, multihour rappelling venture, the upper falls can be accessed from above via Nordhoff Ridge Road (refer to the USGS quad for greater detail).

Route 58 is also accessed from the Rose Valley Campground (via Nordhoff Ridge Road, the usually locked gate situated beside campsite number 2).

Route 67

ROSE-LION CONNECTOR (22W16)

LENGTH AND TYPE:	1.6-mile one-way
RATING:	Easy
TRAIL CONDITION:	Clear
MAP(S):	USGS *Lion Canyon*; Harrison's *Sespe Wilderness*
CAMP(S):	—
HIGHLIGHTS:	Views of Rose Valley and Piedra Blanca and surrounding wilderness; Lion Creek watershed

TO REACH THE TRAILHEAD(S): From the junction of CA 33 and CA 150 in Ojai, drive north along CA 33 approximately 14.5 miles to Forest Road 6N31 (Rose Valley Road). Turn right (south) onto this road and continue east 3.1 miles to the intersection with Rose Valley Lake Road. Turn right (north) here and continue 0.5 mile northward to the **shoulder** (**3,400', 299729E 3823508N**) just south of the Rose Valley Campground road sign. There are restrooms here (on the west side of the road) and in the campground ahead, but no water. A Forest Service Adventure Pass, federal Interagency Pass, or equivalent permit is required to park a vehicle anywhere in the Rose Valley Recreation Area.

TRIP SUMMARY: A pleasant hike with minimal elevation gain, the Rose-Lion Connector makes a pleasant day trip and is a nice alternative approach to the Lion Canyon Trail (22W06).

Trip Description

From the shoulder, walk to the Rose Valley Campground road sign and from there follow the trail eastward under cover of mature cottonwood trees. Very soon you'll cross Rose Valley Creek, which feeds the trio of lakes strung along just downstream of you. Your route follows a well-marked trail (in places defined by handlaid rock borders) along an unnamed drainage until you break from this tributary and climb through a manzanita- and oak-lined path that will lead you up to the **saddle (0.8 mile, 3,700', 300840E 3823300N)** between this drainage and that of Lion Canyon.

From the saddle, you'll descend somewhat steeply at first down the other side, initially along scrub-enclosed trail and then into a sandy, yucca-populated and well-rutted area that ultimately drops you into another drainage. Follow the trail along the banks of this tributary to Lion Canyon another 0.75 mile until you reach the cobblestone-lined wash that is **Lion Creek (1.6 miles, 3,385', 301800E 3823567N)**. The creek banks make for an ideal lunch spot, especially when there is water. The rock outcrop on the canyon wall opposite (which can be seen from a bit of a distance during your descent) is another 150 feet along and marks the **junction (1.6 miles, 3,390', 301858E 3823552N)** with this trail and the Lion Canyon Trail.

Once you've lazed long enough along the banks of the creek, return the way you came. If you've come this way as an alternative to the lower stretches of the Lion Canyon Trail, refer to *Route 87* for the rest of your route.

CHAPTER eleven

Mt. Pinos and Chumash Wilderness

This chapter details the trails of the Mt. Pinos area, including the San Emigdio Mesa and the Chumash Wilderness.

CONSIDERED THE CENTER OF THE UNIVERSE by the Chumash of old, 8,831-foot Mt. Pinos (*Iwihinmu*) is the highest point in Ventura County (and, for that matter, the Los Padres). Though the immediate area (including the Chumash Wilderness) boasts a fairly limited number of trails relative to other areas of the forest, it is a highly regarded recreation destination, particularly in the winter months.

Most visitors to the area focus on the mountain itself. With a well-maintained paved road leading to 8,300 feet and within 2 miles of the peak, it grants uncommonly good access to snow and high-elevation environs. A fire lookout was constructed atop the peak during the Depression and doubled as an airplane spotting station during World War II; today a radio (microwave) transmitter and associated outbuildings dominate the peak (though peak-baggers can access the actual summit).

The old parking lot and former condor observation area just west of the peak is now the jumping-off point for treks into the Chumash Wilderness. From the old condor observation area, views west toward the Transverse Ranges are impressive, and to the north the San Joaquin Valley and the Sierra Nevada can easily be seen (air quality of the valley permitting). The Chumash Wilderness—granted its designation in 1992 as part of the Los Padres Condor Range and River Protection Act also responsible for many of the newer wildernesses in the Los Padres—consists of 38,150 acres and spans from just west of Mt. Pinos to Mt. Abel (Cerro Noroeste). Sawmill Mountain, the high southern flanks over which the Vincent Tumamait Trail (named after a respected Chumash historian and storyteller) travels, is the wilderness's highest point at 8,818 feet.

Wildflower displays atop Mt. Pinos are equally impressive when the spring blooms show (though the north face of the mountain often has snow well into May). The area

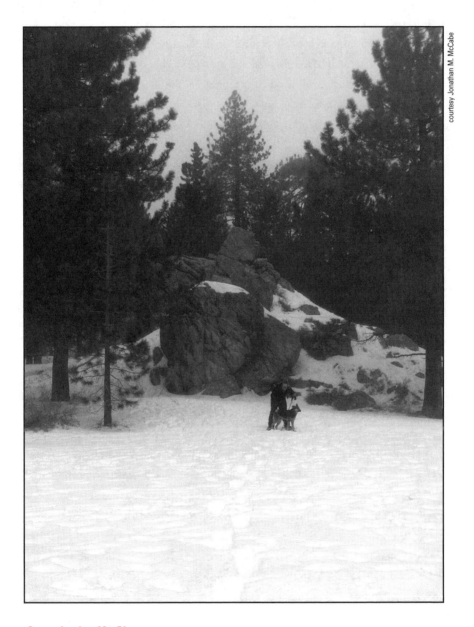

Snowshoeing Mt. Pinos

immediately surrounding the summit has been designated a botanical area by the U.S. Department of Agriculture. The Kern-Ventura County line effectively bisects the mountain, with the actual peak just south of the line (thereby placing it in Ventura County).

The Chula Vista parking area—which for the last two decades has been the farthest passenger vehicles are allowed to travel—is also an extremely popular destination for amateur astronomers, as the elevation and air quality typically allow for stargazing of far greater quality than can be found anywhere else between the Sierra Nevada and the higher peaks of the Angeles. Please bear this in mind if approaching in the evening, as your vehicles' headlights can disrupt stargazing.

When snow has fallen, the Mount Pinos Highway—and the Chula Vista parking area in particular—can be something of a madhouse of families, skiers, and snow revelers all vying for limited parking space. In summer, mountain bikers enjoy the non-wilderness trails, often staging shuttle vehicles at the top and bottom of the mountain. The Kern County Sheriff's Department will close either or both of the road's two snow gates as conditions dictate, so check with either the Mt. Pinos Ranger District at (661) 245-3731 or the Kern County Roads Department at (661) 862-8850 before heading for the mountain during or after significant snow events.

Trailheads

Mt. Pinos Trailhead (8,340', 305455E 3854362N)

From Frazier Park: From the Frazier Mountain Park Road exit (Exit 205) on I-5 in Frazier Park, head west along Frazier Mountain Park Road (after you pass through Frazier Park it will become Cuddy Valley Road) for 12.2 miles to the Y with Mil Potrero Highway at the base of Mt. Pinos. Go left at the Y and continue up the Mount Pinos Highway (FS Route 9N24) another 8.5 miles to the Chula Vista **parking area (8,340', 305455E 3854362N)**.

From Ojai: From the junction of CA 33 and Lockwood Valley Road, head east on Lockwood Valley Road 26.8 miles to the junction with Frazier Mountain Park Road. Turn left (northwest) and continue along Frazier Mountain Park Road (after you pass through Frazier Park it will become Cuddy Valley Road) for 5.1 miles to the Y with Mil Potrero Highway at the base of Mt. Pinos. Go left at the Y and continue up the Mount Pinos Highway (FS Route 9N24) another 8.5 miles to the Chula Vista **parking area (8,340', 305455E 3854362N)**.

There are portable toilets but no other facilities here (better vault toilets are available at the Chula Vista walk-in campground a few hundred yards to the east). A Forest Service Adventure Pass, federal Interagency Pass, or equivalent permit is required to park a vehicle anywhere along the Mount Pinos Highway or atop the parking area during winter.

Note: The lodgelike building at the north end of the Chula Vista parking lot is staffed during the ski season by volunteers of the Mount Pinos Nordic Ski Patrol (**nordicbase.org**). Updates on conditions, maps, and general information are typically available there.

Other trailheads along the Mount Pinos Highway (FS 9N24) include the **McGill Trailhead** (**6,150', 309206E 3856572N**)—which is approximately 0.6 mile south of the Y with the Mil Potrero Highway at the base of the mountain—as well as those originating at McGill and Mt. Pinos Campgrounds.

Cerro Noroeste/Mt. Abel (8,100', 298637E 3856234N)

Just down the road from Campo Alto atop Cerro Noroeste is the western trailhead of the **Vincent Tumamait Trail.** To reach the trailhead, head west from Pine Mountain Club along the Mil Potrero Highway approximately 3 miles to the junction with Cerro Noroeste Road/ FS Route 9N25 (the Apache Saddle Fire Station is easily identifiable here). Turn left (south) at the junction and follow Cerro Noroeste Road another 6.9 miles up the mountain slope to a small turnoff on the right (east) side of the road. (Parking is available along the roadside, but do be careful to park completely off the pavement, as the road is a bit narrow here.)

Toad Springs Trailhead (5,530', 295851E 3859550)

From Pine Mountain Club, head west along the Mil Potrero Highway for approximately 3.8 miles to the turnoff on your left (south) for Quatal Canyon Road, a graded dirt road. Follow Quatal Canyon Road 0.6 mile (passing Toad Springs Campground) to the trailhead. The parking spot just off the road—with room enough for two or three vehicles—is down a steep embankment and not recommended for passenger vehicles.

Nettle Spring Trailhead (4,420', 290040E 3853325N)

This trailhead is less than 0.25 mile down the road from the Nettle Spring Campground. The camp is one of the few remaining car campgrounds in a region that was once host to many (including, Cienega, Yellowjacket, Mud Springs, Blue Rock Spring, and Ozena, now all closed or abandoned) and serves as the western roadhead for the Toad Springs Trail (22W01). There are restrooms but no other facilities here.

From CA 33 in the Cuyama Valley, head northeast along Apache Canyon Road (Forest Route 8N06) 8.3 miles along a well-graded dirt road to the turnoff for Nettle Spring Campground. Four-wheel drive typically isn't necessary (though do mind the creek crossings), but a higher-clearance vehicle is recommended.

Camp Three Falls (5,450', 304665E 3847184N)

From Lockwood Valley Road, follow Boy Scout Camp Road westward 2.8 miles to the camp gate. Operated by the Ventura County Council of the Boy Scouts of America, Camp Three Falls is named for the falls in the three branches of Lockwood Canyon to the north (one of which you'll pass along the North Fork Trail). While non-Scouts are not allowed to park on the grounds proper, one can park outside the camp gates and then walk along the main entrance road. Even if the gate is open, do not enter the camp.

Campgrounds

Three campgrounds are located along the highway heading up Mt. Pinos; two are open seasonally, and the third is a short walk from the Chula Vista parking lot. Situated beneath the magnificent Jeffrey pines that tower over the mountain's slopes, all sites feature tables, stoves, and vault toilets. None have water.

CAMP :: CHULA VISTA

ELEVATION:	8,300'
MAP:	USGS *Cuddy Valley*
UTM:	305735E 3854443N

The only year-round campground on the mountain, Chula Vista is a walk-in camp with 12 sites. The walk in is about 500 feet from the northeast end of the Chula Vista parking area. Established in 1959 (originally as a day-use site), the camp makes an ideal spot to base oneself for multiday ski or snowshoe trips centered around Mt. Pinos.

There is no fee to camp here, though a USFS Adventure Pass, federal Interagency Pass, or equivalent is required to park at the nearby Chula Vista parking area during winter. The site typically isn't cleared of snow in winter, so be prepared to engage in some shoveling after any measurable snows, as the fire rings are typically buried during winter.

CAMP :: MCGILL AND MCGILL GROUP

ELEVATION:	7,500'
MAP:	USGS *Cuddy Valley*
UTM:	307712E 3854429N

By far the largest campground on Mt. Pinos, McGill—open April 15–November 15—consists of 78 sites. The campground, established in 1962, is managed by Rocky Mountain Recreation Company: (877) 444-6777; **rockymountainrec.com** (reservations can also be made through **recreation.gov**). The standard family sites cost $16 per night, whereas the two group sites (60 or 80 people) cost $75 per night. Reservations must be made at least four days in advance for the group sites.

CAMP :: MT. PINOS

ELEVATION:	7,800'
MAP:	USGS *Cuddy Valley*
UTM:	307056E 3854033N

This 19-site campground—often overlooked by those visiting the mountain—is a pleasant spot commanding good views of the valleys to the east. It was established in 1964 and is open May 15–November 1. Sites are $16 per night. Like McGill, this campground is managed by Rocky Mountain Recreation Company: (877) 444-6777, **rockymountainrec.com** (reservations can also be made through **recreation.gov**).

Atop Cerro Noreste (or Mt. Abel) is **Campo Alto**, a dry camp of 15 sites. One only needs a USFS Adventure Pass, federal Interagency Pass, or equivalent to claim a site here. The same holds true for Chuchupate Campground along Frazier Mountain Road to the south of Lockwood Valley. Numerous 4WD/high-clearance camps (Caballo, Marian, Cherry Creek, Pleito Creek, and Salt Creek) dot the massif of San Emigdio Mountain north of the Mil Potrero Highway and the San Andreas Rift.

The western Chumash Wilderness is dominated by the San Emigdio Mesa, a barren and largely empty badland of deep ravines and alluvium draining toward Lockwood Valley and the Cuyama River by its main outlets (Quatal, Apache, and Dry Canyons). Traveling across the piñon-dotted badlands from Toad Springs Campground (five sites) to just down the road from Nettle Spring Campground (nine sites), the Toad Springs Trail bisects the main portion of the wilderness with a largely untouched western portion (over which there are few official or recognized trails, all short and unmaintained).

A quick look at a USGS or Forest Service map of Mt. Pinos reveals numerous trails meandering all about the slopes; many of these are cross-country ski routes and not all are covered herein.

Ski and Snowshoe Routes

Numerous ski and snowshoe routes throughout the Mt. Pinos area—while not formally recognized as hiking routes by the USFS—make fine and relatively short options for easy day trips. Most of the routes follow long-retired service, logging, or sawmill roads and are signed with trail name, distance, and difficulty. A brief summation of the most popular routes is provided on the following pages; detailed maps of the routes are available during the ski season for a small donation at the Nordic Base at the Chula Vista parking area.

If hiking or snowshoeing along the ski routes in the winter, please be considerate of your fellow trail users and adhere to ski trail etiquette. This includes staying out of the ski tracks if you are not using skis, so as to keep the ski route in the best condition.

Fir Ridge (2.4-mile out-and-back)

From the **turnout (7,870', 306859E 3853924N)** 0.2 mile up the highway from Mt. Pinos Campground, follow the old Fir Ridge fire road northward on a surprisingly level route. At the junction with the Harvest Trail, keep right (northeast) to reach the turnaround at 1.2 miles.

Harvest (2-mile out-and-back)

From the Chula Vista parking area, follow the marked trail departing from the northeast corner of the parking area past the campground. Stay straight (east) at the split from the Knoll Loop Trail and follow the occasionally rocky route through the ravine a few times before reaching the junction with Fir Ridge Road.

Inspiration Point (2.4-mile out-and-back)

This may very well be the most popular day trip atop Mt. Pinos. From the Chula Vista parking area, follow Forest Route 9N24 west toward Mt. Pinos, climbing steadily but not too aggressively for nearly a mile to the first of two meadows. Head north to the vista from there.

Iris Point (2.2-mile out-and-back)

Iris Point heads south from the spur road leading to Mt. Pinos Campground, following an old roadbed and crossing the upper headwaters of Seymour Creek before reaching its namesake point atop the ridge dividing the Seymour and Amargosa drainages, just on the edge of the Chumash Wilderness. At 0.9 mile the fork is simply the split leading back on itself; staying left will lead you directly to the fantastic vantage point, including unique views of Alamo, Frazier, and Pine Mountains, and—when visibility cooperates—the Topatopa Mountains looming above the Sespe far away.

Knoll Loop (0.9-mile one-way)

From the Chula Vista parking area, follow the marked trail departing from the northeast corner of the parking area past the campground. Turn right (south) at the split from the Harvest Trail and continue along the easy grade before a slightly steeper drop leads you to a turnout on Mount Pinos Highway. The actual loop entails hiking back along the road nearly

0.5 mile back to the parking area. You may wish to opt for turning back the way you came and avoid sharing your hike with motor vehicles.

South Ridge (2-mile one-way)

This route heads north from the turnoff for Mt. Pinos Campground, roughly paralleling the bend in the highway, and then meeting the road on the other end of that bend. This is a popular snowshoe route, frequented by mountain bikers in the summer. You'll note several berms, which make for ideal jumps for those riders, so do exercise caution when sharing the trail with more ambitious riders.

Whitethorn Nature Trail (1-mile out-and-back)

This extremely easy route is ideal for trips with the very youngest hikers in your crew. The trailhead is situated on the left (west) side of the lower McGill parking area, and after a brief initial climb, you'll enjoy a level route above camp, with placards describing the characteristics of various flora along the route. The trip is a great primer for those interested in the plant life of the Mt. Pinos region.

In the early 1990s, approximately 0.25 mile of the route was rebuilt to make it accessible to visitors in wheelchairs. This included a fair portion of hard-surfacing, making the route not only ADA-compliant but also easy hiking for the very young. Also note throughout McGill Campground the various groups of giant sequoias, planted there in the 1970s as a foresting experiment.

■ ■ ■ ■ ■ ■ ■ ■ ■ ■ ■ PINE MOUNTAIN CLUB

Five miles from the Y with the Mil Potrero Highway is Pine Mountain Club, a private community of approximately 2,000. Many of the homes in the area are second/vacation homes or rental properties, and the population increases notably during the summer and on holiday weekends. In addition to offering markets, lodging, and other services, the community is also one of the few enclaves in the Los Padres with a fuel station, which, given some of the distances between trailheads in the region, can facilitate more complicated shuttle logistics than other such ventures elsewhere in the forest. (Fuel is also available approximately 25 miles to the east in Frazier Park.)

The Mt. Pinos Ranger District contains the vast majority of OHV routes and motorcycle-friendly trails within the southern Los Padres. Many of these trails make for excellent hikes, but as the focus of this guide leans toward foot trails, most of those on which motorcycles or ATVs are allowed are not covered here. If you're interested in exploring options beyond those presented within this guide, discuss trail options north of Cuddy Valley (Tecuya Ridge, Sam Emigidio Mountain, and many other excellent routes) and within Lockwood Valley (Lockwood Peak, San Guillermo Mountain, etc.) with the rangers at Chuchupate Station.

Route 68

TOAD SPRINGS (22W01)

LENGTH AND TYPE:	5.8-mile out-and-back from Nettle Spring Trailhead to San Emigdio Mesa meadow; 6.6-mile out-and-back from Toad Springs Trailhead to northern edge of meadow; 7.1-mile one-way from Nettle Spring Trailhead to Toad Springs Trailhead
RATING:	Moderate
TRAIL CONDITION:	Passable to clear (unmaintained former 4WD and motorcycle trail)
MAP(S):	USGS *Sawmill Mountain* and *Apache Canyon*
CAMP(S):	—
HIGHLIGHTS:	Expansive piñon forest; San Emigdio Mesa; fascinating geology; eroded geography

TO REACH THE TRAILHEAD(S): Use the Nettle Spring and Toad Springs Trailheads to access this route.

TRIP SUMMARY: This traverse of the Cuyama badlands and San Emigdio Mesa follows the Toad Springs OHV route (closed now for years to motor traffic) through some unique geology and high desertlike piñon and sage forest. This narrative describes the route from south to north.

Trip Description

From the **Nettle Spring Trailhead (4,420', 290040E 3853325N)**, follow the retired 4WD route in a counterclockwise arc to the southeast and along the northern edge of private property, eventually heading northeast and away from the Apache Canyon drainage. Most of the flora accompanying you here are piñons, some scrub and live oaks, junipers, and a hearty complement of sage. The soil is composed largely of granitic alluvium, and while a bit sandy in spots, it makes for easy trekking. A **grass hedge (0.5 mile, 4,460', 290635E 3853351N)** often obscures the route here and leads some to follow an old road that dead-ends shortly up the canyon. When you reach the grasses, keep right and pass through them, easily gaining the proper route again just up the slope to where the trail joins the **drainage (0.7 mile, 4,520', 290712E 3853496N)**; you'll follow toward San Emigdio Mesa.

Follow this drainage easily toward the east, enjoying the shade it provides on warmer days; within the first 0.25 mile of this narrower route you'll pass through the old **road gate** (**0.9 mile, 4,630', 290960E 3853577N**). Continue on a steady but very mild grade, coming out of the ravine after about 2 miles and hiking along a stretch of road that has largely been spared the erosion of the early portion just hiked. Here views of Mt. Abel (Cerro Noroeste) to your east and surrounding environs steadily improve, and you gain altitude beneath the mature and fairly widely spaced piñons and junipers.

Stay left (north) at the first junction with the old **road** (**2.7 miles, 5,100', 293043E 3854779N**), and soon you'll enter the magnificent **meadow** (**2.9 miles, 5,150', 293357E 3854943N**) along the eastern flanks of Mt. Abel. The route heading straight (east) will lead to Mesa Spring Camp; the route to your left (north) is the Toad Springs route. *Note:* Older maps designated this lower route along the base of the meadow as the 22W01 (Toad Springs) route, but the later OHV corridor through the wilderness would direct one right (east) here along the old doubletrack, only to turn left (north) later once along the upper edge of the meadow. The more recent 1:126,750 Los Padres recreation maps (last updated in 2008) depict the current route, which takes the lower (western) edge of the meadow to the junction.

From the junction, follow the route along the base of the meadow and then up its northern edge to the junction with your route and the trail coming in from Mesa Spring, set just beneath the piñons that form the perimeter here. Uncommonly large Mormon tea bushes dot this stretch as you approach the **junction** (**3.8 miles, 5,440', 294117E 3855921N**) with Mesa Spring Trail. From here, your route heads north across the headwaters of several of Quatal Canyon's tributaries, all the while skirting the western flanks of Mt. Abel (Cerro Noroeste). Views of the canyons and steep stretches of badlands are especially impressive along the high points as you hike along 3 miles of seesawing retired motorcycle trail over the ridges and into sandy washes. Despite all the up and down, your progress yields nearly no net elevation gain. Toward the end of this stretch, you descend fairly steeply into a narrow tributary—just as you reach the Quatal watershed, pass through the **wire fence** (**7 miles, 5,500', 295831E 3859475N**) erected by the US Forest Service to keep ATV riders out. The wire fence is usually cut and pulled back by protesting riders, but even when intact it's easy enough to crawl through.

The **Toad Springs Trailhead** (**7.1 miles, 5,530', 295851E 3859550**) along Quatal Canyon Road is just up the slope on the other side of the creek.

In the mid-1990s, a landslide mid-trail was cause for what at the time was considered a temporary closure of the route to ATVs. Whether through lack of funds or a preference to keep the area free of motor vehicles, the repairs were never made and the trail remains closed to ATVs (at least legally).

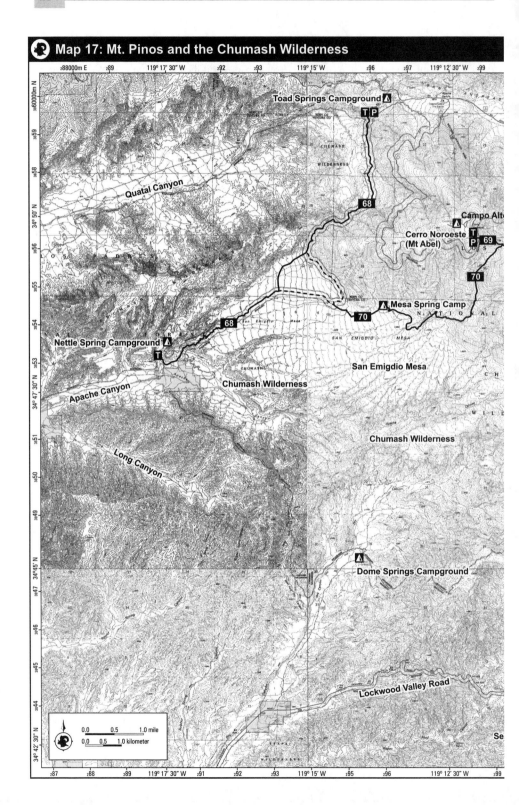

Map 17: Mt. Pinos and the Chumash Wilderness

Toad Springs Campground

68

Campo Alto

Cerro Noroeste
(Mt Abel)

69

70

Mesa Spring Camp

70

68

Nettle Spring Campground

San Emigdio Mesa

Chumash Wilderness

Apache Canyon

Quatal Canyon

Long Canyon

Chumash Wilderness

Dome Springs Campground

Lockwood Valley Road

0.0   0.5   1.0 mile
0.0   0.5   1.0 kilometer

MAP 17 Mt. Pinos and the Chumash Wilderness 285

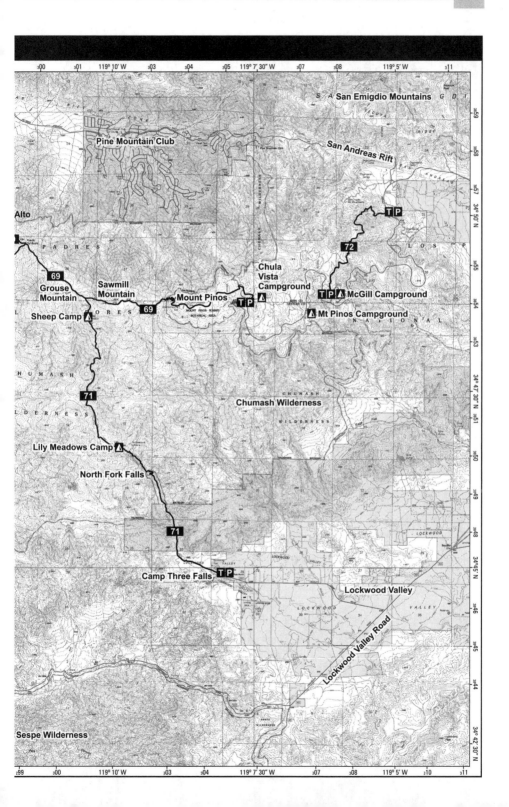

PATHS LESS TRAVELED: CIENEGA TRAIL ▪ ▪ ▪ ▪ ▪ ▪

The 1995 *Apache Canyon* and *Sawmill Mountain* quads (and many downloadable GPS data sets) show the old Cienega Trail (Trail 22W24 on the quads) heading northeast from the end of Apache Canyon Road toward a junction just west of Mesa Spring. In the 1950s, this was the original route to access Mesa Spring. This route is no longer a very viable option—the trail has gone unmaintained for decades, and its lower terminus leads to private property and thereby cannot be exited without trespassing (or some fairly ambitious cross-country trekking).

▪ ▪ ▪ ▪ ▪ ▪ ▪ ▪ ▪ ▪ ▪ ▪ ▪ ▪

Route 69

MT. PINOS TO MT. ABEL (Vincent Tumamait Trail [21W03])

LENGTH AND TYPE:	3.7-mile one-way to junction with North Fork Trail; 5.7-mile one-way to Cerro Noroeste Road
RATING:	Moderate
TRAIL CONDITION:	Clear
MAP(S):	USGS *Sawmill Mountain*
CAMP(S):	—
HIGHLIGHTS:	High-altitude and subalpine trekking

TO REACH THE TRAILHEAD(S): Use the Mt. Pinos Trailhead to access this route.

TRIP SUMMARY: This classic traverse of Mt. Pinos, Sawmill Mountain, and Grouse Mountain to Mt. Abel (Cerro Noroeste) follows an alternately exposed and tree-dotted route, staying above 7,500 feet the entire distance. This is one of the prettiest routes in the forest; winter visits require skis or snowshoes.

Trip Description

From the southwest corner of the **Mt. Pinos parking area (8,340', 305455E 3854362N)**, follow the dirt Forest Road 9N24 north and then west (staying left at both forks) through the Mount Pinos Summit Botanical Area to the old **condor observatory site (1.8 miles, 8,805', 303548E 3854268N)** on the west edge of the mountain. This unique stretch of forest is above 8,500 feet elevation and is home to a unique collection of plants. A four-page guide to the ferns, conifers, and flowering plants found here is available for download from the USFS website.

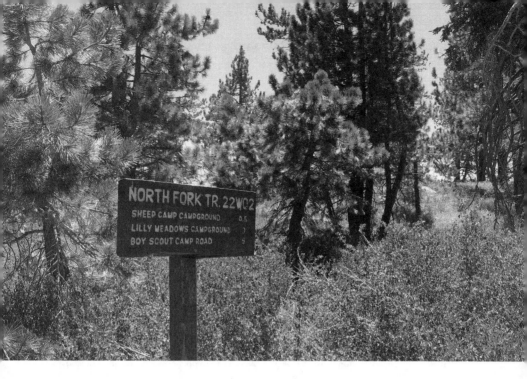

As recently as the early 1990s, this stretch was accessible by passenger vehicle, but it's now only accessible to official vehicles. Views from this vantage point go on for many miles, and the Cuyama badlands lie before you. To the north—air quality permitting—take in views of the southern Sierra Nevada. Interpretive signs detailing the history of the condor, Mt. Pinos's role in Chumash culture, and a brief biography of Vincent Tumamait are all posted. There are some benches and spots to enjoy lunch around the old parking area as well, but no facilities.

From the old parking lot, follow the singletrack through open, granite-strewn terrain and down the slope of Mt. Pinos. As late as May snow can be found on the north-facing slopes (in winter, this route is buried under feet of snow), and you'll pass through white firs, Indian paintbrush, white thorn ceanothus, and stands of Jeffrey pines as you drop into a small **saddle (2.4 miles, 8,390', 303054E 3854451N)** between Pinos and Sawmill. Climb the eastern flank of Sawmill (note the lightning-blasted treetops along this stretch), heading almost due west. Though the trail passes to the south of the actual peak (8,818 feet), many peak-baggers make the quick jaunt northward to sign the register.

A gradual descent from atop Sawmill will deposit you at the upper junction with the **North Fork Trail (3.7 miles, 8,500', 300990E 3854562N)**; see *Route 71*. Continue west here, making easy progress under the old pines and firs on a rolling stretch over the north edge of Grouse Mountain (8,582 feet; the peak proper is to the south of the trail for those interested) and then drop somewhat steeply into the **Puerta del Suelo (5.2 miles, 7,620',**

299408E 3856010N). The trail dropping to the left (south) is Mesa Spring Trail; see *Route 70*. It's a short but fairly steep climb from here to **Cerro Noroeste Road/Forest Road 9N25 (5.7 miles, 8,090', 298628E 3856235N)**. Campo Alto is just up the road.

Route 70

MESA SPRING (22W21)

LENGTH AND TYPE:	7.2-mile out-and-back to Mesa Spring Camp via Puerta del Suelo; 4.6-mile one-way to junction(s) with Toad Springs Trail
RATING:	Moderate
TRAIL CONDITION:	Passable to clear (unmaintained former 4WD and motorcycle trail)
MAP(S):	USGS *Sawmill Mountain*
CAMP(S):	Mesa Spring
HIGHLIGHTS:	Conifer forest; excellent views; San Emigdio Mesa; fascinating geology; eroded geography

TO REACH THE TRAILHEAD(S): See Map 17 to determine your approach; this route must be approached first along the Tumamait Trail (*Route 69*) or the Toad Springs Trail (*Route 68*).

TRIP SUMMARY: A steady descent from Puerta del Suelo leads into the upper San Emigdio Mesa and badlands. A brutally hot excursion in the summer once into the lower piñon- and scrub-dotted sections, this is an excellent trip with few visitors.

Trip Description

From **Puerta del Suelo (7,620', 299408E 3856010N)** between Mt. Abel and Grouse Mountain, follow the singletrack south. Views—though at times obscured by the massive pines and firs here—are impressive to the south when there is a break in the trees. The upper stretch of this descent is shaded by the tall conifers that dominate this area, but gradually the terrain changes as you lose elevation. You'll cross the main drainage along which this trail meanders a handful of times, passing through oaks, manzanitas, yuccas, and then the classic scrub, sage, and piñons that so define the San Emigdio.

After 1.5 miles of drop, the descent begins to level some, and you'll make the curve westward, leaving much of your cover as you break into the northern edge of **San Emigdio Mesa (1.7 miles, 6,500', 298218E 3854048N)**. Shortly beyond, this drainage of Apache Canyon cuts southward again, but your route will continue westward, working across several usually dry tributaries toward the sage-carpeted **clearing (1.9 miles, 6,010', 296393E 3854382N)** just before Mesa Spring Camp, where two old doubletrack roads—plainly visible in the clearing here—

split. Follow the right (north) fork toward some oaks and piñons at the base of the hill, where you'll find the old spring tank and **Mesa Spring Camp (3.8 miles, 6,000', 296035E 3854550N)**.

CAMP :: MESA SPRING

ELEVATION:	6,000'
MAP:	USGS *Sawmill Mountain*
UTM:	296035E 3854550N

This old 4WD site, now deep in the Chumash Wilderness, is seldom used due to its unique terrain, yet never seems to become overgrown or lost in the brush. The old tables here are still serviceable, and the old spring tank here ensures water year-round (treat first). Though the old post requests that you sign the register, there hasn't been a register here in decades—don't feel the need to hunt for it.

From camp, follow the trail along the western **edge (4.1 miles, 5,800', 295772E 3854272N)** of this clearing southward. Once on the western edge of the clearing where the piñons rear up again, navigating for the correct trail can be a bit tricky, especially in snow or poor weather. First, take the right (northwest) of the two forks here—heading left will lead along the old and abandoned Cienega Trail (22W24), a former 4WD route that is still surprisingly clear but dead-ends at private property farther down the canyon (though several use trails lead off this trail and head north to reconnect with the official US Forest Service route).

Following the upper route will lead you to the larger expanse of the western mesa meadow. Some use trails cut in and out and through the drainages along old singletracks and 4WD routes here; most lead to the meadow trail for something of a shortcut, but the easiest way from this direction is to stay on the fixed route to reach the **eastern edge (4.8 miles, 5,575', 295043E 3854631N)** of the massive meadow.

From here, heading right (north) leads toward Quatal Canyon along the Toad Springs route; heading left (west) leads toward Nettle Spring (the lower Toad Springs route). See *Route 68* for your options.

Route 71

NORTH FORK LOCKWOOD CREEK (22W02)

LENGTH AND TYPE:	10.1-mile one-way to Chula Vista parking area via Vincent Tumamait Trail (shuttle); 7.5-mile round-trip to Lily Meadows Camp from Camp Three Falls
RATING:	Strenuous (south to north); moderate (north to south)
TRAIL CONDITION:	Clear; heavy snow in winter and early spring

MAP(S):	USGS *San Guillermo Mountain* and *Sawmill Mountain*
CAMP(S):	Lily Meadows and Sheep Camp
HIGHLIGHTS:	Badland and conifer forest trekking; excellent views; great training hike for Sierra preparation

TO REACH THE TRAILHEAD(S): Use the Camp Three Falls and/or Chula Vista (Mt. Pinos) Trailheads to access this route.

TRIP SUMMARY: This trail makes for a great weekend or a moderately long shuttle day trip (a round-trip just to Lily Meadows Camp is also a great and easy weekend trip). Because of its proximity to Camp Three Falls (a Boy Scout camp) and the relatively easy first leg, this trail is popular with groups, and you can expect company on portions of the trail (especially on holiday weekends). With its relatively easy access but higher elevation and steady climb, the route makes an excellent training route for those preparing for a Sierra trip, climbing nearly 3,500 feet over the course of 8 miles from Camp Three Falls in Lockwood Valley to near the summit of Mt. Pinos. Conversely, it also makes a great downhill trip starting at Mt. Pinos.

Trip Description

From the end of Boy Scout Camp Road (**5,450', 304665E 3847184N**), follow the private road to the Camp Three Falls parking area. Continue through the edge of the parking area to the chain gate marking **Forest Road 8N31 (0.2 mile, 5,500', 304237E 3847353N)**.

Follow this dirt and decomposed granite service road through the barren singleleaf piñon– and juniper-dotted scrubland northwest along the edge of the Scout camp, meandering along the banks of the North Fork of Lockwood Creek (crossing once just on the outskirts of camp) to a **rock formation (1.1 miles, 5,630', 303338E 3848006N)** with a small collection of Chumash pictographs. Onward, the volcanic-looking fins looming on your left (west) are, in geologist parlance, subaqueous fan delta deposits. The road continues northward, crossing the creek a few times (as well as a number of usually dry tributaries) before reaching the **junction (2.5 miles, 5,950', 302654E 3849896N)** with the North Fork Trail.

Before heading up the singletrack, consider a quick visit to the base of **North Fork Falls (6,025', 302531E 3849915N)**, another 500 feet up the main road and around the canyon. A guerrilla camp beneath a towering ponderosa just short of the falls makes a nice lunch spot (frequently used by Scouts as well).

From the junction, the trail climbs steeply above the falls, crossing the formal boundary of the Chumash Wilderness along this steep and exposed (but quite short) climb to a **saddle (2.7 miles, 6,250', 302565E 3849968N)**, providing expansive views of Lockwood Valley and Frazier Mountain to the south. From the saddle, follow the creek as the ravine begins to narrow. Immediately the cover begins to change from piñons and scrub to scattered live oaks and numerous Jeffrey pines. Sugar pines and bigcone Douglas-firs dot the ridgeline high on your left.

It's a steady but not strenuous climb to **Lily Meadows** (**3.7 miles, 6,610', 301582E 3850700N**), a thin slice of fairly level ground wedged into a wide swath of the steep, tree-clad canyons. The trail camp here is ideal for an easy overnight.

Note: The camp is directly on the right (east) side of the trail, nowhere near as far up the ravine as indicated on the *Sawmill Mountain* quad.

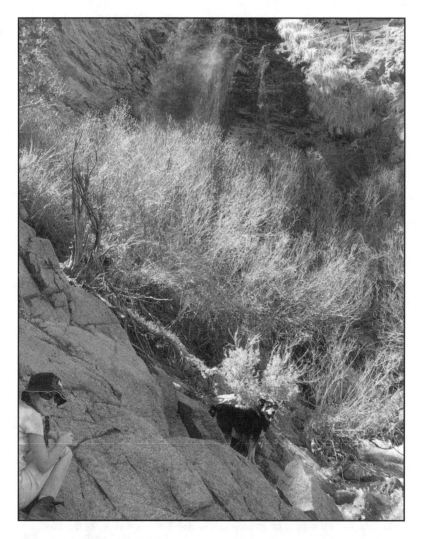

Refreshing North Fork Falls

CAMP :: **LILY MEADOWS**

ELEVATION:	6,610'
MAP:	USGS *Sawmill Mountain*
UTM:	301582E 3850700N

Though the various breeds of wild onions growing in the area are of the lily family, one cannot help but surmise the outdoorsman who gave Lily Meadows its current name mistook the plentiful irises growing in the summer meadows for lilies (various signs in the Los Padres spell it both "Lilly" and "Lily"). Lily Meadows is a pleasant site with a fire ring but no stove. For years a table remained at the site, but it was dismantled sometime in 2009. A handful of guerrilla sites are around the area, and water can typically be had in the creek (though in drier seasons it's often a bit of a walk back down-canyon along the willow-lined ravine before the water returns to the surface). Snow can often be found along the surrounding north- and east-facing slopes in all but the warmest summer months.

Local woodpeckers seem to especially enjoy hammering the lightning-blasted upper boughs of Jeffrey pines up-canyon, as their furtive pecking can often be heard in the midmorning.

From Lily Meadows, continue northward along the flanks of Sawmill Mountain, crossing the creek a handful of times before reaching a **gap (5.2 miles, 7,294', 301091E 3852754N)** that marks the real beginning of your climb. (From this gap a thread of a trail heading east can sometimes be seen; the falls of the Middle Fork of Lockwood Creek is accessible through the shallow drainage and over a small ridge.)

The trail continues climbing through the pine forest another mile to **Sheep Camp (6.4 miles, 8,221', 301052E 3854063N)**.

CAMP :: **SHEEP**

ELEVATION:	8,221'
MAP:	USGS *Sawmill Mountain*
UTM:	301052E 3854063N

When not overrun by Scouts or other youth groups, Sheep Camp is one of the great trail camps of the Los Padres. At 8,221 feet above sea level, it is also (by far) the highest trail camp in the Los Padres. Water here is available year-round from a small spring seeping through the porous, decomposed granite of Sawmill Mountain's southwest slopes. At its edge the camp offers sweeping westward views of the San Emigdio Mesa.

Used by San Joaquin Valley ranchers in the early 20th century, Sheep contains three sites; the northernmost is a small affair set beneath a cluster of pines and contains one stove. A second (and generally the least desirable) site is situated closest to the spring, and the largest site is on the lower flat overlooking the mesa. Great horned owls often sit sentinel in these mature woods at night, hooting under some of the clearest night skies found anywhere this side of the deserts.

From Sheep Camp, the trail climbs to another iris-laden spring, and beneath lightning-blasted pines it leads you to the **junction (6.8 miles, 8,500', 300990E 3854562N)** with the Vincent Tumamait Trail (*Route 69*). Heading left (west) here leads toward Grouse Mountain and Cerro Noreste (Mt. Abel), as well as the junction with the Mesa Spring Trail (see *Route 70*) at Puerto Suelo.

Heading right (west) here will lead along the Tumamait over Sawmill Mountain to Mt. Pinos.

Route 72

McGILL TRAIL (21W02)

LENGTH AND TYPE:	3.7-mile one-way
RATING:	Easy south to north (downhill); moderate north to south (climb)
TRAIL CONDITION:	Clear (well maintained and popular mountain bike route)
MAP(S):	USGS *Cuddy Valley*
CAMP(S):	—
HIGHLIGHTS:	Excellent views; conifer forest

TO REACH THE TRAILHEAD(S): Use the McGill Trailhead to access this route.

TRIP SUMMARY: From McGill Campground, this easy-to-follow route drops toward the edge of Cuddy Valley along Mount Pinos Highway. It is described from south to north (downhill).

Trip Description

This is one of the most popular mountain bike routes in the area, so the trail is in very good condition throughout the year (except when snowed-over). Be mindful of downhill riders, who often take this route at speed.

From the **trailhead (7,520', 307687E 3854422N)**, follow the trail southward up the hill and through a gap to the **junction (0.2 mile, 7,590', 307734E 3854738N)** with the alternate trail and old road. Benches are set beneath the shady stretches here. Head right here along the singletrack beneath mature Jeffrey pines and white firs; to your right are the short and well-maintained trails of the McGill grounds, including the Whitethorn Nature Trail and the sequoia trees planted there in 1972.

From here you'll begin the descent above the Cuddy Creek drainage, roughly following the ridgeline separating Cuddy and San Emigdio Creeks for a ways until committing to the Cuddy drainage and curving eastward. Massive conifer specimens and the occasional outcrop of granite provide very pleasant scenery, and the views down toward the valley and across to Frazier Park are usually superb.

Small oaks and piñon pines enter the mix along your descent to meet the lower signed **trailhead and parking area** (**3.7 miles, 6,250', 309177E 3856637N**).

For those interested in a marginally longer trek, the trail does continue another 0.5 mile here alongside the road to a second, **lower trailhead** (**4.1 miles, 6,050', 309127E 3857169N**) just up from the old San Emigdio pines plantation.

Pine Mountain

*This chapter details routes along, leading to,
or leading from Pine Mountain.*

A POPULAR CAMPING, CLIMBING, AND RECREATION AREA, Pine Mountain is an east-west trending massif spanning from Pine Mountain summit (5,160 feet) along CA 33 on the western edge to the gap between the Piedra Blanca and Beartrap watersheds on the east. It marks the boundary between the Mt. Pinos and Ojai Ranger Districts in this area.

To reach the road from Ojai, follow CA 33 31.5 miles north to the turnoff to your right (east) at the summit. From Lockwood and Cuyama Valleys, follow CA 33 south to the summit.

Forest Service Road 6N06 traces the mountain's spine. It was originally graded by the Shell Oil Company in the 1930s, but the prospective wells near Reyes Peak didn't yield enough oil to prove profitable, and the road eventually became the province of the US Forest Service (USFS). The road receives little maintenance these days, and while (usually) passable by passenger cars, it is better suited to high-clearance or 4WD vehicles. The road is typically closed from the first snow of the season until about Memorial Day.

Though rather sparse along the initial approach, as the road continues eastward and gains elevation, massive ponderosa and sugar pines begin to appear. There is no water along Pine Mountain Road, but restrooms are located at both campgrounds, as well as at the Reyes Peak Trailhead (at road's end).

Two car camps avail themselves to hikers—**Pine Mountain Campground (6,650', 286729E 3835510N)** and **Reyes Peak Campground (7,030', 287698E 3835385N)**. Both have only six sites, so they do tend to fill up quickly on weekends. A Forest Service Adventure Pass, federal Interagency Pass, or equivalent is required to park anywhere within the campground area (the pass doubles as your site fee). The campgrounds also happen to be situated adjacent to the most popular bouldering spots along the mountain.

Five of the six sites that comprise Pine Mountain are situated in a bowl (often referred to as "The Dustbowl" in dry summers) shaded by massive pines and firs. Just past the first

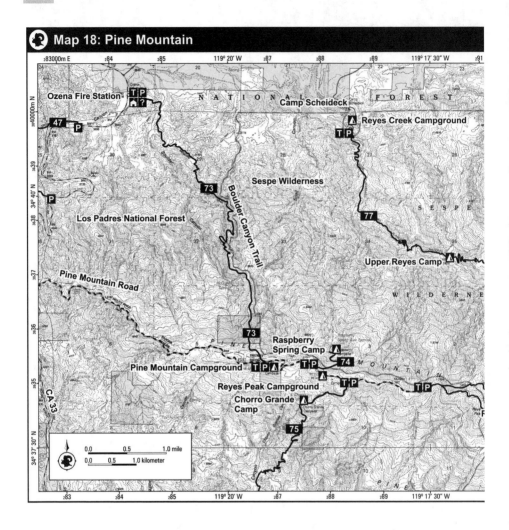

Map 18: Pine Mountain

site in camp is a small parking area and a use trail leading to the formation on the southern edge of the bowl known as "The Picnic Area." A sixth campsite is farther along the road, at the hairpin in the road near an old corral.

Reyes Peak Campground, its sites spread out alongside the road, features popular rock formations such as Happy Hunting Ground, The Keep, and Enlightenment Ridge, the latter perhaps being the most popular and situated just on the edge of the easternmost campsite. This is the site climbers look to secure first for a weekend of bouldering. Refer to Steve Edwards's *Rock Climbing Santa Barbara and Ventura* for detailed descriptions of the routes.

MAP 18 Pine Mountain   297

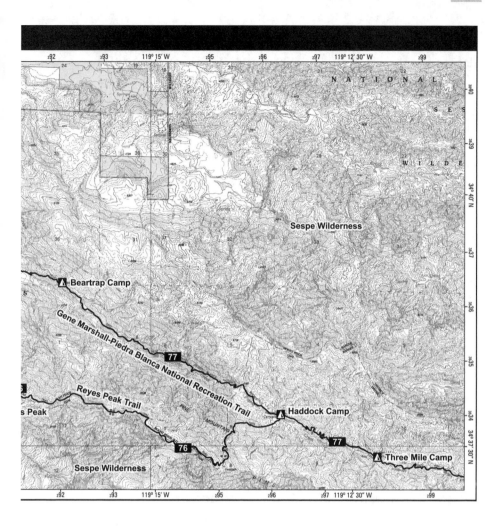

Pine Mountain Trailheads

FOUR TRAILHEADS are located along Pine Mountain Road: Boulder Canyon, Raspberry Spring, Upper Chorro Grande, and Reyes Peak.

Boulder Canyon Trailhead (6,650', 286729E 3835510N)

Located directly across the entrance to Pine Mountain Campground, the trailhead is 4.8 miles up Pine Mountain Road from the highway. Hikers typically park in the campground. From Pine Mountain summit, drive 4.8 miles to the Pine Mountain Campground. A small parking area ideal for day use is immediately to the left (east) of the camp entrance. A

Forest Service Adventure Pass, federal Interagency Pass, or equivalent is required to park in the camp; a restroom is available here. The trail leads to the Ozena Fire Station; see *Route 73* for the trail description.

Raspberry Spring Trailhead (7,030', 287698E 3835385N)

Located on the north side of Pine Mountain Road, the trailhead is just as one enters Reyes Peak Campground (5.7 miles from CA 33). A Forest Service Adventure Pass, federal Interagency Pass, or equivalent is required to park here; the campground's restroom is just up the road. The trail leads to Raspberry Spring Camp; see *Route 74* for the trail description.

Upper Chorro Grande Trailhead (7,160', 288335E 3835096N)

This trailhead is located on the south side of the road just beyond the last site of Reyes Peak Campground (6.1 miles from CA 33). There is only room for two vehicles here, but some parking can be had along the road as needed. No passes are required to park here, and there are no facilities. The trail leads southward toward Chorro Springs and Oak Camps and the highway; see *Route 75* for the trail description.

Reyes Peak Trailhead (6,980', 289829E 3834936N)

This trailhead is located at the end of Pine Mountain Road (7.1 miles from CA 33). No passes are required to park here, and there is a restroom. The trail here leads across the ridge via Haddock Mountain to the Gene Marshall–Piedra Blanca National Recreation Trail, as well as to Reyes Peak; see *Route 76* for the trail description.

Other Pine Mountain–Area Trailheads

Lower Chorro Grande Trailhead (4,085', 285821E 3831061N)   From the junction of CA 33 and CA 150 in Ojai, drive 25.5 miles north along CA 33 to a large dirt parking area on the left (south) side of the highway. Signage on both sides of the highway indicates that the trail's start is directly across the road. There are no facilities here.

Ozena Trailhead (3,570', 284289E 3840432N)   From Pine Mountain summit, 31.5 miles north of Ojai, continue 5.6 miles north along CA 33 to the Ozena Fire Station. Park here.

Potrero John Trailhead (3,660', 291918E 3829366N)   From the junction of CA 33 and CA 150 in Ojai, drive north along CA 33 approximately 21 miles to a small parking area on the right (north) side of the highway, just past the bridge over Potrero John Creek. The parking space has room enough for two vehicles; there are other spots along the south side of the road farther along, and a much larger space is on the Sespe side of the highway south of the Potrero John Trailhead.

Reyes Creek Trailhead (4,000', 288450E 3839739N) From the junction of CA 33 and CA 150 in Ojai, drive north along CA 33 (beyond the Pine Mountain summit) approximately 37 miles to Lockwood Valley Road. Proceed 3.5 miles east along Lockwood Valley Road to Forest Road 7N11 and turn right (south). Almost immediately the road crosses the Cuyama River; exercise caution (the road is not passable after heavy rain). Travel 1.75 miles through Camp Scheideck and into Reyes Creek Campground. Stay right and follow signage to the trailhead parking area. There are restrooms but no water available here.

Route 73

BOULDER CANYON (23W03)

LENGTH AND TYPE:	2.2-mile out-and-back to McGuire Spring; 5-mile one-way to Ozena Fire Station (shuttle)
RATING:	Easy south to north; moderately strenuous north to south (climb)
TRAIL CONDITION:	Clear along McGuire Trail; clear to passable on McGuire Spring spur trail
MAP(S):	USGS *Reyes Peak*; Harrison's *Sespe Wilderness*
CAMP(S):	McGuire Spring
HIGHLIGHTS:	Stands of sugar pines in the upper elevations and classic chaparral trekking at the lower elevations; excellent views of the San Emigdio badlands and Cuyama River Valley

TO REACH THE TRAILHEAD(S): Use the Boulder Canyon and/or Ozena Trailheads to access this route.

TRIP SUMMARY: From Pine Mountain car camp, this trail descends Boulder Canyon through high alpine conifer forest, oak woodland ravines, and hard chaparral to reach the Ozena Fire Station in Lockwood Valley.

Trip Description

From Pine Mountain car camp, cross Pine Mountain Road to the **Boulder Canyon Trailhead** (**6,650', 286729E 3835510N**), which is marked by a wooden sign that reads BOULDER CYN TR. Follow the trail for perhaps 100 yards under cover of massive Jeffrey pines and white firs before all climbing on this route is effectively ended and you drop onto the north-facing slope of the mountain. The area here is the fantastic landscape for which Pine Mountain is known—far cooler climes than the lower stretches of the forest, towering conifers (including numerous majestic sugar pines), and panoramic views of Lockwood Valley, the San Emigdio badlands, and the Cuyama drainage. Follow the route easily on the at-times steep descent toward an exposed knoll at the end of the low ridge you've been traversing. You'll begin to leave the tall pine forest for the more classic chaparral and scrub dotted with manzanitas, oaks, and mountain mahoganies and zigzag down an easy series of long switchbacks with great views of the deep cleft that is Boulder Canyon to your left (west) before crossing the east fork of **Boulder Creek (2.1 miles, 5,010', 286060E 3837739N)**. Your progress along the north- and east-facing slopes of the drainages here will be shaded by heavy oak woodlands (watch the leaves and acorns, as they can make portions of the track rather slippery), and the exposed portions are rocky with yuccas, high grasses, and hard chaparral. This section makes for a fairly steep descent.

After crossing another tributary to Boulder Creek, you'll continue to drop rather quickly—alternately along exposed rocky ridges and scrub-laden slopes—until reaching the junction with the old **Ozena (or Snail Canyon) Trail (2.9 miles, 4,100', 285885E 3838560N)**. In decades past this trail—the old 23W29—led to Ozena Campground and an eastward connector led to Camp Scheideck and the Reyes Creek Trailhead. Be sure to stay left (south) here and not drop into the Snail Canyon drainage (unless that is your intended route; Snail Canyon is not detailed herein).

From the Snail Canyon junction, a very short climb allows you to gain a series of easy ridges and drop farther into the Boulder drainage; if you listen carefully you can often hear the fire station's public address system squawking farther down the canyon. Impressive stands of manzanitas with waist-thick trunks usher you into a small sage-carpeted **basin (3.6 miles, 4,000', 285514E 3839241N)**. Here the trail levels out considerably and leads you along the drainage to a crossing of the main branch of **Boulder Creek (4.5 miles, 3,670', 284880E 3840211N)**. Cattle sometimes gain access to this portion of the trail and can be found grazing; make every attempt to not spook them if you encounter them on this stretch. From the creek, you'll climb easily to a **gap (4.6 miles, 3,700', 284801E 3840324N)** with a view of the Ozena Fire Station.

It's an easy drop to the **livestock gate (4.8 miles, 3,650', 284660E 3840374N)**—marked with another wooden BOULDER CYN TR sign—and into the wide field occupied by the fire station, and then on to the **parking area (5 miles, 3,570', 284289E 3840432N)** in front of the station.

Route 74

RASPBERRY SPRING (23W02)

LENGTH AND TYPE:	1-mile out-and-back
RATING:	Moderate (steep return)

TRAIL CONDITION:	Clear
MAP(S):	USGS *Reyes Peak;* Harrison's *Sespe Wilderness*
CAMP(S):	Raspberry Spring
HIGHLIGHTS:	Lunch spot; stands of sugar pines; excellent views of the San Emigdio badlands and Cuyama River Valley

TO REACH THE TRAILHEAD(S): Use the Raspberry Spring Trailhead to access this route.

TRIP SUMMARY: From Reyes Peak car camp, the Raspberry Spring Trail (23W02) descends through mature conifer stands to the Raspberry Spring Camp and namesake spring.

Trip Description

This short and very pleasant hike begins at the parking area on the western edge of Reyes Peak Campground. From the trailhead, proceed eastward down the well-shaded trail. Steep at times, the trail opens to a small meadow shortly, and then switchbacks westward. Jeffery pines, white firs, and towering sugar pines dominate the forest here. After another series of well-spaced and rather casual switchbacks, the view opens to reveal a wide expanse of the Cuyama Valley and drops you into **Raspberry Spring Camp (0.4 mile, 6,640', 288021E 3835588N)**.

Raspberry Spring proper (**0.5 mile, 6,600', 287970E 3835636N**) is another 0.1 mile west along the trail, at the very beginning of a steep ravine. Here you'll find a lush and narrow little

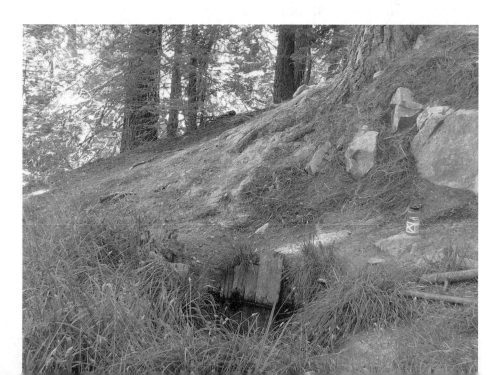

ledge with an old spring casing at the base of several white firs. The water should be filtered, but this spring is usually a reliable source. And as the name states, a number of raspberry brambles can be found along the spring's watershed; the berries typically grow in midsummer.

The return to camp from the spring is quite steep.

CAMP :: RASPBERRY SPRING

ELEVATION:	6,640'
MAP:	USGS *Reyes Peak*
UTM:	288021E 3835588N

A secluded camp set among mature Jeffery pines, white firs, and sugar pines, Raspberry Spring Camp is situated on a narrow strip of trailside forest and the last fairly level space before the north slope of Pine Mountain drops precipitously. There are three camps: one is a barren spot with two stoves mere feet off the trail; the second is just downslope along a short spur trail; and the third (and perhaps best) is to the right (east) of the trail before the drop into the "main" camp. Veer right (east) off the trail just prior to entering the obvious camp and trek 50 feet to a seldom-used site with ample space and a comfortable cooking area.

Route 75

CHORRO GRANDE (23W05)

LENGTH AND TYPE:	5.1-mile one-way
RATING:	Moderate north to south; strenuous south to north
TRAIL CONDITION:	Clear
MAP(S):	USGS *Reyes Peak* and *Wheeler Springs;* Harrison's *Sespe Wilderness*
CAMP(S):	Chorro Springs and Oak
HIGHLIGHTS:	Great views of the Sespe watershed; unique geology

TO REACH THE TRAILHEAD(S): Use the Upper and/or Lower Chorro Grande Trailheads to access this route.

TRIP SUMMARY: From Reyes Peak car camp, the Chorro Grande Trail (23W05) descends through conifer forest, chaparral, and willow-laden streambeds to the lower trailhead alongside CA 33. This trip can be modified a number of ways; for an easy trip, Oak Camp can be accessed from the lower Chorro Grande Trailhead in only 1.7 miles; Chorro Springs Camp is accessible in 0.8 mile from Reyes Peak. This trip can also be done in reverse (south to north) for a challenging climb of 3,000 feet vertical gain.

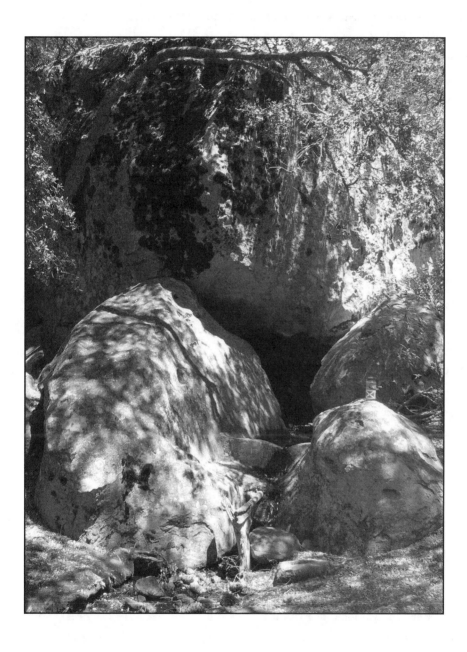

Trip Description

From the **Upper Chorro Grande Trailhead (7,160', 288335E 3835096N)**, quickly descend through scrub and the lower reaches of the mountain's sugar pine stands amid fascinating boulder formations into **Chorro Springs Camp (0.8 mile, 6,440', 287417E 3834736N)**. Here you'll find a massive boulder with a reliable spring bubbling from beneath. The large oaks make for an ideal rest spot.

CAMP :: CHORRO SPRINGS

ELEVATION:	6,440'
MAP:	USGS *Reyes Peak*
UTM:	287417E 3834736N

Chorro Springs Camp is a great spot for picnickers and campers alike. The main site is situated among gnarled interior oaks; a second—and more private—site is just west, in a narrower side canyon beneath large ponderosa pines. A few yards down-trail, you'll find a third kitchen area with a New Deal–era ice can stove still intact.

From camp, continue southward along a series of switchbacks, quickly leaving the forest for the more exposed chaparral of Pine Mountain's southerly flank. The views here of the Sespe drainage are expansive, and ceanothus, mountain mahoganies, and manzanitas dominate the hillsides, interrupted only by occasional stands of bigcone Douglas-firs and bare rock. For much of the next few miles you'll have a view of the Sespe and the highway where your second vehicle is parked. The going is rocky and steep in places.

After passing through an exposed knoll of small boulders, another series of switchbacks leads you to the **intersection (2.8 miles, 4,740', 286500E 3833300N)** with Gypsum Mine Road (a dirt service road popular with field geologists and fossil hunters that cuts westward along Pine Mountain's flanks) and a spur trail leading eastward toward Burro and Munson Creeks. Just up-canyon is the riverside flat where once stood Three Pines Camp, flooded out in 1973 and never replaced.

Your route here picks up an old jeep trail, and as a result the going is far more level than what you've just come down. Pass through a glade of low scrub and tall grass to the trail marker on the right indicating **Oak Camp (3.4 miles, 4,650', 286404E 3832790N)**, a pleasant site set beneath (appropriately enough) a large coppice of interior oaks. *Note:* Many maps— among them the USGS *Wheeler Springs* 7.5-minute and the USFS Los Padres National Forest (South) maps—incorrectly place this camp to the east of the trail.

CAMP :: OAK

ELEVATION:	4,650'
MAP:	USGS *Wheeler Springs*
UTM:	286404E 3832790N

Oak Camp is a pleasant series of three sites set beneath a canopy of interior live oaks. Chorro Grande runs along the western edge of camp, providing semi-reliable water in all but the driest periods. Three stoves are here; the nicest is the one farthest up-canyon, set comfortably beside the creek.

From Oak Camp, the final 1.7 miles down the drainage takes you across formations of unique Sespe sandstone, crossing the creek and tributaries a handful of times and cutting across sand and conglomerate rock at many points. The final 0.5 mile of your trek is along rolling hillside trail as you descend back to the **parking area** across CA 33 (**5.1 miles, 4,085', 285799E 3831052N**).

Route 76

REYES PEAK TRAIL (23W04)

LENGTH AND TYPE:	5.8-mile one-way to Haddock junction; 2-mile out-and-back to Reyes Peak
RATING:	Moderate
TRAIL CONDITION:	Clear
MAP(S):	USGS *Reyes Peak, Lion Canyon,* and *San Guillermo Mountain;* Harrison's *Sespe Wilderness*
CAMP(S):	—
HIGHLIGHTS:	Old lookout site atop Reyes Peak; fantastic views of the Cuyama Valley, Mt. Pinos, and the Pacific; conifer forest

TO REACH THE TRAILHEAD(S): Use the Reyes Peak Trailhead to access this route. As of early 2012, a Forest Service Adventure Pass is not required to park at the Reyes Peak Trailhead (but it or an equivalent is necessary to park within the boundaries of the two campgrounds farther down Pine Mountain Road). There is a restroom but no other facilities here.

TRIP SUMMARY: This route traverses the central stretch of the Pine Mountain massif from Reyes Peak and across Haddock Mountain through mature high-elevation pine forest. It terminates at the saddle dividing the Beartrap and Piedra Blanca watersheds (the junction with the Gene Marshall–Piedra Blanca National Recreation Trail).

Trip Description

From the **Reyes Peak Trailhead (6,980', 289829E 3834936N)**, follow the trail (formerly a service road) eastward and over a rise approximately 250 yards to a **split (0.15 mile, 7,000', 290048E 3834992N)**. The right (southern) fork that winds southward down the slope along the retired road will lead you to an old flat, but *not* to Reyes Peak (this is a common mistake). To reach Reyes Peak, follow the middle fork (sometimes poorly defined at this junction) that heads southeast up the flank of the mountain and refer to the "Reyes Peak" sidebar below.

REYES PEAK ▦ ▦ ▦ ▦ ▦ ▦ ▦ ▦ ▦ ▦ ▦ ▦

"The top of Reyes Peak was lit by the fire of sunset, and a soft wind from the sea moved through the pines."

Louis L'Amour, *The Californios*

There is no longer an *official* system trail to reach Reyes Peak—the highest point along Pine Mountain—but the use trail receives frequent use from peak-baggers and hiking groups. This route was established by Forest Service rangers and used heavily during the life of the Reyes Peak Lookout (1927–1932).

From the **junction (0.15 mile, 7,000', 290048E 3834992N)** with the old road and Reyes Peak Trail, follow the middle of the three trails to the southeast and up a rather steep 0.25 mile through the sandstone outcrops, towering ponderosa pines, and white firs before leveling off. Continue rather easily along a ridgeline with fantastic views of the Cuyama and badlands to the north and the Sespe drainage and beyond to the south. A second short climb will lead you to a glade situated between a tree-shaded peak to the north and a cluster of rocks to the south. Follow the track through the grass to the base of those projecting rocks.

An easy scramble up these rocks will bring you to the top of **Reyes Peak (1 mile, 7,514', 290941E 3834467N)**. Just to the northeast of the USGS monument, you'll spy the remaining timbers and bolts where once stood the Reyes Peak fire lookout, destroyed by the infamous Matilija Fire in 1932.

▦ ▦ ▦ ▦ ▦ ▦ ▦ ▦ ▦ ▦ ▦ ▦ ▦ ▦ ▦ ▦

To traverse the length of the Reyes Peak Trail eastward toward Haddock Mountain and the junction with the Gene Marshall–Piedra Blanca National Recreation Trail, follow the left (northeast) fork at the early split and continue beneath the towering sugar and ponderosa pines. In short time you'll pass into the Sespe Wilderness while traversing the northern flank of Reyes Peak. The terrain here is well shaded, lush, and quite simply one of the most beautiful stretches in the southern Los Padres. The massive firs and ponderosa, sugar, and Jeffrey pines will remind you why this area was named Pine Mountain—this is the stretch of forest that bears it out.

Once beyond the slopes of Reyes Peak, the vistas open and views of the Cuyama, Lockwood Valley, and points north are impressive. The first 1.5 miles of this route pass quickly; it is overall quite level and the tread is in fine shape. Shortly you'll begin an undulating series of false summits, with the south- and southwest-facing strata of Haddock Mountain looming ahead. On a clear day, views can reach from the Channel Islands to your south and the southern Sierra Nevada to your north as you pass out of the thicker trees into a more open land of sandstone formations and grass clearings. Every so often the trail passes very close to the sheer drop-offs that are the very upper headwaters of the Derrydale drainage, so do mind any four-legged companions.

As you continue eastward, the actual peak of **Haddock Mountain** is some 50 feet south of the trail (**4 miles, 7,431', 294573E 3833584N**), not to be confused with the nearby survey marker by the same name shown on topographic maps. Farther on are some more rock formations and guer-

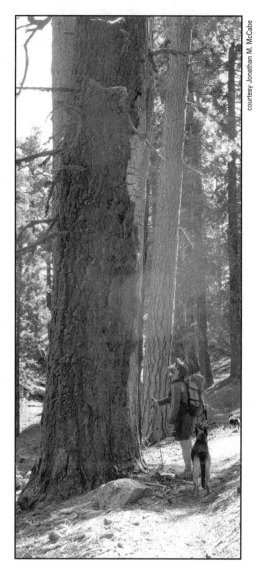

Along the Reyes Peak Trail

rilla campsites used in decades past. Just as you pass a very old wooden sign informing you that you are indeed on Haddock Mountain, the trail begins the descent toward the Piedra Blanca Trail. More exposed than much of your earlier route, this stretch of trail switchbacks along some pretty steep terrain, but all the while with excellent views (primarily of Beartrap Canyon and points north), ushering you to the **junction** (**5.8 miles, 6,110', 296097E 3834276N**) with the Gene Marshall–Piedra Blanca National Recreation Trail; see *Route 77*.

Route 77

GENE MARSHALL–PIEDRA BLANCA
NATIONAL RECREATION TRAIL (22W03)

LENGTH AND TYPE:	18.5-mile one-way (shuttle)
RATING:	Moderate to strenuous
TRAIL CONDITION:	Clear to Beartrap Camp; passable between Beartrap Camp and Haddock Saddle (seasonal); clear between Haddock and Sespe
MAP(S):	USGS *Reyes Peak*, *San Guillermo Mountain*, and *Lion Canyon*; Harrison's *Sespe Wilderness*
CAMP(S):	Upper Reyes, Beartrap, Haddock, Three Mile, Pine Mountain Lodge, Twin Forks, and Piedra Blanca
HIGHLIGHTS:	Expansive views of the Cuyama Valley and Sespe River drainage; incense cedar and sugar pine stands; the Piedra Blanca formation

TO REACH THE TRAILHEAD(S): Use the Reyes Creek and Piedra Blanca Trailheads for this shuttle.

TRIP SUMMARY: The Gene Marshall–Piedra Blanca National Recreation Trail (NRT) follows Raspberry Creek (officially unnamed) up and over into the Reyes Creek drainage, and then again into the Beartrap Creek watershed. The trail ascends the north slope of Pine Mountain, reaching its crest at a saddle just south of the Reyes Peak Trail, and then descends into the scrub and rock formations of the Piedra Blanca and Sespe watersheds.

Trip Description

Begin this hike at the southwest corner of the **parking area** (4,000', 288450E 3839739N) adjacent to Reyes Creek Campground. Almost immediately you'll cross the creek (there is often poison oak here) and climb gradually into the Sespe Wilderness along the Raspberry drainage's west banks. A few switchbacks under the cover of oaks provide your initial elevation gain, and then a gentler ascent leads along the drainage, crossing the main watershed a handful of times before veering southeast to follow a thinner and steeper drainage fork after about 1.5 miles.

The drainages here are dominated by alders, oaks, and mixed conifers. The ascent out of the watershed and toward the exposed saddle between Raspberry and Reyes is classic chaparral, dotted with yuccas and singleleaf piñons.

Continue climbing to a **saddle** (2.5 miles, 4,900', 289463E 3837540N). Across the canyon, the switchbacks that will lead you out of Reyes Creek can be spotted zigzagging up the mountainside. From this initial saddle, the trail descends quickly into the Reyes Creek drainage. The trail crosses a tributary to the main Reyes Creek and then enters a stretch of thicker conifers—predominantly incense cedars—and soon leads to **Upper Reyes Camp** (**3 miles, 4,675', 290236E 3837319N**). The creek here is year-round and accessible just up the trail (the crossing also makes an ideal lunch spot).

CAMP :: UPPER REYES

ELEVATION:	4,675'
MAP:	USGS *Reyes Peak*
UTM:	290236E 3837319N

The first established camp as one hikes south along the trail, Upper Reyes consists of two sites, one on each side of the creek. The first site—and that preferred by most backpackers—is situated west of the creek within a small coppice of mature incense cedars and includes a stove. Occasionally used by horse packers, this spot has room enough for a few tents in the main area of camp and on a higher flat area just west of the kitchen.

The other site also possesses a single stove and is about 200 feet farther along the trail and across Reyes Creek beneath a large and multitrunked inland oak. This site isn't quite as comfortable and has less usable level space, but it's a suitable alternative if the main site is already occupied.

From Upper Reyes, your ascent out of the watershed begins quickly, and the switchbacks climb immediately after the second camp. In the spring the thick scrub and buckthorns here can be an impediment. After a steady climb—often dotted with mariposa lilies in the spring and early summer—you'll reach the **saddle** (**4.5 miles, 5,380', 291409E 3836961N**) between the Reyes and Beartrap Creek watersheds.

The descent toward Beartrap Creek is steep at points and is a marked contrast from the exposed and rocky slopes of Reyes Creek just hiked. Here the conifers and oaks, along with the canyon's steeper slopes, provide ample shade and are usually much cooler. A small **saddle** (**4.7 miles, 5,200', 291937E 3836855N**) provides a vantage point from which the main Beartrap Camp area can easily be identified below—a lone ponderosa pine stands sentinel among the incense cedars.

From this saddle, drop into the shaded and tree-covered creek bed. The trail here crosses Beartrap Creek and then bears right (south). The main **Beartrap Camp** (**4.8 miles, 5,100', 292052E 3836763N**) is on a flat just upstream from the crossing, but there are two small sites ideal for solo trekkers or a pair just downstream (left of the trail). These sites are seldom used, but both have stoves and room enough for a small tent.

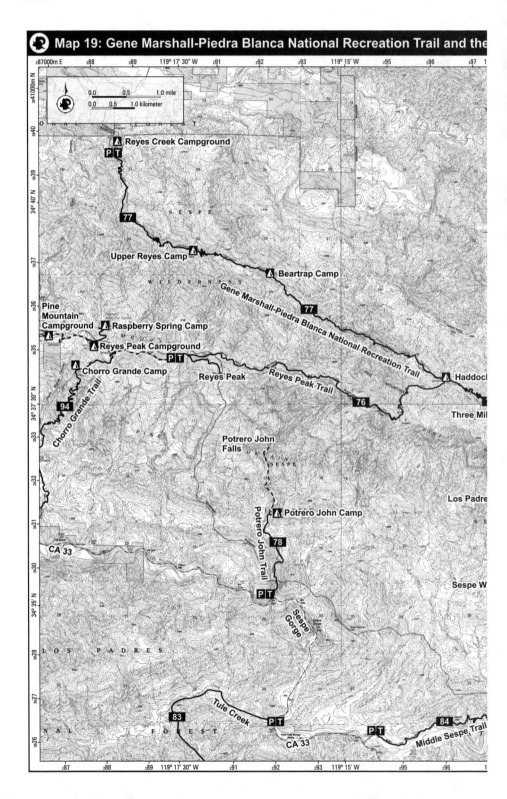

Map 19: Gene Marshall-Piedra Blanca National Recreation Trail and the

MAP 19 Gene Marshall–Piedra Blanca NRT and the Upper Piru 311

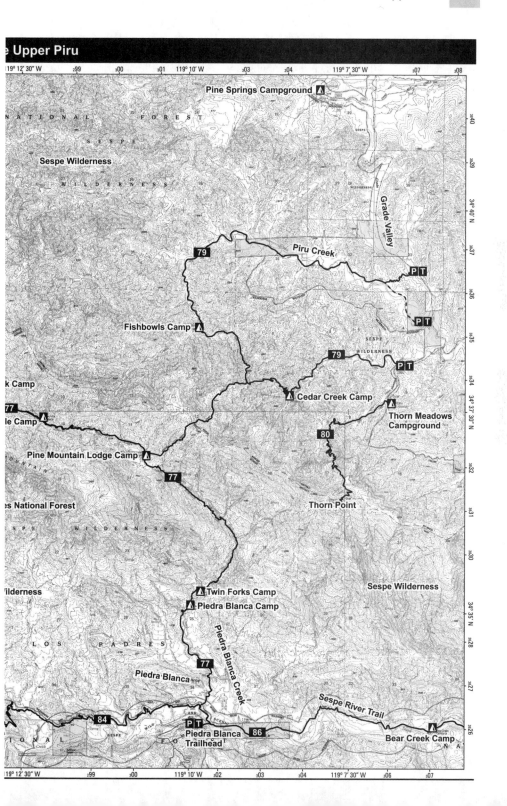

Upper Piru

119° 12' 30" W   ₂99   ₃00   ₃01   119° 10' W   ₃03   ₃04   119° 7' 30" W   ₃07   ₃08

Pine Springs Campground

NATIONAL   FOREST

SESPE

Sespe Wilderness

WILDERNESS

₃₆40

₃₆39

34° 40' N

Grade Valley

79   Piru Creek   ₃₆37

P T   ₃₆36

Fishbowls Camp   P T   ₃₆35

SESPE
WILDERNESS

79   P T   ₃₆34   34° 37' 30" N

k Camp

77   Cedar Creek Camp   Thorn Meadows
Campground

le Camp

Pine Mountain Lodge Camp   80   ₃₆32

77

es National Forest   Thorn Point   ₃₆31

SESPE   WILDERNESS

ilderness   ₃₆30

Sespe Wilderness

Twin Forks Camp   34° 35' N

Piedra Blanca Camp   ₃₆28

LOS   PADRES

Piedra Blanca Creek

₃₆27

Piedra Blanca   77

Sespe River Trail

84   ₃₆26

P T   Piedra Blanca   86   Bear Creek Camp
Trailhead   N A

IONAL   SESPE   FO

119° 12' 30" W   ₂99   ₃00   119° 10' W   ₃02   ₃03   ₃04   119° 7' 30" W   ₃06   ₃07

Named for the hunting activities conducted in this area in the late 19th century, Beartrap Creek is a perennial creek, and the main camp is situated within a narrow and lush portion of the canyon.

CAMP :: BEARTRAP

ELEVATION:	5,100'
MAP:	USGS *Reyes Peak*
UTM:	292052E 3836763N

Beartrap Camp actually consists of three camp areas, with a total of five cooking areas. The main camp is situated on a large flat along the creek's east bank, buttressed by two large incense cedars and immediately recognizable by the towering ponderosa pine near the base of the eastern hillside. The lower of the two cooking areas here possesses two stoves (one of these is quite possibly a stove from the old Beartrap No. 2 campsite up-canyon, which was washed out in the 1974 floods).

Two smaller camps are downstream from where the trail crosses the creek, west of the creek and about 100 yards from the main sites. These are seldom used and quite secluded, under cover of bigcone Douglas-firs and incense cedars.

The fifth cooking area is about 300 yards upstream on a flat on the creek's west bank, beneath a group of fire-scarred incense cedars. Its stove is likely the other survivor from Beartrap No. 2.

From the main clearing, continue upstream (south) toward Pine Mountain and the Haddock Saddle. This, the least-traveled section of the trail, is often overgrown (especially in late spring) and entails numerous stream crossings. A mile from camp is the clearing where once stood the **Beartrap No. 2 sites (6 miles, 5,320', 293291E 3835681N)**, washed out in 1974. The trail climbs easily as the canyon narrows, eventually reaching the drier headwaters of the creek. Here there are numerous rock formations on the canyon's left (east) side.

From these rocks, the switchbacks lead steeply up. Sugar pines, after which Pine Mountain is named, begin to appear along the western slopes; their long, distinctive cones are often scattered along the trail.

After the trail **summits (7.6 miles, 6,262', 295351E 3834764N)**, you'll descend gradually into the Piedra Blanca Creek drainage. Here manzanitas begin to reappear, and stands of pines dominate much of the terrain.

Three quarters of a mile from the trail summit is the junction with trail 23W04, which leads nearly 6 miles west along Haddock Mountain and Reyes Peak to the Reyes Peak Trailhead (see *Route 76*). Just beyond this junction is **Haddock Camp (8.3 miles, 6,110', 296150E 3834286N)**.

■ ■ ■ ■ ■ ■ ■ ■ ■ EAST FORK BEARTRAP

Until the mid-1960s, there was another trail roughly parallel to the main trail now known as the Gene Marshall–Piedra Blanca NRT. Trail 23W01—East Beartrap Trail— climbed from the saddle between the Beartrap and Piedra Blanca drainages, heading north along the Ojai and Mt. Pinos Ranger District boundary to gain the ridge between these drainages and those leading to Piru Creek in the east. The route then followed this ridge in a generally northwesterly direction, before dropping into the watershed of Beartrap Creek's eastern fork just as one was directly above Beartrap Site No. 1.

The route then followed the east fork to its confluence with the main fork, and then westward and finally south again to meet the Cuyama River at Dry Canyon. The lower (northern) portion of this traverse isn't practical any longer, as the area is quite over-grown, but the hearty (and ambitious!) can still make a trek of the higher ridge between Haddock Saddle and Beartrap No. 1; with care it's possible to descend into the main fork of the creek along those rock formations set along the camp's eastern edge.

■ ■ ■ ■ ■ ■ ■ ■ ■ ■ ■ ■ ■ ■ ■ ■ ■

CAMP :: HADDOCK

ELEVATION:	6,110'
MAP:	USGS *San Guillermo Mountain*
UTM:	296150E 3834286N

A spacious site situated on a grass-covered flat along Piedra Blanca Creek, Haddock possesses four recent-model stoves. The primary kitchen is the first encountered from the north, beneath a large ponderosa and some Jeffrey pines, with easy access to the creek. The second is northwest along the flat. The site can accommodate larger groups.

From Haddock, continue southeast through mixed conifer terrain. You'll note increasing numbers of white firs and enjoy a fairly level trail for 2 miles. What elevation is gained is lost in a quick descent just before **Three Mile Camp** (**10.2 miles, 5,900', 298016E 3833385N**), set comfortably beside the increasingly reliable Piedra Blanca Creek.

CAMP :: THREE MILE

ELEVATION:	5,900'
MAP:	USGS *Lion Canyon*
UTM:	298016E 3833385N

A comfortable creekside site with three stoves and an aged picnic table, Three Mile is surrounded by a handful of mature incense cedars.

From Three Mile Camp continue east up and over a series of four knolls over the course of 2 miles, moving away from the main Piedra Blanca Creek drainage.

Just beyond the easternmost tributary to the main fork of Piedra Blanca Creek lies the **Pine Mountain Lodge** campsite (**12 miles, 6,000', 300395E 3832665N**). The junction of the Cedar Creek Trail (21W10) is in the very center of camp (see *Route 79*).

CAMP :: PINE MOUNTAIN LODGE

ELEVATION:	6,000'
MAP:	USGS *Lion Canyon*
UTM:	300395E 3832665N

An exposed and overused site, Pine Mountain Lodge is named after the cabin built in this area in the 1890s by a group of hunters and outdoorsmen known as the Sisquoc Rangers. The lodge was accidentally destroyed in the mid-1940s during a failed attempt by the Forest Service to fell some diseased trees nearby, and over the decades its remnants have been dismantled and scattered.

Four fire rings are in the main site, the most popular situated beneath a pair of mature incense cedars. A fifth ring is a short walk east down the Cedar Creek Trail. Nearby in a grassy meadow is the more remote and original Pine Mountain Lodge camp, complete with an old picnic table and stove.

Though it can reduce to a trickle in the summer, the spring just north of camp can generally be relied upon. It issues from a narrow crevice in the large rocks situated upstream. Signage at the campsite is antiquated and displays older trail designations but overall remains accurate.

Just beyond the small meadow south of the camps, you'll enter a final pine flat, and then drop quite steeply into the drainage of the North Fork of Piedra Blanca Creek. The conifers give way to oaks and chaparral quickly, and large rocks inlaid with Eocene-era molluscan fossils litter the trail.

In 3 miles the trail drops nearly 2,400 feet, and on this exposed southerly aspect, it can make for a very hot descent (or ascent, for the hardy) in the summer months. After 2.5 miles the trail meets the North Fork's creek bed and levels out to follow the creek toward the confluence with the main Piedra Blanca Creek. Among the varied flora, Matilija poppies begin to appear. Be mindful that in spring, poison oak becomes abundant along this stretch. Alders populate the creek banks and provide opportunities for shade.

Just upstream from the confluence of Piedra Blanca Creek's north and main forks, a short spur trail leads left (east) over the creek and up to **Twin Forks Camp** (**15.3 miles, 3,620', 301609E 3829485N**).

CAMP :: TWIN FORKS

ELEVATION:	3,620'
MAP:	USGS *Lion Canyon*
UTM:	301609E 3829485N

Twin Forks is a small site set on a flat above the creek. There is one stove at the main site, but little room for tents. Sleeping space is available on another flat behind camp, near a squat mature oak.

Another site downstream from the main camp has a fire ring and sandier soil but less shade. The site's access to the creek is often obstructed by poison oak in the spring.

From Twin Forks, it is approximately 0.25 mile downstream along the trail to **Piedra Blanca Camp** (**15.6 miles, 3,550', 301345E 3829173N**).

CAMP :: PIEDRA BLANCA

ELEVATION:	3,550'
MAP:	USGS *Lion Canyon*
UTM:	301345E 3829173N

A wide, relatively flat site dominated by massive oaks, Piedra Blanca is popular with day-trippers. Both the main site (two stoves) and a smaller site (one stove) just downstream continue to recover from fire damage. Easy access to the creek and space enough for large groups make this a comfortable first night in for youth groups.

From Piedra Blanca, the trail is typically well traveled and free of the overgrowth that can often define the previous stretches of trail.

Heading toward the Sespe River, the going is quite easy as the trail parallels the creek along its right (west) bank for approximately 1.5 miles, and then angles away from the creek toward the **Piedra Blanca formation** (**17 miles, 3,300', 301781E 3827334N**).

The trail crosses another tributary and then quickly gains about 150 feet before leveling out in the rock formations that are the region's landmark. For approximately 0.75 mile, you'll bisect the formation before opening into the chaparral along the Sespe.

At the **junction** (**17.7 miles, 3,100', 301539E 3826834N**) of the Middle Sespe Trail (22W04)—see *Route 84*—bear left (southeast) and then after another 0.5 mile bear right (southwest) at the next **junction** (**18.1 miles, 3,000', 301843E 3826401N**; see *Route 86*), heading toward the trailhead and parking area across the river.

In the trail's present configuration, you'll cross the Sespe River three times to double back and wind your way up to the old Lion Campground, now the **Piedra Blanca Trailhead** (**18.5 miles, 3,040', 301320E 3826437N**).

Route 78

POTRERO JOHN (23W06)

LENGTH AND TYPE:	3.4-mile out-and-back to campground; 6.2-mile out-and-back to falls
RATING:	Easy
TRAIL CONDITION:	Clear
MAP(S):	USGS *Wheeler Springs*; Harrison's *Sespe Wilderness*
CAMP(S):	Potrero John
HIGHLIGHTS:	Easy day hike; great backpacking route for first-timers; waterfall beyond camp

TO REACH THE TRAILHEAD(S): Use the Potrero John Trailhead to access this route.

Approaching Potrero John Camp

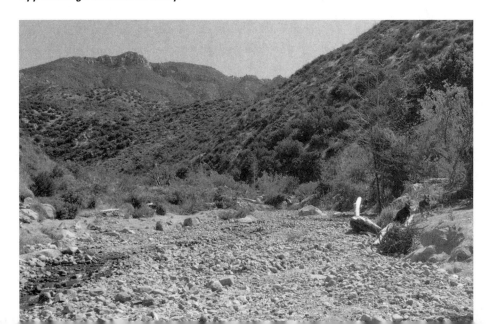

The large rock wall just downstream from the confluence of Potrero John and Sespe Creeks is the well-known Sespe Wall, popular with climbers the world over. Climbers can often be seen on the large (southern) wall on weekends, and more casual climbers often scramble around the Potrero John and Black Walls just upstream (near the Derrydale confluence).

TRIP SUMMARY: From the turnout along CA 33, this easy hike follows Potrero John Creek from its confluence with the Sespe to a campsite set beneath large live oaks. A more challenging rock-hop beyond camp leads to a series of waterfalls. The canyon is named for John Power, who lived in the area in the late 19th century.

Note: In January 2010 a flash flood tore through the canyon, scouring the streambed and washing out several portions of the old trail; in the years following there are likely to be numerous permutations and side trails based upon the old route, which had largely been static for decades. While there are some reports of the lower trail having totally vanished, such hyperbole has not proven to be the case; Potrero John is still very easy to navigate. Simply know the specific route will be in flux for the foreseeable future.

Trip Description

From the **parking area (3,660', 291918E 3829366N)** just west of the bridge, follow the trail eastward behind the highway railing and toward the creek (be especially cautious of poison oak here). The trail quickly cuts left (north) to lead you along an easy creekside flat. Approximately 500 feet from the parking area you'll cross a large jumble of **rockfall (500 feet, 3,680', 291974E 3829459N)**. Dropping down off the other side of the jumble will lead you along a pleasantly shaded stretch and then drop down into the first of numerous creek crossings. In the drainage is where damage from the flash flood is most apparent; logjams and debris are still present.

Drop from the rocky jumble back onto the easy trail, and soon you'll make your first crossing and ascend the opposite bank to a guerrilla camp set on a high flat in this narrow portion of the canyon. A large incense cedar and several oaks populate the trailside here; on either side of the canyon bigcone Douglas-firs cling to the fairly steep and rocky canyon walls, while cottonwoods, live oaks, and alders line your route along the stream channel. In the spring, Matilija poppies and mariposa lilies are among the numerous trailside flora.

From the guerrilla camp, drop back into the creek to cross again and climb the other side amid blackberry brambles and more poison oak. This crisscrossing continues a handful of times (you'll pass the post marking the Sespe Wilderness boundary, and numerous wading pools make for tempting rest stops) until you reach the namesake potrero (often said to be Spanish for "meadow" but perhaps more accurately "grazing pasture for horses") after nearly a mile. This stretch was high enough and far enough from the debris flow that it has remained intact post-flooding.

Follow the easy trail toward a solitary oak at the far end of the potrero, where you'll find the **spur trail (1.6 miles, 4,210', 291931E 3831372N)** leading across the creek to **Potrero John Camp (1.7 miles, 4,200', 291959E 3831374N)**.

CAMP :: POTRERO JOHN

ELEVATION:	4,200'
MAP:	USGS *Wheeler Springs*
UTM:	291959E 3831374N

A pleasant site set beneath a cluster of mature live oaks and nestled beside a steep rock escarpment, Potrero John Camp is an easy destination for first-time backpackers and little legs. One main kitchen in the lower part of camp consists of a large grill, and there are usually makeshift log benches. There is room enough for two or three tents; above camp there are some additional spots.

Water can usually be had from the creek in all but the driest of times. Once lined by alders along the creek, the camp now meets the cobble-strewn shore of the "new-look" (post-flood) wash; this site is popular with Scout groups on weekends.

POTRERO JOHN FALLS ▦ ▦ ▦ ▦ ▦ ▦ ▦ ▦ ▦ ▦ ▦

For those interested in a longer day than the easy trip into Potrero John Camp, the falls upstream are a good exercise in rock-hopping and riparian cross-country trekking. In the years before 2010's flood, accessing the falls generally entailed following an unofficial trail—the condition of which varied greatly depending on season and whether any industrious volunteers had recently worked the route—and scrambling along old debris piles. All that has changed, and the pleasant, bigcone Douglas-fir shaded stretches of trail will likely fall into disuse, while the channel bed remains clear and easily accessed.

From the **junction (1.6 miles, 4,210', 291931E 3831372N)** with the main trail and the trail into camp, continue northward along the track as it curves through low yerba santas, manzanitas, and mountain mahoganies for 0.25 mile until it reaches the edge of the **wash (2.1 miles, 4,260', 291953E 3831778N)** along an east-west dogleg in the drainage. From here it's just as easy to follow the drainage as to try and stay along the trail, especially as the canyon narrows considerably and it curves back toward the north. Continue following the drainage to a stretch of exposed rock—an excellent naturally carved stone wading **pool (2.9 miles, 4,610', 291831E 3832736N)** is here.

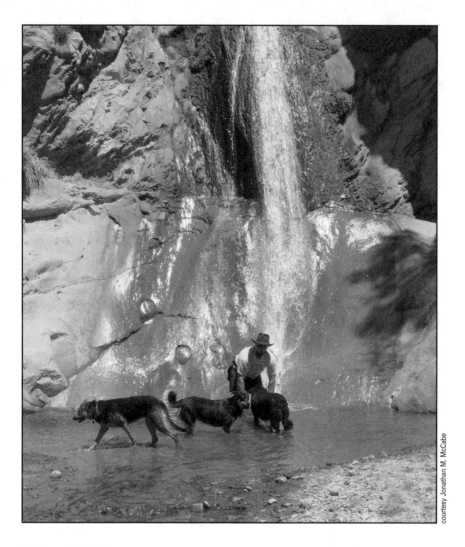

Potrero John Falls

Follow the rocks to a 90-degree **bend (3 miles, 4,635', 291906E 3832765N)** in the creek coming in on the left (north). Scramble or chimney up the short vertical wall to access the lower falls and pool here; a steep but short trail to the left of the lower pool curves up and around to the main **Potrero John Falls (3.1 miles, 4,675', 291907E 3832793N)** and pool.

Grade Valley, Mutau, and the Upper Piru

This chapter details the routes within the Mt. Pinos Ranger District south of Lockwood Valley Road along Grade Valley, including those along the Piru and Mutau Creek drainages, as well as the Thorn Point Lookout.

LONG A CATTLE-GRAZING AREA, Grade Valley still features many inholdings and leases, but this well-treed area—sections of which received heavy damage from the 2006 Day Fire—remains largely accessible to forest users. OHV riders especially take advantage of the numerous trails that originate here and head east out through Lockwood Valley and toward the Hungry Valley State Vehicular Recreation Area.

Off-road enthusiasts, hunters, and those collecting fuelwood are common encounters en route to any of the trailheads. In addition to the private holdings along this stretch, the area has been home to small-scale mining activity, dating back to the 1830s. The entire area is usually closed to motor vehicles in winter, as snow falls heavily here.

Grade Valley Trailheads

Cedar Creek Trailhead (4,850', 306347E 3834516N)

Follow the directions to the Fishbowls Trailhead, on the next page. From the Fishbowls Trailhead, continue south along Mutau Flat Road. After 1.25 miles the road crosses Piru Creek; even in drier seasons the water here can be deep enough to prevent crossing, especially for passenger cars (there is a small parking area just before the crossing if this is the case). If passable, continue across Piru Creek and stay right (west) at the fork just beyond. Continue another mile to a small parking area on the left (south) side of the road. The trailhead is 100 feet back along the road, creekside. There are no facilities here.

Fishbowls Trailhead (4,880', 306773E 3836771N)

From the junction of Lockwood Valley Road and Grade Valley Road (Forest Road 7N03) in Lockwood Valley, bear south onto Grade Valley Road toward Mutau Flat. Continue along this road (which turns to dirt after 2 miles) for 5.7 miles.

The Fishbowls Trailhead (the old Grade Valley Campground) is on your right. There are restrooms, but no water is available. The original trailhead to the Fishbowls Trail **(4,850', 306932E 3835595N)** is just south of the new trailhead, and is little more than a dirt turnaround at the end of a field. Its route follows Piru Creek directly, connecting with the newer length of trail about 0.5 mile in.

Johnston Ridge Trailhead (4,900', 311602E 3835396N)

From the junction of Lockwood Valley Road and Grade Valley Road (Forest Road 7N03) in Lockwood Valley, bear south onto Grade Valley Road toward Mutau Flat. Continue along this road (which turns to dirt quickly) for 11.1 miles (three creek crossings) to the turnoff to the Johnston Ridge Trailhead. There are restrooms but no other facilities here. Many of the parking spots have hitching posts.

Little Mutau Trailhead (6,750', 320450E 3835279N)

Though not in Grade Valley, this trailhead is an important shuttle point for trips following the Little Mutau Trail (*Route 82*).

From I-5 (Golden State Freeway) south of the CA 138 junction, take Exit 195 for Smokey Bear Road and head west to the junction with old US 99. Make the quick dogleg to the left (south), and then make a quick right onto the graded dirt road heading into the Hungry Valley State Vehicular Recreation Area.

Note: This is a fairly long (20-plus miles) drive along a largely unpaved route. This road is usually accessible to two-wheel drive passenger vehicles, but a higher-clearance vehicle would be better suited. Four-wheel drive isn't necessary except in the most extreme conditions, in which case either California State Parks or the US Forest Service (USFS) will likely have closed the roads or have cautions posted. Call the Mt. Pinos Ranger District at (661) 245-3731 to check road conditions during or immediately after any measurable precipitation.

At 1.2 miles is a California State Parks kiosk, where visitors are charged $5 for day use of the forest areas beyond the state land. A Forest Service Adventure Pass, federal Interagency Pass, or equivalent will also suffice; inform the ranger you are heading for the forestlands beyond, and either pay or present your pass.

From the kiosk, continue along Hungry Valley Road 3.9 miles to the intersection with Gold Hill Road (Forest Road 8N01). Follow this road (paved for quite a stretch) another

12.5 miles (passing the turnoffs for Kings and Gold Hill Camps and crossing Piru Creek once) toward the Big Spring junction. Follow the signage to continue south from this junction another 4 miles along Forest Road 7N01 to the Little Mutau Trailhead. There is a vault toilet but no water or other facilities here.

Thorn Meadows (Snedden) Campground (5,000', 306183E 3833701N)

From the junction of Lockwood Valley Road and Grade Valley Road (Forest Road 7N03) in Lockwood Valley, bear south onto Grade Valley Road toward Mutau Flat. Continue along this road (which turns to dirt quickly) for 5.7 miles. The Fishbowls Trailhead (the old Grade Valley Campground) is on your right; there are restrooms but no water or other facilities here. Continue south along Mutau Flat Road. After another 1.25 miles the road crosses Piru Creek; even in drier seasons the water here can be deep enough to prevent crossing, especially for passenger cars (there is a small parking area just before the crossing if this is the case). If passable, continue across Piru Creek and stay right (west) at the fork just beyond onto Thorn Meadows Spur Road (Forest Road 7N03C).

Traveling along the spur road another 1.5 miles, you'll pass the corral, the trailhead for Cedar Creek (see *Route 79*), and the old Thorn Meadows Guard Station in quick succession just before reaching Thorn Meadows Campground (formerly/also known as Snedden Campground).

Thorn Point Trailhead is at the northeast corner of camp. There are no facilities here, but there is an outhouse, and three campsites with tables and stoves—each under a large incense cedar, ponderosa pine, or inland oak, respectively—are available for day and overnight use.

The Snedden moniker comes from a family of homesteaders and cattle ranchers who operated in Lockwood Valley, Mutau Flats, and as far north as Santa Barbara Canyon along the Cuyama in the late 19th century. In 1916 the children of the original homesteaders formed the Snedden Land and Cattle Company after their father's passing. Over the years, Thorn Meadows and Snedden Campground have been largely interchangeable in referring to the USFS site established here in 1961.

Note: On busy weekends, if not camping at Thorn Meadows, it's probably more appropriate to park at the old Thorn Meadows Guard Station about 200 feet down the road.

Grade Valley Campgrounds

In addition to Thorn Meadows (Snedden) Campground detailed above, two other campgrounds avail themselves to Grade Valley visitors.

First is **Pine Springs,** a rustic (read: dry) 12-site campground located 0.8 mile up Forest Road 7N03A (turn off 2.6 miles from Lockwood Valley Road). It tends to be frequented by

OHV users, as the turnoff for 7N03A is very close to both Piano Box/Yellowjacket OHV route departures. Second is **Halfmoon Campground**, some 10 miles along Grade Valley Road from Lockwood Valley Road, then another 0.25 mile along 7N03C. The Piru Creek Trail (an old OHV route) is at the east end of this 10-site campground.

Both sites are well shaded by pines and have restrooms, but they do not have water. A Forest Adventure Pass, federal Interagency Pass, or equivalent is required to claim a site at either camp.

Route 79

FISHBOWLS–CEDAR CREEK LOOP (21W05 and 21W10)

LENGTH AND TYPE:	13.5-mile loop
RATING:	Moderate
TRAIL CONDITION:	Clear
MAP(S):	USGS *Lockwood Valley* and *San Guillermo Mountain*; Harrison's *Sespe Wilderness*
CAMP(S):	Fishbowls and Cedar Creek
HIGHLIGHTS:	Fishbowls formation and swimming holes; giant conifers; magnificent views of Mutau Flat and Lockwood Valley

TO REACH THE TRAILHEAD(S): Use the Cedar Creek and/or Fishbowls Trailhead for this loop.

TRIP SUMMARY: From the Fishbowls Trailhead, this loop follows the rugged but easily traveled Piru Creek drainage through the fire-scarred pines and sage to the confluence of Piru Creek's main tributaries and then southward into the conifer- and oak-shaded canyons of the Fishbowls area. From the Fishbowls, the route climbs nearly 1,000 feet out of the Piru watershed before dropping steeply into the Cedar Creek drainage and back to the second parking area and road.

Trip Description

This loop trip makes a comfortable and fairly easy one- or two-night backpack or a long day trip. If you have two vehicles in your party, one can be parked at either trailhead and—at the end of the hike—used to shuttle back to the first vehicle. If you're using only one vehicle, you can either park it just before the Piru Creek crossing (advisable if a passenger car), the Fishbowls Trailhead (easiest, but you'll have to cover the distance on foot at the end of the hike), or at the Cedar Creek Trailhead (ideal, as you can cover the distance while your legs are fresh). The gap is an easy 2.5-mile walk along the road with virtually no elevation gain/loss.

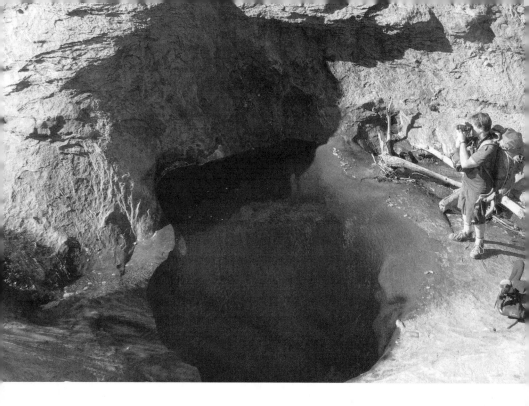

Once at the **Fishbowls Trailhead (2.5 miles, 4,880', 306773E 3836771N)**, follow the trail through the center of the old Grade Valley Campground (now a parking and day-use area) opposite the restrooms and pass through a shallow wash into a small pine-shaded amphitheater before climbing 100 vertical feet to a low ridge. From here, you can see the broad drainage of Piru Creek, and damage from the 2006 Day Fire is immediately apparent in the form of fire-blackened pines that stretch for miles along the Piru watershed. From this small ridge the trail leads into the drainage, eventually converging with the older portion of the trail.

Much of your route here follows an old jeep trail upstream, crossing coarse sand and gravel alluvium in an easy and meandering hike. The limit of the old jeep trail is marked by an abandoned gate strung with heavy-gauge cable, installed decades ago to keep off-road enthusiasts from the forest beyond.

Continue to the **convergence (4.3 miles, 5,120', 301418E 3837038N)** of two forks of Piru Creek; head left (south) into a lush canyon lined with ferns, pines, incense cedars, and black oaks. Follow the meandering drainage another 1.25 miles to the main **Fishbowls** site (**5.6 miles, 5,210', 301704E 3835445N**), set comfortably beside huge boulders and incense cedars.

CAMP :: FISHBOWLS

ELEVATION:	5,210'
MAP:	USGS *San Guillermo Mountain*
UTM:	301704E 3835445N

A series of four campsites set alongside Piru Creek, Fishbowls is a comfortable spot for camping, picnicking, and general relaxation. The swimming holes just upstream from camp are refreshing, and the main swimming hole is quite deep and can accommodate four to six bathers easily. The main site, an old jeep camp with a tidy kitchen area and room enough for a pair of tents, is set downstream from the fork where the trail cuts south to follow a minor tributary. The other three sites are across the creeks' fork along a flat that leads to the swimming holes.

From Fishbowls Camp, the popular Fishbowls formation for which the camp is named is another 0.8 mile westward along the main canyon (you'll pass the other three Fishbowls campsites on your way). This series of pools is a lovely area to enjoy any time, but during warm weather they are especially inviting.

To continue your loop, return to the trail between the first and second camps and head south. After 0.5 mile of easy climbing and a short series of switchbacks, you'll find yourself along an exposed **crest (6.1 miles, 5,500', 302313E 3835730N)** with superb views of the canyon from which you've come (to the north), the eastern slopes of Pine Mountain to the west, and Lockwood Valley to the east. From this lookout continue climbing steadily southward along a conifer- and scrub-covered ridgeline until you reach the junction with **Pine Mountain Lodge Trail (7.1 miles, 5,925', 302791E 3834256N)**. Expansive views continue along the eastern edge—the Cedar Creek drainage is now in view toward the southeast—and heavy stands of sugar pines dot the slopes.

■ ■ ■ ■ ■ ■ ■ **SIDE TRIP: PINE MOUNTAIN LODGE TRAIL**

From the junction of the **Cedar Creek and Pine Mountain Lodge Trails (5,925', 302791E 3834256N)**, the route to Pine Mountain Lodge heads off toward the southwest, paralleling high above the South Fork of Cedar Creek for a steady but not overly strenuous ascent to the **saddle (1.1 miles, 5,960', 301381E 3833254N)** between the Piru/Cedar and Piedra Blanca drainages. Views here are fantastic. The route then drops through the rockier slopes of the North Fork of Piedra Blanca Creek to **Pine Mountain Lodge Camp (2.4 miles, 6,000', 300395E 3832665N)**.

■ ■

From the junction, stay left (southeast) and enjoy the view while you switchback down along a sandstone ridge and then drop steeply into the lush drainage of Cedar Creek's south fork and **Cedar Creek Camp (8.7 miles, 5,080', 303775E 3833940N)**.

CAMP :: CEDAR CREEK

ELEVATION:	5,080'
MAP:	USGS *San Guillermo Mountain*
UTM:	303775E 3833940N

A well-shaded site set beside its namesake, Cedar Creek Camp is situated beneath an array of towering ponderosa pines and incense cedars. Protected during the 2006 Day Fire, the site's trees and amenities escaped unscathed, while trees and terrain no more than a hundred feet along its immediate periphery are charred and lay in ruin. Once the end of an old jeep trail, this site has four kitchens and water is usually available.

From Cedar Creek Camp, the trail picks up another old jeep trail and follows Cedar Creek downstream. Your route here is again quite level, traveling through the wash at times amid fern-covered meadows and sandstone gullies cut by the creek. The trail cuts across the creek a final time to lead you back to the **Cedar Creek parking area** (**11 miles, 4,850', 306347E 3834516N**).

It's another 2.5 miles along the road to the **Fishbowls Trailhead** (**13.5 miles, 4,880', 306773E 3836771N**) if you haven't left a vehicle here.

Route 80

THORN POINT (21W07)

LENGTH AND TYPE:	7-mile out-and-back
RATING:	Moderately strenuous (climb)
TRAIL CONDITION:	Clear
MAP(S):	USGS *Lockwood Valley, Topatopa Mountains,* and *Lion Canyon*; Harrison's *Sespe Wilderness*
CAMP(S):	—
HIGHLIGHTS:	Outstanding views; historic fire lookout

TO REACH THE TRAILHEAD(S): Use the Thorn Meadows (Snedden) Campground to access this route.

TRIP SUMMARY: This steady climb leads from Thorn Meadows to the abandoned Thorn Point fire lookout through chaparral and then conifer trail. The elevation gain is just less than 2,000 vertical feet.

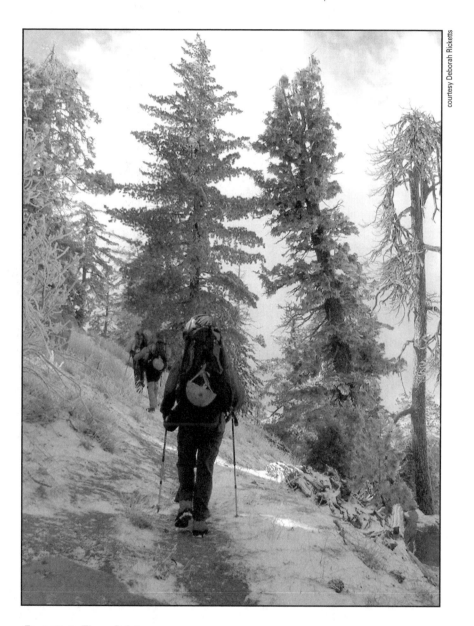

courtesy Deborah Ricketts

En route to Thorn Point

Trip Description

From the **Thorn Meadows Trailhead** (**5,000', 306164E 3833696N**), follow the track down into the shallow ravine and back out, and then hike approximately 100 yards to the Sespe Wilderness boundary and sign. From there, head upstream along the easy trail with good views of the sandstone formations and mature conifers of the upper meadows. Ferns hem the lower stretches of the trail as you follow the drainage of Cedar Creek's southernmost fork. Some damage from the 2006 Day Fire is apparent, but the route beyond your initial approach here escaped largely unscathed compared to other nearby areas. Ponderosa pines and incense cedars mix with oaks to provide ample stretches of shade as you make easy crossings of the creek and tributaries before you reach an intermittent **tributary** (**0.9 mile, 5,150', 304968E 3833229N**), marking the start of your ascent.

Cross the streambed here and embark on a series of switchbacks, all the while gaining fantastic views of the complex and rather impressive sandstone formations separating this drainage and that of Mutau Creek to your south. Views of Frazier Mountain and Grade and Lockwood Valleys begin to open up as you work toward a short **gap** (**1.4 miles, 5,360', 304696E 3833069N**) with views on both sides of the trail. Here, as you head southward along a ridgeline, the larger conifers (white firs, sugar pines, and the like) begin to enter the mix, and soon you'll leave the chaparral behind altogether in favor of the crushed and crumbly sandstone trail under cover of huge, well-spaced conifers. The lookout tower is visible from a view of the switchbacks here, providing motivation for those who need it.

After some steady climbing, a sandstone **outcrop** (**2.2 miles, 6,040', 304852E 3832481N**) on your left (east) makes for an excellent rest spot and provides outstanding views of those sandstone formations that loomed above at your start. From the outcrop, follow the switchbacks farther (at times quite steeply) before reaching a more level and occasionally **grassy stretch** (**2.6 miles, 6,440', 304948E 3832115N**) for something of a respite. Along this ridge above the Cedar and Mutau drainages, there are some outcrops of mollusk fossils from the Eocene era inset directly in the trail along the way. Follow this pleasant stretch for nearly 0.25 mile—crossing the **headwaters** (**2.8 miles, 6,460', 305015E 3831824N**) of Mutau Creek along the way—before embarking on another series of switchbacks leading to the **ridgeline** (**3.2 miles, 6,715', 305161E 3831588N**) that forms the boundary of the Mt. Pinos and Ojai Ranger Districts, as well as the divide between the Piru and Sespe drainages. Here you'll have your first views of the Sespe, Topatopa Mountains, and numerous points south. The vegetation here becomes a bit of a mix again, with some chaparral (notably bigberry manzanitas) reentering the mix due to the southern aspect of portions of the route here. This stretch was also touched by the 2006 Day Fire, and stands of poodle-dog bush still dot the trailside, so exercise caution.

Huge sandstone boulders line your climb to the southwest until you reach **Thorn Point** (**3.5 miles, 6,935', 304865E 3831468N**) and the abandoned fire lookout. This is one of the few lookouts in the southern Los Padres not only still standing but also still accessible. (See "Lookout!" on page 12 for more information about the legacy of the old fire lookouts in the southern Los Padres.) Immediately to the southwest of the lookout is the old civilian Aircraft Warning Service (AWS) observer cabin. In March 1944, toward the end of World War II, the AWS was disbanded (transformed somewhat into the Ground Observer Corps, which in turn was canceled by the U.S. Air Force in the late 1950s).

Below and to the south of Thorn Point are the headwaters of Trout Creek, which drains into the Sespe. The terrain here drops off steeply into the myriad drainages. It's easy to see why the US Forest Service and Air Corps chose this site for observation, as views as far as the Oxnard Plain and the Pacific are easily had.

Return the way you came.

MEANWHILE, UPSTAIRS . . . ■ ■ ■ ■ ■ ■ ■ ■ ■ ■ ■

The concrete-and-steel staircase ascends the 20-foot open brace steel tower and leads to the 14-foot-square cab that opens a visitor's eyes to a fascinating piece of history. The interior of the old lookout is something of a shambles, but it still contains old Forest Service records, including lightning strike forms, maps, and accoutrements of life in the tower (e.g., stove, bunk, and even a telephone). The old green wooden cabinet at the center of the space once held an alidade table fitted with the USFS-specific Osborne Fire Finder to determine distance and location of wildfires.

Please respect the historical significance of this unique piece of forest history.

■ ■ ■ ■ ■ ■ ■ ■ ■ ■ ■ ■ ■ ■ ■ ■ ■ ■ ■ ■

Route 81

STONEHOUSE (20W35)

LENGTH AND TYPE:	9.4-mile out-and-back
RATING:	Easy
TRAIL CONDITION:	Well maintained (former service and motorcycle road) to clear (unmaintained but open route)
MAP(S):	USGS *Lockwood Valley*; Harrison's *Sespe Wilderness*
CAMP(S):	Stonehouse
HIGHLIGHTS:	Easy navigation; pleasant willow- and pine-dotted terrain

TO REACH THE TRAILHEAD(S): Use the Johnston Ridge Trailhead to access this route.

TRIP SUMMARY: This rather easy hike leads along a portion of the Johnston Ridge Trail (a former motorcycle route) to Mutau Creek, and then easily along Mutau Creek to a camp near the Alamo/Mutau/Piru confluences.

Trip Description

From the **Johnston Ridge Trailhead (4,900', 311602E 3835396N)**, pass through the motorcycle barriers and head north along the singletrack for 0.5 mile until the trail connects with the old Johnston Ridge motorcycle and **service road (0.4 mile, 4,920', 311918E 3835334N)**. Follow the old road easily down into the Mutau drainage and to the junction with the **Stonehouse Trail (1.4 miles, 4,780', 312829E 3834865N)**. On your right (south) through the gate is the private road leading toward Mutau Flat; occasionally you'll spot cattle (or, more often, their leavings) in this vicinity. The route straight (east) leads across Mutau Creek and toward the Little Mutau and Johnston Ridge routes (*Routes 82* and *89*, respectively). Damage from the 2006 Day Fire is apparent along many swatches of the forest here.

Follow the Stonehouse (northerly) route here, an easily navigated affair along an old sandy wash road. For about 1.5 miles you'll stay on the west side of the creek before reaching a wide sandy **wash (3.1 miles, 4,650', 314268E 3836798N)**. Cross here to gain the other side, only to progress another few hundred yards downstream and cross again. Keep an eye out for western pond turtles along this stretch, as they enjoy basking in the sun and (slowly) waddling through the willow saplings creekside.

You'll keep to the west side for the remainder of the route until you reach the **Mutau-Alamo confluence (4.7 miles, 4,500', 315197E 3838619N)**. Cross the creek here to gain the bank and **Stonehouse Camp.**

CAMP :: STONEHOUSE

ELEVATION:	4,500'
MAP:	USGS *Lockwood Valley*
UTM:	315241E 3838614N

Named for an old stone miner's cabin built in the late 19th century that once stood near the Mutau-Alamo confluence, this site gets very little use and stopped appearing on US Forest Service maps in the 1990s (it never seemed to appear on USGS quads). The old stoves here have been washed away by storms in the past few decades, but some of the 10-foot-long foundation of the old cabin is still visible. Camping may be more comfortable along the pine-dotted flat a bit farther downstream.

Beyond camp, the trail drops a bit more steeply for 0.75 mile toward the Piru Creek confluence. Though not detailed herein, the Piru Trail (an OHV route) can be followed back toward Halfmoon Campground, 4.5 miles upstream.

Route 82

LITTLE MUTAU (20W10)

LENGTH AND TYPE:	9.4-mile one-way from Johnston Ridge Trailhead to Little Mutau Trailhead; 12.2-mile out-and-back to Little Mutau Camp
RATING:	Moderate
TRAIL CONDITION:	Clear to passable
MAP(S):	USGS *Lockwood Valley* and *Alamo Mountain*; Harrison's *Sespe Wilderness*
CAMP(S):	Little Mutau
HIGHLIGHTS:	Solitude; expansive views of the Sespe drainage and Topatopa Mountains; conifer forests

TO REACH THE TRAILHEAD(S): Use the Johnston Ridge Trailhead and/or Little Mutau Trailhead to access this route. The narrative describes the route west to east (Johnston to Little Mutau Trailheads).

TRIP SUMMARY: This route follows the Little Mutau Creek watershed from Johnston Ridge Trailhead to the creek's headwaters and the Little Mutau Trailhead. This trip is an out-and-back or a rather long (and somewhat complicated) shuttle.

Trip Description

From the **Johnston Ridge Trailhead (4,900', 311602E 3835396N)**, pass through the motorcycle barriers and head north along the singletrack for 0.5 mile until the trail connects with the old Johnston Ridge motorcycle and **service road (0.4 mile, 4,920', 311918E 3835334N)**. Follow the old road easily down into the Mutau drainage and to the junction with the **Stonehouse Trail (1.4 miles, 4,780', 312829E 3834865N)**. On your right (south) through the gate is the private road leading toward Mutau Flat; occasionally you'll spot cattle (or, more often, their leavings) in this vicinity. The route to your left (north) leads along Mutau Creek toward Stonehouse and the Piru confluence (see *Route 81*). Damage from the 2006 Day Fire is apparent along many swatches of the forest here.

Follow the trail down into the sandy, willow-dotted wash to the **Mutau Creek crossing (1.5 miles, 4,770', 312998E 3834876N)**. Cross here and climb the slope—entering the Sespe Wilderness—on the other side and into the draw to the junction with the **Johnston Ridge**

Trail (**2.2 miles, 4,950', 313722E 3834442N**). Continue straight here; see *Route 89* for the drop into the Sespe. Though by this point you're well into the Sespe Wilderness, and despite the barriers in place, motorcycle tracks can still occasionally be seen on this stretch.

Follow the trail through fire-scarred chaparral and sage dotted with piñons, climbing fairly steeply at times to gain a **gap** (**3.5 miles, 5,729', 315074E 3834826N**) along the ridge separating the Mutau and Little Mutau drainages. Despite the fire damage, many of the fields between clusters of pines exhibit fine displays of lupines and numerous other meadow flowers in spring and early summer. Here, descend into the Little Mutau drainage, and then follow the occasionally arid alder- and pine-shaded canyon upstream to **Little Mutau Camp** (**4.5 miles, 5,250', 316745E 3834567N**).

CAMP :: LITTLE MUTAU

ELEVATION:	5,250'
MAP:	USGS *Alamo Mountain*
UTM:	316745E 3834567N

This seldom-visited camp is set beneath a cluster of towering conifers largely spared damage from the fires and contains a small fire ring and some old ice cans. Water is reliable in all but the driest seasons.

From camp, continue upstream for nearly 1.5 miles to the junction with **Alder Creek Trail** (**6.5 miles, 5,790', 318965E 3833606N**). The upper Alder Creek route here has been effectively abandoned by the US Forest Service since the 2006 Day Fire, but for the hardy it makes a viable route. The old trail leads a rough 7 miles to the main and east fork confluence to the still-maintained route between the Sespe and Dough Flat (*Route 90*).

From this junction, continue along your route and proceed along the at-times steep 2-mile climb along the ridge separating the Little Mutau and Alder Creek watershed. As the climb begins to top out, you'll reach a somewhat faint **doubletrack** (**8.1 miles, 6,850', 320335E 3834744N**). (The portion heading off to your right [east] is part of an old service road—as well as the original 20W10 trail—and leads toward McDonald Peak before connecting to the road east of the peak.) Continue straight through the open glades and pines along this old roadbed to the **Little Mutau Trailhead** (**8.5 miles, 6,750', 320450E 3835279N**).

The Sespe

*This chapter details trails traveling along
or leading to or from Sespe Creek.*

Sᴇsᴘᴇ Cʀᴇᴇᴋ ɪs ᴀᴛ ᴏɴᴄᴇ ᴀ ᴍᴀɢɴɪꜰɪᴄᴇɴᴛ sᴛʀᴇᴛᴄʜ of boulder-strewn gorges, rock walls, and deep emerald pools, but also a stark reminder of man's impact upon a stretch of river to which many have laid claim and over which many have clamored through the centuries. It begins its 55-mile descent toward the Santa Clara River from a series of springs along the Potrero Seco just north of what is now the Matilija Wilderness.

Named for a Chumash village (Sek-pe), the creek was for decades a haven for campers, horse packers, and (later) 4WD enthusiasts (but also unsavory elements) and received heavy use. Only after the storms of 1978 and the decision to close the old Sespe Road to vehicular traffic did the modern Sespe begin to emerge, though numerous derelict outbuildings, and even the occasional road sign and gatepost, can be spotted along what is now a long route unfettered by motorized or mechanized traffic.

The Sespe Wilderness, a wide swath of nearly 220,000 acres established in 1992, also includes the renowned 53,000-acre Sespe Condor Sanctuary (formed in 1947 and expanded in 1951, and into which human entry is prohibited). More than 30 miles of the Sespe runs through the wilderness, and the main trails through this region follow the enigmatic riverbed for more than 20 miles before the Sespe cuts southward through the condor sanctuary (an older and now-abandoned route follows this stretch through narrow slot canyons and fantastically desolate country). But long before it was protected under so many designations, it had a long history of use—and, yes, abuse—from all those who'd entered.

Bradley Monsma put it succinctly in his *The Sespe Wild*:

> *The Sespe bears a remarkably rich layering of natural and cultural history. Though most of it has been officially designated both wilderness and wild and scenic river, it has never been "untrammeled." The indigenous Chumash, the Spanish padres and*

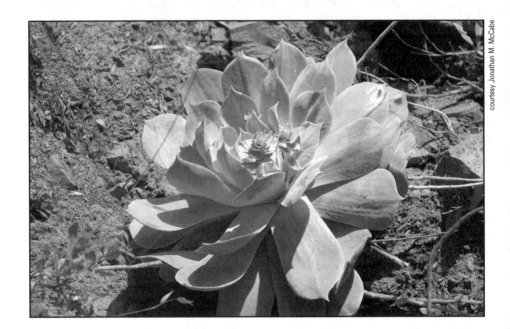

Canyon liveforever (Dudleya cymosa)

soldiers, ranchers, hunters, "anthropologist" grave robbers, serious ethnographers, geologists, miners, oil drillers, dam speculators, pioneering rock climbers and kayakers, hot-springs neopagans, and wilderness activists have all contributed to the stratification of stories.

The Sespe watershed is a rallying point for conservationists the state and world over, often termed the "last free river" in Southern California, and the watershed as a whole is also home to numerous endangered species, most notably the arroyo toad, steelhead trout, and California condor.

Sespe and Sespe Wilderness Trailheads

Buck Creek Trailhead (6,500', 324025E 3834614N)

From I-5 (Golden State Freeway) south of the CA 138 junction, take Exit 195 for Smokey Bear Road and head west to the junction with the old US 99. Make the quick dogleg to the left (south), and then make a quick right onto the graded dirt road heading into the Hungry Valley State Vehicular Recreation Area.

Note: This is a fairly long (20-plus miles) drive along a largely unpaved route. This road is usually accessible to two-wheel drive passenger vehicles, but a higher-clearance vehicle would be better suited. Four-wheel drive isn't necessary except in the most extreme conditions, in which case either California State Parks or the US Forest Service (USFS) will likely have closed the roads or have cautions posted. Call the Mt. Pinos Ranger District at (661) 245-3731 to check road conditions during or immediately after any measurable precipitation.

At 1.2 miles is a California State Parks kiosk, where visitors are charged $5 for day use of the forest areas beyond the state land. A Forest Service Adventure Pass, federal Interagency Pass, or equivalent will also suffice; inform the ranger you are heading for the forestlands beyond, and either pay or present your pass.

From the kiosk, continue along Hungry Valley Road for 3.9 miles to the intersection with Gold Hill Road (Forest Road 8N01). Follow this road (paved for quite a stretch) another 12.5 miles (passing the turnoffs for Kings and Gold Hill Camps and crossing Piru Creek once) toward the Big Spring junction. Follow the signage to continue south from this junction another 4 miles along Forest Road 7N01 to the **Little Mutau Trailhead (6,750', 320450E 3835279N)**. There is a vault toilet but no water or other facilities here.

It is another 3 miles east along the road to the **Buck Creek Trailhead**. There are no facilities here.

Dough Flat Trailhead (2,840', 326001E 3821693N)

From Fillmore, follow Goodenough Road to its northern end, and then follow Forest Route 6N16 approximately 10 miles to the Dough Flat Trailhead and parking area. The road is rough in places, intermittently paved the first 3 miles to Oak Flat and graded dirt the remaining 7 miles. The parking area has restrooms and informational signs.

Dry Lakes Trailhead (3,720', 294313E 3824470N)

From the junction of CA 33 and CA 150 (the "Y") in Ojai, drive north along CA 33 approximately 15.6 miles (past the Rose Valley turnoff) to a parking area on the left (west) shoulder of the highway, just before the road begins to drop into the Sespe drainage. Exercise caution crossing the road here, as it's a fairly blind corner and the highway is especially popular with motorcyclists on weekends. Numerous trail threads access the trail, but the best trailhead to use is the **old route (3,720', 294303E 3824519N)** guarded with large boulders just north of the turnout. There are no facilities here.

Frenchman's Flat (2,050', 340159E 3831869N)

From I-5 (Golden State Freeway) in Castaic, take Exit 183 for the Templin Highway (Forest Road 6N32). Head west from the off-ramp to the old Golden State Highway (formerly US 99) and continue north approximately 5.1 miles to the **parking area (2,050',**

340159E 3831869N). There are restrooms a short distance up the old road from here and trash receptacles near the gate, but no facilities.

A Forest Service Adventure Pass, federal Interagency Pass, or equivalent permit is required to park a vehicle at this trailhead.

Johnston Ridge Trailhead (4,900', 311602E 3835396N)

From the junction of Lockwood Valley Road and Grade Valley Road (Forest Road 7N03) in Lockwood Valley, bear south onto Grade Valley Road toward Mutau Flat. Continue along this road (which turns to dirt quickly) for 11.1 miles to the turnoff for the Johnston Ridge Trailhead. There are restrooms but no other facilities here. Many of the parking spots have hitching posts.

Juan Fernandez Boat Launch (Lake Piru) (1,100', 338307E 3817566N)

From CA 126 in Piru, take the Main Street exit and head north through the town of Piru (at the north end of town as the road begins to head east, it becomes Piru Canyon Road) for 7 miles to the tollbooth. As of this writing, there is a $12 day-use fee to park or pass through the area—though within the national forest, because the Lake Piru Recreational Area is under the jurisdiction of the United Water Conservation District, neither a USFS Adventure Pass nor a federal Interagency Pass will suffice. There are restrooms, a snack bar, bait shop, and market here.

Continue along the road another 2.3 miles to the Juan Fernandez Boat Launch, which has in recent years effectively become the trailhead for hikes into the forest beginning along Piru Creek. *Note:* During winter, the stretch of road leading from the Reasoner Creek parking area to the Fernandez Boat Launch is usually closed. This will entail an additional 1.5-mile walk each way.

Little Mutau Trailhead (6,750', 320450E 3835279N)

From I-5 (Golden State Freeway) south of the CA 138 junction, take Exit 195 for Smokey Bear Road and head west to the junction with the old US 99. Make the quick dogleg to the left (south), and then make a quick right onto the graded dirt road heading into the Hungry Valley State Vehicular Recreation Area.

Note: This is a fairly long (20-plus miles) drive along a largely unpaved route. This road is usually accessible to two-wheel drive passenger vehicles, but a higher-clearance vehicle would be better suited. Four-wheel drive isn't necessary except in the most extreme conditions, in which case either California State Parks or the USFS will likely have closed the roads or have cautions posted. Call the Mt. Pinos Ranger District at (661) 245-3731 to check road conditions during or immediately after any measurable precipitation.

At 1.2 miles is a California State Parks kiosk, where visitors are charged $5 for day use of the forest areas beyond the state land. A Forest Service Adventure Pass, federal Interagency Pass, or equivalent will also suffice; inform the ranger you are heading for the forestlands beyond, and either pay or present your pass.

From the kiosk, continue along Hungry Valley Road for 3.9 miles to the intersection with Gold Hill Road (Forest Road 8N01). Follow this road (paved for quite a stretch) another 12.5 miles (passing the turnoffs for Kings and Gold Hill Camps and crossing Piru Creek once) toward the Big Spring junction. Follow the signage to continue south from this junction another 4 miles along Forest Road 7N01 to the Little Mutau Trailhead. There is a vault toilet but no water or other facilities here.

Los Alamos Trailhead (2,980', 333256E 3841892N)

From I-5 (Golden State Freeway) south of the CA 138 junction, take Exit 195 for Smokey Bear Road and proceed south along Pyramid Lake Road for 1.5 miles to the turnoff for Hard Luck Road. Turn right (west) here and follow Hard Luck Road for 2.7 miles—passing the Los Alamos Campgrounds—to the small parking area at the junction with the fire station spur road. There are no facilities here; the nearest restrooms and potable water can be found at Los Alamos Campgrounds 0.5 mile back along the road. *Note:* Most maps (those printed before 2010) show Hardluck car campground as the start for this area; this is no longer the case.

Middle Lion Campground (3,160', 301226E 3825202N)

From the junction of CA 33 and CA 150 (the "Y") in Ojai, drive north along CA 33 approximately 14.5 miles to Forest Road 6N31 (Sespe River Road) in Rose Valley. Turn right (south) onto this road and continue east 4.7 miles to a road indicating Middle Lion Campground. Turn right (south) here and continue 0.8 mile southward to Middle Lion Campground. A Forest Service Adventure Pass, federal Interagency Pass, or equivalent grants you access to one of the campgrounds (parking can be a bit awkward anywhere else). There is no water here, but there are restrooms.

Middle Sespe Trailhead (3,300', 294062E 3826024N)

From the junction of CA 33 and CA 150 (the "Y") in Ojai, drive north along CA 33 approximately 16.7 miles (passing the Rose Valley turnoff) to the old Beaver Campground turnoff. Turn right (northeast) toward the river. It's another 100 yards to the parking area beside the locked gate. There are no facilities here, nor is a USFS Adventure Pass necessary to park here.

Piedra Blanca Trailhead (3,040', 301320E 3826437N)

From the junction of CA 33 and CA 150 (the "Y") in Ojai, drive north along CA 33 approximately 14.5 miles to Forest Road 6N31 (Sespe River Road) in Rose Valley. Proceed 5.6 miles along this road to the parking area at the Piedra Blanca Trailhead (site of the old Lion car camp). The trail is on the northeast edge of the parking area's second loop. There are restrooms here, but no water is available.

A Forest Service Adventure Pass, federal Interagency Pass, or equivalent permit is required to park a vehicle at this trailhead.

Tule Creek (3,400', 291891E 3826415N)

From the junction of CA 33 and CA 150 (the "Y") in Ojai, drive north along CA 33 approximately 18.4 miles (out of the North Fork Matilija watershed and into the Sespe watershed, passing a very noticeable slide area on your left) to a small parking area on the right (east) shoulder of the road near the confluence of Tule and Sespe Creeks. The trail begins on the other side of the road, and there are no facilities here.

Campgrounds Along the Sespe

Though there were once nearly a dozen campgrounds along the Sespe accessible by car or 4WD, all are now shuttered, have been removed, and have been converted to trail use. Use Middle Lion or Rose Valley Campgrounds for camping near the Sespe trails; see Chapter 10.

Route 83

TULE CREEK (23W17)

LENGTH AND TYPE:	5-mile out-and-back to Tule Flat; 4-mile one-way to Dry Lakes Ridge Trail junction
RATING:	Moderate to the flat; strenuous to Dry Lakes Ridge
TRAIL CONDITION:	Passable to difficult (unmaintained use trail)
MAP(S):	USGS *Wheeler Springs* (this route does not appear on current maps)
CAMP(S):	—
HIGHLIGHTS:	Arroyo willow and chaparral; solitude along a historic route

TO REACH THE TRAILHEAD(S): Use the Tule Creek Trailhead to access this route.

TRIP SUMMARY: This long-abandoned but still somewhat navigable route follows TuleCreek from the Sespe-Tule confluence to a wide sage-covered flat. A slightly clearer route then ascends the northern slopes of Dry Lakes Ridge to join the old firebreak trail there.

Trip Description

From the **parking area (3,400', 291891E 3826415N)** beside CA 33, walk across the road and drop into the drainage from the **access (3,275', 291830E 3826426N)** on the southwest edge of the bridge. Follow the old trail/runoff to the cobbled bed of Tule Creek and cross to the north bank. Here the remnants of the old 23W17 trail are still in fairly good repair—the Tule drainage is still visited by hunters with enough frequency to keep the route in marginally decent tread (there are a few sections of low clearance, and it's brushy, but it's usually doable).

Follow the trail along a very easy grade, wandering away from the immediate creekside and quickly gaining views of the northern slopes of Dry Lakes Ridge to your left (south), and passing through a few sections of the tule reeds that give this drainage its name. Mature willows line much of the upper stretches, and thin willow saplings line your progress closer to the trail. As the canyon narrows, the trail cuts to just above the creekside; the wash here nearly always has water. Continue through the drainage of a small **tributary (0.7 mile, 3,450', 290984E 3826874N)** and on toward a rise, which on the other side drops you into a side wash; pick up the trail just on your left and pass through a short section of dry, exposed terrain. Quail seem especially abundant along this stretch (and spent shotgun and rifle shells are perhaps testament to this having been the case for years). Shortly you'll approach and then cross the **stream (1 mile, 3,480', 290685E 3827160N)** again in a dark, alder-lined ravine choked with blackberry vines.

From the crossing, the trail leads through a short marshy stretch before opening into a wide and exposed expanse of sage and iron-stained rock. To the north, you'll spot the towering alders and cottonwoods that mark the meandering Tule Creek. The trail triangulates back toward the creek, finally leading you to the water again in a narrow slot of shale and eroded marine layers. Scramble around a coppice of thick willow along the old track here, but rather than crossing again, parallel the root- and sapling-strewn creek to another (often-dry) **tributary (1.1 miles, 3,545', 290105E 3827216N)** on your left (south) and follow the drainage a few hundred yards before cutting to the right where the trail departs the drainage to regain the hillside.

From here the trail begins to get thicker, and as you head toward the creek once more, poison oak begins to rear its ugly head. The trail is far more overgrown here, and the next **crossing (1.7 miles, 3,860', 289831E 3827157N)**—dark, shady, and even in the driest years usually running—is as fine a spot as any to break for lunch.

For those who wish to continue the often-bloodletting trek toward Dry Lakes Ridge, you have only another mile or so before you reach the flats and the turn up-canyon, but be advised it involves a bit of bushwacking, route-finding, and sometimes even crawling on one's knees beneath hedges of impassive whitethorn ceanothus. From the crossing, continue along the deteriorating track for a lush stretch, and then cross the creek once more directly across a generous **seep** (**1.8 miles, 3,600', 289730E 3827143N**)—this can make for a mucky ascent into the hard chaparral above, even in summer.

Work through this wide thicket of ceanothus to the main flat where numerous tributaries converge in a wide flat of braided streams, old cottonwoods, and willows. Follow the drainage and track a bit to the left (south) to the **base of the ridge** (**2.4 miles, 3,720', 289176E 3896599N**), which marks the start of the rather brutal and fairly brushy ascent. Pants and long sleeves are a must; gloves aren't a bad idea.

Ascend the ridge along the decades-old fire cut southward up the slope. Here you're following an old cut that in places—while sometimes steep—is wide and graded well enough to look more like an old roadbed than just a firebreak or dozer line. As such it makes the navigation easier than one might expect, but there are still several sections where you'll push through impassive manzanitas or heavy clumps of mountain mahoganies and ceanothus. And it's a steep affair, so you'll be grateful to finally emerge at the **junction** (**4 miles, 4,900', 290232E 3824665N**) with the Dry Lakes Ridge fire cut.

From here it's 1.2 miles to your left (east) to the main Dry Lakes Basin and camp and 3.5 miles along the ridge back to CA 33 (see *Route 85*); to your right (west), the fire cut follows the ridgeline another 2 miles to meet the Ortega Trail (see *Route 52*), where you can access CA 33 either at Wheeler Gorge (south) or Cherry Creek junction (north).

OFF THE MAP ▨ ▨ ▨ ▨ ▨ ▨ ▨ ▨ ▨ ▨ ▨ ▨ ▨ ▨ ▨

There's a bit of a gap in terms of legacy cartographic coverage for this route; none of the various *Wheeler Springs* 7.5-minute topographic maps show the route, and by the mid-1990s map updates, both the Tule Creek and Dry Lakes Trails had been long-abandoned. The 1:126,720 scale national forest visitor maps of the 1960s did depict the Tule Creek route, but trails shown in maps of that era were notoriously "approximate" and often quite inaccurate (and certainly not suitable for navigation). Oddly enough, the best map for those new to Tule Creek during that era often proved to be the 1975 Los Angeles 1x2 (1:250,000 scale) quadrangle, as it showed the contours—albeit in 100-foot intervals—and allowed the backcountry trekker some semblance of navigation using visible topographic features.

▨ ▨ ▨ ▨ ▨ ▨ ▨ ▨ ▨ ▨ ▨ ▨ ▨ ▨ ▨ ▨

Route 84

MIDDLE SESPE TRAIL (22W04)

LENGTH AND TYPE:	8.6-mile one-way (final 0.9 mile along Piedra Blanca–Gene Marshall and Sespe River Trails); shuttle
RATING:	Moderate (distance)
TRAIL CONDITION:	Clear
MAP(S):	USGS *Lion Canyon*; Harrison's *Sespe Wilderness*
CAMP(S):	—
HIGHLIGHTS:	Arroyo willow and chaparral trekking; views of the Sespe and Pine Mountain

TO REACH THE TRAILHEAD(S): Use the Piedra Blanca and Middle Sespe Trailheads for this shuttle.

TRIP SUMMARY: This 8.6-mile route—with perhaps the easiest shuttle in this guide—parallels Sespe Creek from the former Beaver Campground (now the Middle Sespe Trailhead) to the Piedra Blanca Trailhead through arroyo willow streambed, chaparral, and sandstone boulder fields. Because the trail is not within the wilderness boundary, mountain bikers may occasionally be encountered.

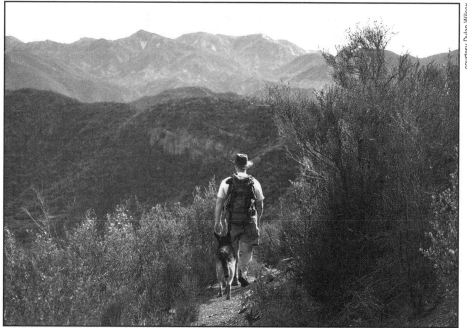

courtesy Dylan Wilcox

Trip Description

From the Middle Sespe **parking area (3,300', 294080E 3826031N)**, follow the trail eastward. On your left (west) is the old Beaver Campground, situated at the Briggs-Sespe confluence and closed in 1999 to protect natural habitats, most notably those of the endangered arroyo toad. Once a pleasant campground of 11 sites situated on an oak- and cottonwood-shaded flat between CA 33 and Sespe Creek, the old grounds are now an occasional destination for lax target shooters and idle day-trippers not inclined to clean up after themselves. The sad irony is that in closing this site to protect the endangered aquatic species, the US Forest Service has (inadvertently) given rise to a dumping ground littered with detritus and the shattered remains of shotgun-blasted computer monitors and other impromptu targets.

Follow the singletrack down into the Sespe **drainage (0.2 mile, 3,225', 294999E 3826022N)**, crossing the creek amid a wide swath of grasses and reeds (in the summer this is typically a simple rock-hop, but after rains and in the spring this can entail some wading). On the other side, follow the easy track while several drainages come in from your left (north). Part of your progress here is along the old road grade; as a result the going is easy and the trail—while no longer frequented by motor vehicles—remains quite clear.

Very subtly the track leaves the **old route (1.4 miles, 3,200', 295879E 3826355N)** and begins a switchbacking ascent (formerly, the Middle Sespe Trail followed the creek bed here all the way to beyond both the Rock Creek and Howard Creek confluences). The switchbacks lead you up along and then across a **drainage (2 miles, 3,525', 296482E 3826542N)**, laying out the cottonwood- and fir-lined bend in the Sespe below. On the more exposed stretches you'll likely notice the burned remains of older flora—these are the slow-healing scars of the 1985 Wheeler Fire. Views of the Sespe below, as well as Nordhoff Ridge to your south, become clearer as you traverse this stretch.

At the top of your climb, you'll cut diagonally across a short rocky ridge and glimpse your first expansive views of not only Rock Creek to your left (north) but also the Howard Creek confluence and Rainbow Ranch property. The old Howard Creek Campground was once located at the northern end of Howard Creek Road beside the confluence; the campground was abandoned in 1978 after heavy floods damaged the grounds beyond "reasonable" repair. Though the route is long-abandoned, it is still physically accessible.

Follow the easy switchbacks down the slope here northward, finally gaining a drainage that leads to the crossing with **Rock Creek (3.8 miles, 3,275', 297203E 3826801N)**. There are some minor patches of poison oak here.

Rock Creek typically has water even in the driest years (and was the site of Jeff Howard's infamous run-in with Basque sheepherder Alphonso Urtasan). As it marks the halfway point of your journey along this route, it also makes a fine lunch or rest spot.

From Rock Creek, follow a short series of switchbacks up to a low ridge and continue eastward along a low and fairly barren ridge littered with large sandstone boulders, undulating between sparsely vegetated and rocky stretches and lengths of trail hemmed in by high chaparral. Several minor (and usually dry) creek crossings lead you down into the private inholding; please respect private property and stay on the trail (several posted signs request the same).

From this point, the trail alternates between a near-level route weaving in and out of the drainages coming off the southern flanks of Pine Mountain to your left (north) and wide, rocky stretches across riverside plateaus one might swear were once roads (some of these sections are in fact wider and easier going than many service roads). Your views to the right (south) provide a unique perspective of this stretch of the Sespe.

In time, the looming white sandstone of the Piedra Blanca formation begins to come into view, and the road leading down from Rose Valley to the Piedra Blanca Trailhead (easily discerned due to its telltale cluster of pines) is visible here; the distance, however, is somewhat deceiving, as you must go beyond the parking area to reach the junction with the **Gene Marshall–Piedra Blanca National Recreation Trail (7.7 miles, 3,110', 301843E 3826401N)**. Take the right fork, and then the junction with the **Sespe River Trail (8.2 miles, 3,000', 301845E 3826398N**; another right here).

Follow the Sespe River Trail 0.5 mile eastward to the **Piedra Blanca Trailhead (8.6 miles, 3,050', 301320E 3826437N)** and your shuttle vehicle.

■ ■ ■ ■ ■ ■ ■ ■ ■ ■ ■   **HOW WILD IS "WILD"?**

It's just beyond the Sespe's confluence with Rock Creek and Howard Creek where the upper reach of its Wild and Scenic designation begins. A dam was proposed near the Howard Creek confluence in the 1970s, but it was never realized. Federal reports concede that subsequent wilderness designation of the nearby stretches of the Sespe watershed preclude the likelihood of the region ever being dammed, as new pipelines would not be allowed in the Sespe (nor would tunneling through the nearby mountains to Ojai be allowed). Further, numerous endangered species' reliance on the Sespe's waters all but doom any future aspirations to divert this unique watershed.

■   ■   ■   ■   ■   ■   ■   ■   ■   ■   ■   ■   ■   ■   ■

Route 85

DRY LAKES RIDGE (23W18)

LENGTH AND TYPE:	4.8-mile out-and-back to Basin 3; 5.2-mile one-way to Ortega Trail (23W08)
RATING:	Moderate (initial climb is strenuous; thereafter fairly easy)

TRAIL CONDITION:	Clear (old firebreak) to passable (some minor bushwhacking)
MAP(S):	USGS *Lion Canyon* and *Wheeler Springs*; Conant's *Matilija & Dick Smith Wilderness*
CAMP(S):	Dry Lakes West (abandoned)
HIGHLIGHTS:	Solitude; relictual stands of pine; sagebrush basins

TO REACH THE TRAILHEAD(S): Use the Dry Lakes Ridge Trailhead to access this route.

TRIP SUMMARY: Though officially long-abandoned, this route climbs from CA 33 along a firebreak to Dry Lakes Ridge, a unique botanical region.

Note: Basin naming conventions used along the Dry Lakes Ridge (e.g., Basin 2A and Basin 4) are based upon the works of David Magney, botanist and biologist, whose research along the Dry Lakes Ridge is the authority of the area.

Trip Description

From the **roadside (3,720', 294303E 3824519N)**, follow the thin trail past the boulders through a grassy culvert and through gaps in the roadside brush to the base of a rough dozer cut. From there climb steeply northwest up the firebreak through bush poppies, chamises, and the bleached limbs of long-cut brush to reach the adjoining **firebreak (0.5 mile, 4,400', 293916E 3825066N)** along the ridgetop.

Follow this break left (westward) along the still-rough but far-less-steep cut toward the Dry Lakes Ridge Botanical Area, **topping out (1.1 miles, 4,800', 292976E 3825013N)** just north of a knoll and with the first basins well in view below. Views here of Lake Casitas, the Channel Islands, and the Pacific to the south and west and Piedra Blanca, the Sespe watershed, and Pine Mountain to the east and north are fantastic, and from a perspective few others have the opportunity to enjoy. From here you can also distinguish where the firebreak diverges into three distinct cuts near the first basin—bear this in mind as you approach the junction, as what seems to be the obvious route effectively dead-ends and is not the most effective route for traversing this ridge.

Following the dozer line down toward the basins, take special care to veer right off the "main" cut at a **junction (1.3 miles, 4,750', 292756E 3824984N)** where a second, less-worn cut heads right (northwest). This proves the easiest route to navigate and will lead you through all the basins.

Drop easily along the cut into the Great Basin sage and diminishing manzanitas and ceanothus, where your route becomes a better-defined doubletrack road as you enter the first basin (Basin 1). The route here is very easy to follow as you pass through the first series of sage-blanketed basins and into the second. You'll then begin to angle toward a cluster of fire-scarred ponderosa **pines (1.75 miles, 4,700', 292156E 3824924N)** set along the lip of Basin 2A and just below where the dozer cut opened the barrier of vegetation separating this from the higher Basin 2B to the southwest. That the route you now walk is still in such good repair is a testament to the slow recovery of some of the plant types in this unique environment.

Continue westward through Basin 2B past a trio of mature ponderosas and then past another pair of equally impressive pines before passing through another cut down a short but fairly steep grade to the eastern edge of **Basin 3 (2.3 miles, 4,500', 291418E 3824694N)**.

At Basin 3, the vegetative cover lacks the sage that dominates the previous basin and is instead blanketed by grasses and butter lupines. A New Deal–era ice can stove can be found near the dense cluster of pines along the basin's western edge, and some debris (ranging from gas and oil cans to Sterno canisters and heavy-gauge cable) likely left behind decades ago after fire suppression efforts dot the periphery of the meadows.

From the camp at Basin 3, the trail continues nearly 3 miles west toward the Ortega Trail. Follow the cut just north of the stove and cluster of pines and continue west into another small (and the final) basin, where Dry Lakes Ridge West trail camp once stood. From this final basin, follow the cut west as it doglegs out of a small watershed to lead you into a shallow **drainage (3.1 miles, 4,470', 290903E 3824590N)** lined with oaks and willow saplings. From here, the cut ascends steeply, leaving the botanical area and cresting at the **junction (3.5 miles, 4,900', 290232E 3824665N)** with the old Tule Creek Trail.

Cutting to your right (north) here will lead down the Tule Creek drainage, where you can pick up the remnants of the old Tule Creek Trail and follow the drainage out to the highway (have a shuttle vehicle awaiting you) at the Sespe-Tule confluence; see *Route 83* for this route.

Continue another 1.5 miles west along the rough cut with sweeping views laid out beneath you on both your left and right to join with the **Ortega Trail (5.2 miles, 4,780', 287509E 287509N)**.

THE RIDGE THAT TIME FORGOT ▨ ▨ ▨ ▨ ▨ ▨ ▨ ▨ ▨

Built in the mid-1950s after the 1948 Wheeler Fire cleared much of the undergrowth and chaparral, the Dry Lakes Ridge Trail (formerly 23W18) was a popular but still fairly strenuous route, as it was a dry camp and something of a climb for those approaching from the east (as the route described here does). The route was maintained for about 20 years, until the federal fiscal crisis marked both the two sites atop the ridge and the trail proper for removal and/or abandonment.

In the decade that followed, the ridge received very few visitors, and it wasn't until the Wheeler Fire of 1985 and the fire cuts that resulted that a few visitors again began to frequent the area (but even they are typically die-hard geocachers or dedicated botanists and naturalists interested in the flora atop the ridge). Since the 1985 recut, the Dry Lakes Ridge line and the cut west (adjacent to the Ortega Trail) have continued to serve as fire lines; both the Ortega and Dry Lakes dozer lines were utilized again during the 1993 Wheel Fire as well as during the 2002 Wolf Fire.

The term "Dry Lakes" is a bit of a misnomer, as it is generally held that the depressions atop this ridge were never lakes, but rather porous sandstone depressions largely incapable of retaining water, even after heavy rains.

The part that is *not* a misnomer is the "dry"—there is no reliable water along the ridge, so be sure to carry enough for your trip (the drainage on the north side of the saddle beyond Basin 4 is intermittent at best and shouldn't be relied upon).

Dry Lakes Ridge Botanical Area—406 acres set aside by the USFS—is one of five such areas in the Los Padres.

■ ■ ■ ■ ■ ■ ■ ■ ■ ■ ■ ■ ■ ■

Route 86

SESPE RIVER TRAIL (20W13 and 20W30)

LENGTH AND TYPE:	8.8-mile out-and-back to Bear Creek Camp; 10.6-mile out-and-back to Oak Flat Camp; 8.7 miles one-way to junction with Red Reef Trail; 10.2-mile out-and-back to Willett Hot Springs; 30.4-mile out-and-back to Sespe Hot Springs (includes 1.5 miles along Johnston Ridge Trail); 16.9-mile one-way to junction with Alder Creek Trail
RATING:	Moderate (for creek crossings and distance)
TRAIL CONDITION:	Well maintained (former 4WD route; heavily traveled)
MAP(S):	USGS *Lion Canyon, Topatopa Mountains,* and *Devils Heart Peak*; Harrison's *Sespe Wilderness*
CAMP(S):	Bear Creek, Timber Canyon (abandoned trail camp), Oak Flat, Sycamore (abandoned car camp), Thacher (abandoned car camp), Willett, Hartman (abandoned car camp), and Coltrell Flat
HIGHLIGHTS:	Fascinating geology; swimming holes; hot springs; potential condor sightings

TO REACH THE TRAILHEAD(S): Use the Piedra Blanca Trailhead to access this route.

TRIP SUMMARY: This extremely popular route follows the old Sespe River Road, with the main attraction being the numerous swimming spots, Willett Hot Springs, and Sespe Hot Springs (the hottest springs in California).

Trip Description

From the **trailhead** (**3,040', 301320E 3826437N**), follow the trail downstream, crossing the creek three times (after rains this may entail wet feet!) to the **junction** (**0.5 mile, 3,000', 301843E 3826401N**) with the Middle Sespe and Gene Marshall–Piedra Blanca Trails.

Head right (east) here and follow the old road along a comfortable grade. You'll cross **Piedra Blanca Creek (0.9 mile, 2,980', 302498E 3826326N)** as you hike through the private easement that includes Patton's Cabin (also known as Thacher Cabin); be sure to stay on the trail and respect private property. Once out of the easement, you enter the Sespe Wilderness.

Your route continues along the north banks of the Sespe for another 3.5 miles on a fairly level route with a few climbs and descents (all quite minor). The landscape is still recovering from the 2006 Day Fire; portions of the terrain either side of the trail consist primarily of wide swaths of low scrub. When the Sespe is running (in all but the driest months), numerous swimming and wading opportunities present themselves whenever the trail is close to the riverbank.

You'll hike into the sandy, cottonwood-shaded **Bear Creek Camp (4.4 miles, 2,810', 307139E 3826267N)** just before your next crossing.

CAMP :: BEAR CREEK

ELEVATION:	2,810'
MAP:	USGS *Topatopa Mountains*
UTM:	307139E 3826267N

A former car camp, Bear Creek Camp is a bit worn-down but still a good spot if you're looking for a short day out. There are numerous guerrilla fire rings and log benches set beneath the huge cottonwoods, and the site is along the creek, so water is easily accessed. The concrete vault from the old outhouse is still visible on the northwest edge of camp, and the old barrier posts can be seen in the wash west of the site. The 1971 Bear Fire was so named because it originated at this camp.

Note: The *Topatopa Mountains* USGS 7.5-minute quad incorrectly shows Bear Creek Camp on the south side of the Sespe.

Just past Bear Creek Camp is your next **creek crossing (4.5 miles, 2,820', 307207E 3826288N)**. Once across mind your bearings a moment; the trail actually takes a quick jog to your right (upstream) before heading back in your direction of travel. This little dogleg is often cause for the occasional unwarranted rock-hop down the Sespe before hikers realize they've missed something.

From the crossing, follow the trail as it climbs a short distance and then skirts a rocky slide area above the creek before entering intermittently riparian spots spared by the fires. There is a short stretch through an inholding as you pass seeping portions of trail beneath Kerr Springs—you may also spot a few remnants of the outbuildings that once dotted this area (including the brick walls and old latrines).

After a mile of easy hiking, you'll find yourself at another wide **crossing (5.7 miles, 2,740', 308682E 3826474N)**—this is the infamous stretch where in 1969 six youths and four adults perished attempting to cross a storm-swollen Sespe. From here the old road will lead you through a wide area populated by brilliant wildflower displays in the spring and up a steady grade to a wonderful overlook of a bend in the Sespe, now far below. From this vantage point you'll be able to make out Oak Flat Camp (the tables are admittedly a dead giveaway) across Sespe Creek, and you'll have a good view of the geologic layers where Rincon shale, Vaqueros sandstone, and the Sespe formation overlay one another in close quarters.

SAVAGE SESPE ■ ■ ■ ■ ■ ■ ■ ■ ■ ■ ■ ■ ■

Everybody who grew up with the Sespe in their life—or raised children with the Sespe in their life—knows this tale in one form or another. It has become something of a myth in Sespe lore—the story of six boys, their chaperone, and three of their would-be rescuers and how they were consumed by the usually calm and often predictable Sespe. The case has been recounted often enough that it needn't be set to type again here. A heart-wrenching account of the tragedy ("Hell in High Water") was published in the February 2008 issue of *Outside* magazine; that article and other accounts can be found online.

■ ■ ■ ■ ■ ■ ■ ■ ■ ■ ■ ■ ■ ■ ■ ■ ■

Follow the road back down to the drainage—passing through the Kimball Canyon (see "Timber Canyon Spur" on the next page)—and quickly you'll come upon the (easily missed) **junction (7.1 miles, 2,660', 310290E 3826317N)** to Oak Flat Camp. This spur trail receives very little use (and even less maintenance), so it can often be a matter of route-finding and avoiding obstacles to reach the creekside where, again, you'll often need to ford. It's 0.25 mile from the junction to **Oak Flat Camp (2,640', 310476E 3826149N)**.

CAMP :: OAK FLAT

ELEVATION:	2,640'
MAP:	USGS *Topatopa Mountains*
UTM:	310476E 3826149N

Oak Flat is, as its name suggests, situated beneath a pleasant pair of live oaks on a creekside flat just downstream from the confluence of Sespe, Kimball, and Timber Creeks. The primary site provides two old concrete-and-wood plank tables, as well as a serviceable fire pit. A few guerilla sites can be found westward along the flats, the nicest spot perhaps being at the base of the geological layers observed earlier from across the creek. This site is set on a sandy flat beneath numerous cotton-woods. Numerous guerrilla sites are also east of the main site, along the banks of the Sespe where it begins around the flat.

Note: The *Topatopa Mountains* USGS 7.5-minute quad incorrectly shows Oak Flat Camp on the northwest side of the Sespe.

▪ ▪ ▪ ▪ ▪ ▪ ▪ ▪ ▪ TIMBER CANYON SPUR

Until the early 1970s, a trail led to a small campsite known as Timber Canyon. The spur trail and campsite were among those that became casualties of the mid-1970s closures, but the site's amenities (specifically, the stoves) were never removed, and the old Timber Canyon still makes a suitable spot for those looking for a bit more solitude and/or privacy than the trailside camps provide but who perhaps don't wish to endeavor clearing a new kitchen or building a new fire ring. Three stoves still avail themselves for those who take this path less traveled, and while one of the oaks in the area has come crashing down since the 2006 fire swept through, there is still space aplenty on the grassy flat east of the kitchens. Best of all, the site is not visible from the trail.

To access Timber Canyon, head downstream along Kimball Creek (the drainage just before the turnoff to Oak Flat) from the trail through the red Sespe sandstone and to the creekside. There are wind- and water-eroded rock formations and excellent swimming holes here. Just downstream of the Timber Creek confluence is a flat with a handful of mature live oaks and the old camp. Enjoy!

▪ ▪ ▪ ▪ ▪ ▪ ▪ ▪ ▪ ▪ ▪ ▪ ▪ ▪ ▪ ▪ ▪ ▪

Whether staying the night at Oak Flat or continuing on, it's another 1.5 miles from the spur junction to the **Red Reef Trail junction (8.7 miles, 2,640', 311519E 3827096N)**. See *Route 88* for this route.

Some remnants of the old Sycamore car camp (given up when the road was formally closed in 1979) remain just downstream across the same flat the Red Reef Trail crosses; the old site (still quite serviceable as an overnight site) is about 0.2 mile from the junction, beneath the stand of cottonwoods on the north banks of the creek.

From the Red Reef junction, continue eastward, quickly crossing the often-dry Syca-more Creek and heading up to yet another flat overlooking the Sespe, as you head toward Ten Sycamore Flat and Willett Hot Springs. Especially in the years since the Day Fire denuded the hills along the Sespe drainage, you'll note the scars of several old service and oil exploratory roads ascending the mountains to your south; routes followed portions of Red Reef and even Park Canyon but have been since lost to the ages. (Similarly, another trail—20W01A—once ascended the Sycamore Creek drainage to meet with the Johnston Ridge route. It is now little more than a curious thread winding its way up the drainage, with numerous slides covering the old route after about 3 miles up.)

As you round the flat above Ten Sycamore Flat, directly below you'll be able to pick out some of the old spots that were once the Thacher campsites. To reach the camps there, follow one of the few spur trails leading toward the flats just before you reach the Sespe and backtrack about 200 yards back upstream to **Thacher Camp (2,520', 312213E 3827143N)**.

CAMP :: THACHER

ELEVATION:	2,520'
MAP:	USGS *Topatopa Mountains*
UTM:	312213E 3827143N

While neither recognized nor currently maintained by the Forest Service, the old Thacher site is now commonly referred to as Ten Sycamore Flat, though that name is actually applied to the riverside flat across and a bit farther downstream. The site contains a handful of old stoves and fire rings, and—especially nice—some of the old concrete picnic tables still dot this area. Even after the decimation of the Day Fire, a cluster of hearty live oaks still provide shade, and water is easily accessed in the creek.

Note: This site no longer appears on USGS or USFS maps, but it is shown on Harrison's *Sespe Wilderness*, as well as the Sespe-area trailhead signs based on Harrison's map.

Continuing eastward along the main trail, you'll make your next **crossing (9.5 miles, 2,500', 312088E 3827381N)** of the Sespe through willow- and cottonwood-hemmed banks, and along the other side the route is more of a genuine singletrack along the usually cool and shaded south bank until you reach the **junction (9.7 miles, 2,490', 312433E 3827581N)** for Willet campsite and the hot springs.

To gain the Willet sites, follow the spur to the left (north) and cross the creek bed (wider here; there may be several water crossings) to the junction with the Willett use **trail (0.1 mile from the main trail, 2,500', 312431E 3827696N)**. A half mile to your left (west) are the **Willett Hot Springs (0.7 mile from the main trail, 311833E 3827922N)**, and in both directions you'll find numerous sites suitable for making camp. See the following entry for details.

CAMP :: WILLETT

ELEVATION:	2,500'
MAP:	USGS *Topatopa Mountains*
UTM:	312431E 3827696N (trail junction; site is spread out on both sides)

Named for the homesteader who settled near and developed the springs here in the late 19th century, Willett is a sprawling location with plenty of space. Tables, fire pits, and old tool and tackle sheds abound, but so too do a handful of cabins. Some of the best—including the one truly decent remaining first-come, first-serve cabin—are just off to the right (east) of the trail junction after you've crossed the Sespe. A local horse-mounted guide service often makes use of this camp.

The route from camp to the hot springs is a bit of a climb—gaining about 250 feet of elevation in that 0.5 mile from camp—but one that has continued to prove popular over the decades. A large plastic tub has been in place for the last several years. The springs are nowhere near as hot (nor sulfuric) as those at Sespe Hot Springs some 5 miles distant and are in a somewhat less foreboding setting.

Please do not camp near the tub; allow others to enjoy its use.

From the Willett junction back on the south side of the Sespe, it's less than a mile to lightly used **Hartman Camp** (**10.5 miles, 2,480', 313414E 3827240N**).

CAMP :: HARTMAN

ELEVATION:	2,480'
MAP:	USGS *Topatopa Mountains*
UTM:	313414E 3827240N

Named for a squatter who once occupied the site but was of no relation to the Hartmans of Ojai nor the ranch nearby, this camp was once the site of a USFS guard (field) station built in the mid-1920s. Subsequent years saw it converted into the popular '60s- and '70s-era car campground. Little is left of the Hartman site save the old concrete table and scavenged fire rings from that tenure decades ago. A group of mature live oaks (damaged from the 2006 fire) provide some shade here.

Note: This site no longer appears on USGS or USFS maps but is shown on Harrison's *Sespe Wilderness*, as well as the Sespe-area trailhead signs based on Harrison's map.

From Hartman, the going becomes even more level than the previous 11 miles (though by this point you may be just tired enough to not appreciate the subtle change in difficulty). Gone for the next few miles are the (literal) ups and downs over which the previous stretch undulated. Follow the old road across another pair of stream crossings, and as you begin to cross a series of tributaries on your right (south)—the last of which is Park Creek—you'll be as close to the Sespe Condor Sanctuary as you'll come along this route, as the sanctuary's boundary drives northward from the Topatopa Mountains to within a 0.5 mile of the Sespe here.

". . . AND THE FLAMES WENT HIGHER" ▪ ▪ ▪ ▪ ▪ ▪ ▪ ▪ ▪ ▪

Fire has always played a key role in forming forests' landscapes, and the Los Padres is no exception. One of the more unique instances of its incursion into the backcountry is when recording superstar Johnny Cash accidentally started the Adobe Fire in June 1965.

The singer had driven "Jesse," his now-infamous Chevrolet pickup with camper, along the Sespe Road (now the Sespe River Trail) to near Cottriel (Coltrell) Flat for a spot of fishing. The assistant fire control officer of the Ojai Ranger District—who arrived on the scene after being notified of a fire—found Cash reportedly high on pills and sitting on the side of the road with the truck nearby. The fire officer soon determined a portion of the truck's exhaust pipe had detached from the muffler and ignited the grass beneath the truck.

The fire burned 508 acres, and some accounts claim it also killed 49 of the nearby sanctuary's 53 condors. (Cash later claimed to have proclaimed, in his inimitable style, "I don't give a damn about your yellow buzzards!" when informed of this.) The loss of condors has been disputed by fire personnel and discounted for a lack of evidence (e.g., recovered condor carcasses).

The Adobe Fire required a week of firefighting efforts—including air tanker drops—and for his role in turning a portion of the Sespe black, the Man in Black was fined $82,000.

▪   ▪   ▪   ▪   ▪   ▪   ▪   ▪   ▪   ▪   ▪   ▪   ▪   ▪   ▪

Another pair of crossings usher you up toward a gap set between two knolls on the northern banks of the creek, and then down into Coltrell (Cottriel) Flat and—down toward the creek—the **Coltrell Flat campsite** (**13.3 miles, 2,330', 317043E 3827932N**).

CAMP :: COLTRELL FLAT

ELEVATION:	2,330'
MAP:	USGS *Devils Heart Peak*
UTM:	317043E 3827932N

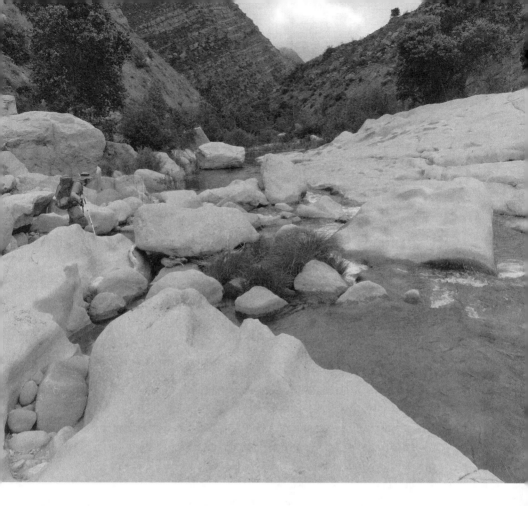

Toward the Devils Gate; courtesy Ventura County Canyoneering

Coltrell (or Cottriel) Flat—named for George W. Cottriel, who patented land here in 1891—has a long and colorful history in the annals of Sespe camping. Scorched in the 2006 Day Fire, the old oaks here still provide shade. Just upstream from camp is an ideal swimming hole, usually a fine spot even during drier seasons.

Note: The Harrison *Sespe Wilderness* map and current USFS recreation maps label this site as "Coltrell Flat"; USGS quads label it as "Cottriel Flat."

An easy 0.5 mile from Coltrell Flat is the signed **junction (13.8 miles, 2,400', 317531E 3827922N)** with the Johnston Ridge Trail (20W12), which follows Hot Springs Canyon to Sespe Hot Spring campsite and then ascends the west side of the drainage and climbs to Mutau Flat. If heading to the hot springs as part of your trek, you'll head left (north) here and continue up Hot Springs Canyon for another 1.5 miles (see *Route 89*).

Now on the stretch of trail officially defined as the Upper Sespe Trail (20W30), cross Hot Springs Creek as it flows into Sespe Creek, and the less-traveled trail here will lead you along the left (north) bank of the creek toward the Alder Creek confluence. The canyons here steepen and begin to close in, and just as the Sespe begins its slow arc southward while your route keeps a roughly eastward bearing, you'll reach the old **Devils Gate junction** (**14.9 miles, 2,220', 318654E 318654N**). The thin route heading right (the old 20W14) follows the Sespe for some 15 miles toward Fillmore, but it's no longer maintained due to the rugged terrain and narrows and private land issues at the southern end.

Continue left/straight here, ascending and dropping down a series of gaps and creek-side knolls as you leave the Sespe behind.

DEVILS GATE

If you can't bear the thought of leaving the Sespe and don't wish to head up toward the plateau dividing this drainage and that of Alder Creek to the east—or if you've planned for a transect of the Sespe from your point of origin to, say, Fillmore—know that there is still a marginally viable route that follows the creek bed to its confluence with Alder Creek. In the 1950s and 1960s two campsites existed along this stretch of the upper Devils Gate route: Sweetwater, situated on a flat between two tributaries coming in from the north slopes of Devils Heart Peak; and Alder Sespe, at the confluence with Alder Creek. Both sites were abandoned as part of the federal budget crunch in the mid-1970s, but the actual sites still have room enough to make camp.

Farther (beyond the Alder-Sespe confluence) are a series of "squeezes," where the Sespe cuts through high canyon walls. Also along some of the canyon walls are the remnants of old roads used by exploratory crews when the viability of damming the Sespe was still being considered. Many folks hike this route, and then—because the original exit via the Van Trees Ranch is no longer allowed—will egress via the old Green Cabins service road along Tar Creek and through the sanctuary. Because the old road is now within the Sespe Condor Sanctuary, hiking it is against the law. Numerous trespassers explore Tar Creek every weekend, whether to rappel, climb, or enjoy the magnificent swimming holes—and the litter and damage continue to mount (as do the number of calls placed to local search and rescue).

As late as the 1980s, the USFS was investigating the possibility of establishing a corridor along the old Green Cabins Road for those wishing to explore this stretch of the Sespe, but nothing came of it.

If you're hearty enough to explore the Sespe Narrows, you can hike back. Please respect the efforts of those working to preserve the condors and keep out of the sanctuary.

Climbing out of the Sespe, you'll reach a small **plateau (16.2 miles, 2,940',
319967E 3828033N)** with excellent views of the lower Alder Creek drainage before dropping
down to the **junction (16.9 miles, 2,410', 320961E 3827547N)** with the lower Alder Creek Trail
(see *Route 90*), marking the formal terminus of the Sespe River Trail. Just beyond is the eastern junction for the old Devils Gate route, and 0.25 mile down Alder Creek is Shady Camp
(see *Route 90* for camp description).

Route 87

LION CANYON

LENGTH AND TYPE:	4.6-mile out-and-back (East Fork); 4.8-mile out-and-back (West Fork); 5.5-mile one-way (Nordhoff Ridge Road)
RATING:	Easy to the forks; moderate to Nordhoff Ridge Road
TRAIL CONDITION:	Clear; passable along portions of the West Fork
MAP(S):	USGS *Lion Canyon*; Harrison's *Sespe Wilderness*
CAMP(S):	East Fork Lion and West Fork Lion
HIGHLIGHTS:	Riparian trekking; numerous swimming and wading holes; waterfalls

TO REACH THE TRAILHEAD(S): Use the Middle Lion Campground to access this route.

TRIP SUMMARY: From Middle Lion Campground, this pleasant and easy hike meanders along
Lion Creek's drainage to the trail junction at the convergence of the creek's east and west forks.
From the junction, you have the option of easy hikes along either fork to relaxing pools, camp-
sites, and waterfalls, or a more strenuous hike up the western canyon to Nordhoff Ridge.

Trip Description

From the **Middle Lion Campground (3,160', 301226E 3825202N)**, hike south through the
campsite at the foot of the road in, and follow the trail to Lion Creek. Cross the creek under
cover of mature alders and continue along the east bank. Opportunities for wading are plentiful here, as there are numerous pools deep enough for wading and general enjoyment.

After an easy 0.5 mile of following the sycamore- and alder-shaded creek, the gorge
narrows and your route begins to climb away from the creek bed, back into the yucca- and
scrub-covered chaparral before rejoining the water's course where the canyon widens just
north of the junction with the **Rose-Lion Connector** trail **(1.3 miles, 3,390', 301858E 3823552N;**
see *Route 67*). A short distance down the connector you can access the creek for a pleasant
water break or lunch spot.

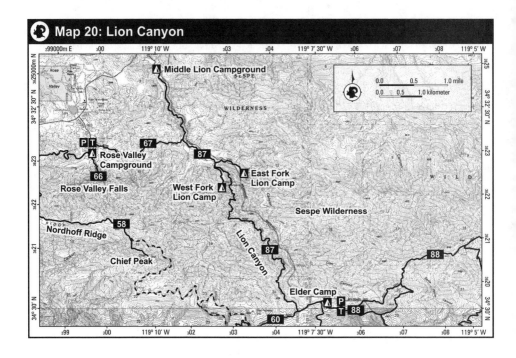

Map 20: Lion Canyon

From the junction, continue southward along the very easy grade another 0.5 mile (passing the actual convergence of the East and West Forks of Lion Creek and crossing the East Fork) until you reach a small meadow at the **Four Points Trail junction** of the Lion Canyon trails (**1.9 miles, 3,430', 302586E 3823042N**).

Here, you have a choice of three paths.

East Fork
The left (easternmost) of the trails presented here leads to East Fork Lion campground in another easy 0.5 mile.

From the junction, follow the trail through the meadow into the creek bed, where your route is lined with arroyo willow for a few hundred feet, and then opens into a wide space alongside the creek, lined with mature sycamores and bigcone Douglas-firs. A number of guerrilla/overflow camps are en route. Where the canyon again narrows and a group of conifers stands along the trail, you'll enter **East Fork Lion campground** (**2.4 miles, 3,470', 303216E 3822842N**). This area is a popular destination for day hikers and local Scout groups, the latter of which make the East Fork Lion a regular destination. As a result, perhaps of some conscientious Scoutmasters' direction, the camp is usually very clean and well tended.

Just beyond are a series of **falls** (**2.5 miles, 3,500', 303300E 3822714N**) and beautiful pools, ideal spots for wading in the summer. The falls spill over a sliver of cobble conglomerate

MAP 21 Sespe River Trail **357**

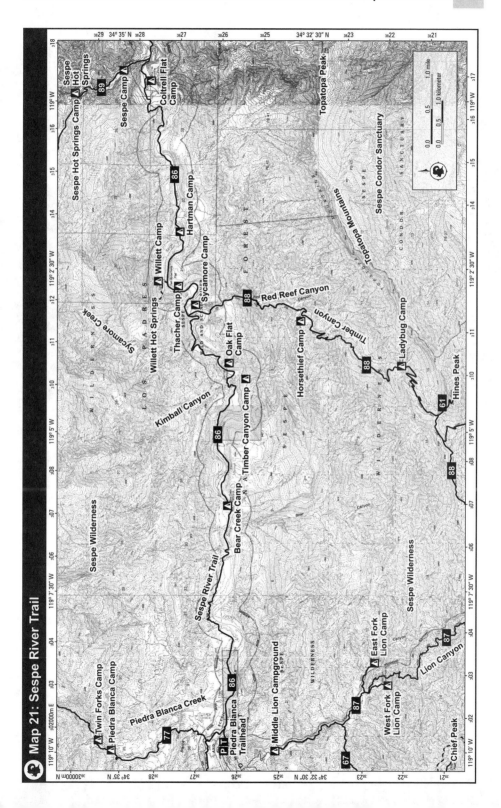

Map 21: Sespe River Trail

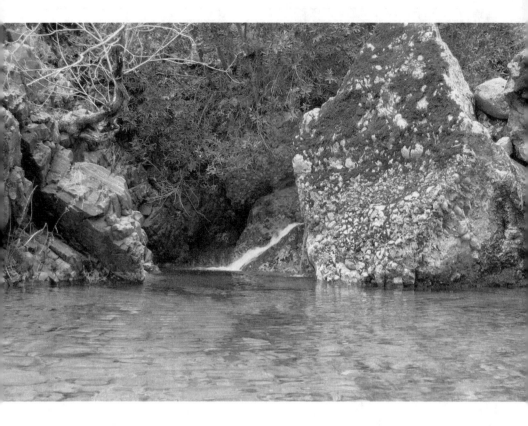

Pools below East Fork Lion Falls

consisting of granitic and quartzitic detritus in an arkosic sandstone matrix; the same layer is crossed by the Lion Canyon Trail en route to Nordhoff Peak, and then again by the West Fork falls (see page 359 for both). Sans conglomerate, this same type of harder sandstone is also found at the falls along Rose Valley Creek (see *Route 66*). These East Fork falls are also littered with large boulders of this conglomerate, many of which are covered with heavy, felt-like green moss. The entire grotto is shaded by numerous alders.

CAMP :: **EAST FORK LION**

ELEVATION:	3,470'
MAP:	USGS *Lion Canyon*
UTM:	303216E 3822842N

This spacious site is set on a pleasant flat on the east banks of the east fork. Formerly known as Spruce Falls Camp, it possesses two kitchens with grills, the nicest of which is situated beneath a pair of huge bigcone Douglas-firs. Grills from other kitchens have been pilfered over the years to augment these two remaining cooking areas. A stretch of sycamores borders the downstream (northern) edge of the camp.

To Nordhoff Ridge

The middle fork of the trails leads 3.5 miles along the west fork to Nordhoff Ridge Road.

From the meadow, follow the trail into the west fork drainage and begin climbing immediately. While not overly steep, there is no break in the chaparral-hedged ascent until you reach the ridge. A handful of springs along the upper half of the route can occasionally be drawn upon for water, but it's best to carry enough and not rely upon these intermittent sources.

The trail climbs along the eastern slopes of the west fork drainage, providing you a view of the sandstone formation over which both forks' falls spill. Ascend for 3 miles with great views of the upper stretches of the canyon—and Chief Peak—before you cross back over a shallow saddle eastward and continue the climb along the western slopes of the east fork. The waters far below can be heard in their rush northward toward the falls, and ultimately for their merger with the Sespe River a few miles farther. Bays and ferns shade the cooler, north-facing corners of the trail, and here too you'll find a number of springs (usually dry).

In the final stretch you'll climb out of the drainage onto the firebreak and **Nordhoff Ridge Road (5.5 miles, 5,140', 304517E 3819606N)**, with magnificent views of the upper Ojai Valley and beyond, as well as (more immediately) Sisar and Wilsie Canyons. Your options from the road are numerous; with shuttle, pickup, or other arrangements, numerous routes detailed in Chapter 10 can all be accessed within a few miles (done in reverse now, as you'll be entering from the high point).

West Fork

The right (westernmost) trail leads 0.5 mile to West Fork Lion campground and the waterfall beyond.

From the junction stay right (west) and continue into the west fork drainage. This trail, the least-used of the three, often entails hiking along a lightly maintained route. While the footing is clear, brush can be overgrown, and a bit of bushwhacking may be the order of the day. About half the route follows the creek bed until stepping to the side for a clear patch until **West Fork Lion campground (2.3 miles, 3,470', 302758E 3822520N)**, which is situated beside a blackberry bramble just before a thick coppice of white alders along the stream.

The **West Fork falls (2.4 miles, 3,520', 302768E 3822400N)** are just beyond and possess the most fascinating example of the area's cobble conglomerate (see the description under the east fork trip on page 356). To access the area above the falls, follow the thread of a trail in

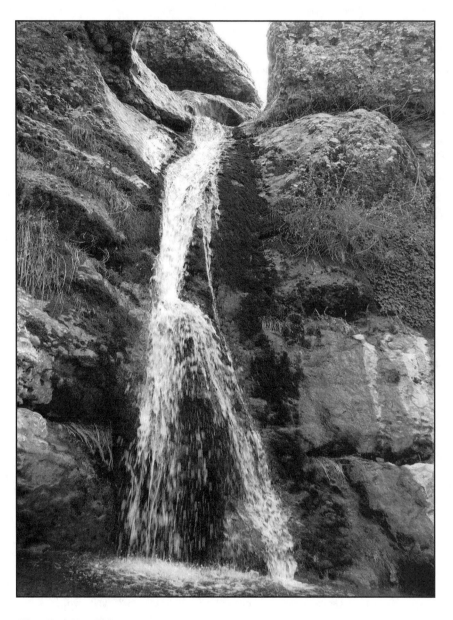

West Fork Lion Falls

the tributary on your left (east of the main pool); it requires a bit of scrambling (using the large bay tree there for leverage can facilitate that scramble).

CAMP :: WEST FORK LION

ELEVATION:	3,470'
MAP:	USGS *Lion Canyon*
UTM:	302758E 3822520N

This site (formerly known as Dynamite Camp)—while comfortable—receives far less use than its east fork twin. Set beneath mature white alders and sycamores, it possesses three kitchens with grills. The main site is directly off the trail on the east bank of the west fork; the second (and much smaller) is just across the creek. A third site can be found on the small "island" just upstream, situated beneath the massive streamside alders. A fourth site—largely forgotten—is along a game trail downstream and on the west bank of the creek. It is situated beneath a coppice of mature sycamores and possesses only a New Deal–era ice can stove.

Route 88

RED REEF TRAIL (21W08)

LENGTH AND TYPE:	26.5-mile one-way (8.5 miles along the Sespe River Trail; 18 miles along the Red Reef Trail and Sisar Road); shuttle
RATING:	Strenuous
TRAIL CONDITION:	Clear to passable from Sespe River Trail to Ladybug; clear from Ladybug to Hines Peak junction; well maintained from Hines Peak junction to White Ledge junction (former and current service roads); clear along lower trail; well maintained along Sisar Road (service road)
MAP(S):	USGS *Topatopa Mountains* and *Santa Paula Peak*; Harrison's *Sespe Wilderness*
CAMP(S):	Horsethief (abandoned), Ladybug, Elder (dry 4WD camp), and White Ledge
HIGHLIGHTS:	Wilderness trekking; fascinating geology

TO REACH THE TRAILHEAD(S): Use the Piedra Blanca and Sisar Canyon Trailheads for this shuttle.

TRIP SUMMARY: This excellent thru-hike—which follows 8.5 miles of the Sespe River Trail before cutting south and up the north slope of the Topatopa Mountains—makes for a wonderful multiday trek, climbing out of the Sespe to the Topatopa Mountains and then descending toward Ojai via Sisar Canyon.

Trip Description

This trip begins at the Piedra Blanca Trailhead in Rose Valley and follows the Sespe River for an easily navigated first leg without great exertion. See *Route 86* for the first 8.5 miles.

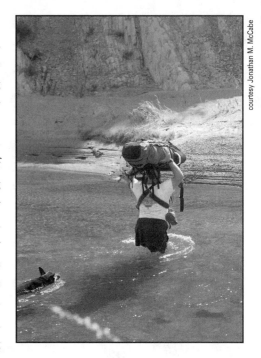

In early 2011, the California Conservation Corps (CCC) reworked the length of the Red Reef Trail, repairing and stabilizing lengthy sections damaged in the 2006 Day Fire. It's a fine example of trail work, and barring any other conflagrations or other disasters should serve hikers for generations to come. There are, however, a few spots where pants or gaiters are still recommended, as resurgent scrub oaks, whitethorn ceanothus, and sundry other unforgiving species encroach upon the tread.

Just another day crossing the Sespe . . .

From the Red Reef and Sespe River Trails **junction (8.5 miles, 2,680', 311519E 3827096N)**, bear right (south) into the grassy meadow and toward the confluence of Red Reef and Sespe Creeks. Through the grasses the trail can be difficult to discern here, but take your bearings on the obvious geologic fractures visible upstream from a stand of mature cottonwoods where another nearby trail leads. (That trail leads into those cottonwoods, where the old Sycamore Campground stands from the days when this stretch of the Sespe Trail was still a 4WD road.)

Staying right, you can follow flagging and rock cairns as they're available over a small rise and down to a sandy **beach (8.8 miles, 2,590', 311633E 3826132N)** situated directly across from where Red Reef Creek pours into the Sespe. If you're still on your first day from the Piedra Blanca Trailhead, this beach area makes for an ideal campsite. (Alternately, you may wish to use the old Sycamore site just downstream, where in decades past there existed another route for accessing this canyon.) The geology here is fascinating; near-vertical layers jut from the mountains on either side and run into the course of the Sespe, at places surfacing along the water like fins. These fins are where the trail and canyon get their name; a formation of red Sespe sandstone cuts across the creek only a few miles up, forming the Red Reef.

When water levels are low, the rock layer forms something of a weir across the Sespe and is often the best place to cross, making a near-bridge for your use. In the spring and after measurable rains, it's best to ford downstream from this line, wading through where the river bottom is an easy base of gravel (upstream is quite rocky and complicated).

Once across the Sespe, the Red Reef Trail ascends the canyon on the right (west) side of the creek, climbing easily through grassy slopes and oak-shaded ledges. Poison oak is common in the shaded areas here. Soon you'll come to your first crossing (**9.5 miles, 3,000', 311990E 3825940N**) of Red Reef Creek, and shortly thereafter you'll pass through **Harris Tunnel** (**9.5 miles, 3,020', 311956E 3825841N**). Note the inscriptions from 1904 on either wall.

Past Harris Tunnel, follow the trail easily along sycamore- and alder-shaded crossings and trail worked by the CCC in 2011. Soon you'll reach the **saddle** (**11 miles, 3,900', 311609E 3824542N**) between the Red Reef and Timber Creek drainages; westward in the grassy flat below you is the old Horsethief campsite. Enjoy the brief downhill you're afforded here, as it is quite literally the *only* downhill you will have until reaching the junction to Ladybug Camp some 3 miles distant. The **spur** (**11.1 miles, 3,800', 311641E 3824344N**) on your right to Horsethief is easy to miss (if you reach the crossing with Timber Creek, you've passed it). Watch for the thin trail at about your 5 o'clock, and then follow it 0.25 mile northward back along the flat to the old site (see opposite).

CAMP :: HORSETHIEF

ELEVATION:	3,840'
MAP:	USGS *Topatopa Mountains*
UTM:	311489E 3824484N

Officially abandoned in 1974 as part of the wide-reaching contraction of services during the fiscal crisis, Horsethief is a very lightly used site with one kitchen and three New Deal–era ice can stoves. While not actually plotted on the 1995 *Topatopa Mountains* quad, the label implies that the site is on the west banks of the creek; rather, it is visible from the Red Reef–Timber Creek Saddle in the grassy area *east* of the creek bend. What little shade was provided by smaller oaks, alders, and sycamores has been lessened in the wake of the Day Fire, but it does make for a pleasant lunch or overnight spot in all but the hottest months.

Beyond the spur is your single **crossing** (**11.2 miles, 3,790', 311577E 3824279N**) of Timber Creek until beyond Ladybug. After crossing you'll approach the remains of a junction; stay right and follow the track as it curves southward along the grassy east banks of Timber Creek. Be mindful not only of your footing here but also of poodle-dog bush. Views of the Topatopa Mountains grow closer and provide encouragement as you continue along another series of switchbacks, while repeating the pattern of an easy ascent that curves in and then out of the tributary ravines.

Soon enough you'll be able to discern the green cluster of trees nestled at the foot of the bluffs and reach the **junction (14.3 miles, 4,800', 310229E 3822139N)** to Ladybug Camp. Even if you're hiking through, the trails meet again, and simply a water break at this pleasant camp is worthwhile. The trail drops steeply here for a few hundred yards until it deposits you beneath the cool shade of mature firs and oaks.

CAMP :: LADYBUG

ELEVATION:	4,760'
MAP:	USGS *Topatopa Mountains*
UTM:	310232E 3822057N

Named for the numerous red-and-black insects that often populate this spot, Ladybug is a very comfortable site that escaped the full brunt of the Day Fire. It is shaded by mature oaks, bays, sycamores, bigcone Douglas-firs, and big-leaf maples that cluster just upstream along the banks of Timber Creek. There is one main kitchen area with two wooden 1960s-era tables and three deteriorating ice can stoves.

The creek is typically reliable, and it is fed by snowmelt and numerous springs higher up along Hines Peak and the Topatopa Mountains. During dry spells and the height of summer, the creek can be dry, but the spring just southeast of camp can typically be relied upon as a source from which to filter or purify water.

From Ladybug, the trail toward the saddle beneath Hines Peak is a consistent climb, gaining more than 1,400 vertical feet in fewer than 2.5 miles. Your efforts are made easier, however, by the magnificent views of the Sespe River now far below, Rose Valley, and the Topatopa Mountains, which now loom over you from the south.

If you have the energy after the ascent to the **saddle (16.6 miles, 6,020', 309046E 3820460N)**, you may wish to consider the side trip to Hines Peak, the highest point in the Ventura County frontcountry. See *Route 61*; the guerrilla trail begins just south of the saddle.

From the saddle, the going is now far less strenuous, as you make your way along the old service road with virtually no mean elevation change. Splendid 360-degree views spread out before you; during clear weather you'll easily be able to spot Mt. Pinos to the north, at least six of the eight Channel Islands, and—once you've distanced yourself a bit from Hines Peak—the skyscrapers of downtown Los Angeles and the snowcapped peak of Mt. Baldy in the San Gabriel Mountains.

The **junction (17 miles, 6,080', 308622E 3821101N)** with the old Last Chance Trail "connector" comes as you begin the first stretch of the old road above Santa Paula Canyon; stay right (southwest) here and continue along the easy westward descent, skirting the very top edges of Lion Canyon. The looming peak on your left (south) that nearly matches Hines Peak in elevation (6,486 feet versus 6,716 feet)—known as No-name Peak—is often mistaken for Topatopa Peak. The confusion of Topatopa Bluffs, Topatopa Lodge, and Topatopa Mountains all on this *Topatopa Mountains* 7.5-minute quad lend to the befuddlement, when Topatopa Peak (6,210 feet) is actually some 5.4 miles farther as the crow flies (and on the *Devils Heart Peak* quad) at the far eastern edge of the range.

West of No-name Peak, you'll find yourself above the headwaters of Santa Paula Creek, and soon you'll pass the high **junction (18.5 miles, 6,050', 306950E 3820198N)** with the Topatopa Bluffs loop. Stay right at this junction as the old road drops steeply toward the edge of the Sespe Wilderness, where a **steel gate (19.5 miles, 5,560', 305843E 3819627N)** marks the wilderness boundary; your route is now a road on which motorcycles, mountain bikes, and permitted autos can legally travel. Continue following the road and quickly you'll pass the other **junction (19.6 miles, 5,460', 305739E 3819569N)** to the Topatopa Bluffs loop (the actual upper trailhead for the Last Chance Trail); the view opens here to display the Upper Ojai Valley, Oxnard Plain, and Pacific.

Descending the road you'll come to the rather bare **Elder Camp (20 miles, 5,260', 305277E 3819648N)** with a stove and table (but no water) just before you head left (south) at the **turnoff (20.1 miles, 5,230', 305145E 3815117N)** to the lower portion of the Red Reef Trail.

CAMP :: ELDER

ELEVATION:	5,260'
MAP:	USGS *Santa Paula Peak*
UTM:	305277E 3819648N

This fairly barren car-camping site—one of three built along Nordhoff Ridge Road in the early 1990s—features little more than a table and fire pit with grill on a flat cleared of brush. No water or facilities are available here, but the views are fantastic, and it's a welcome rest spot for weary Red Reef hikers.

Here the trail follows classic sunbaked chaparral along the descent into Sisar Canyon—popular with local mountain bikers—before dropping into the riparian environs of Sisar Creek and **White Ledge Camp (21.9 miles, 3,880', 304945E 3818139N)**.

CAMP :: WHITE LEDGE

ELEVATION:	3,880'
MAP:	USGS *Santa Paula Peak*
UTM:	304945E 3818139N

Not to be confused with the camp of the same name in the Santa Lucia Ranger District's portion of the San Rafael Wilderness (Santa Barbara County), White Ledge Camp is a very pleasant site shaded under heavy cover of primarily bay trees. The camp is situated at the crux between Sisar Creek and a spring that runs in all but the driest of months. Three stoves are at the site, and the main (center) kitchen has a spacious fire area and makes good use of the site's rocks. Sycamores and live oaks line this site's periphery.

White Ledge is a frequent water or lunch spot for mountain bikers and hikers both.

From White Ledge Camp, the trail crosses the spring on the western edge of camp and then descends easily through lush chaparral and riparian terrain, meeting with the creek after a ways. Follow the singletrack southward until reaching the **road (23.3 miles, 3,300', 304862E 3817310N)** and the terminus of the Red Reef Trail.

Immediately down the road from the junction is a Forest Service gate; continue down the road 3.2 miles to the **parking area (26.5 miles, 1,800', 303946E 3814072N)** at the start of Sisar Canyon Road. See the description of the lower portion of *Route 60* for detailed information of the hike along the road.

Route 89

JOHNSTON RIDGE (20W12) and SESPE HOT SPRINGS

LENGTH AND TYPE:	7.6-mile one-way to junction with Sespe River Trail; 17.2-mile out-and-back to Sespe Hot Springs
RATING:	Moderate north to south; moderately strenuous south to north (climb)
TRAIL CONDITION:	Clear (former motorcycle trail)
MAP(S):	USGS *Lockwood Valley, Topatopa Mountains,* and *Devils Heart Peak*; Harrison's *Sespe Wilderness*
CAMP(S):	Sespe Hot Springs (unofficial) and Sespe (abandoned car camp)
HIGHLIGHTS:	Fantastic views; hot springs; possible condor and bighorn sheep sightings

TO REACH THE TRAILHEAD(S): Use the Johnston Ridge Trailhead to access this route.

TRIP SUMMARY: This trail—once a noisy and dusty motorcycle route until establishment of the Sespe Wilderness in 1992—descends from Mutau Flat into the Sespe drainage and Sespe Hot Springs.

Trip Description

From the **Johnston Ridge Trailhead (4,900', 311602E 3835396N)**, pass through the motorcycle barriers and head north along the singletrack for 0.5 mile until the trail connects with the old Johnston Ridge motorcycle and **service road (0.4 mile, 4,920', 311918E 3835334N)**. Follow the old road easily down into the Mutau drainage and to the junction with the **Stonehouse Trail (1.4 miles, 4,780', 312829E 3834865N)**. On your right (south) through the gate is the private road leading toward Mutau Flat; occasionally you'll spot cattle (or, more often, their leavings) in this vicinity. The route to your left (north) leads along Mutau Creek toward Stonehouse and the Piru confluence (see *Route 81*). Damage from the 2006 Day Fire is apparent along many swatches of the forest here.

Follow the trail down into the sandy, willow-dotted wash to the **Mutau Creek crossing (1.5 miles, 4,770', 312998E 3834876N)**. Cross here and climb the slope—entering the Sespe Wilderness—on the other side and into the draw to the junction with the **Little Mutau Trail (2.2 miles, 4,950', 313722E 3834442N)**. Take the right (south) fork here.

From the Mutau junction you'll climb briefly through oaks and conifers and parallel the northwest headwaters of Hot Springs Canyon to make your way toward Johnston Ridge. Then begins a long 6-mile descent along Johnston Ridge, the length of which offers little cover and no water. Views of Hot Springs Canyon and the greater Sespe drainage are very impressive as you head southward; less impressive are the occasional rusting and discarded motorcycles—some very old—that you're likely to spot beside your route. The tread for nearly the entire descent is in fine shape, given the route's previous life as a motorcycle route. Occasionally—and rather disappointingly—one can still spy recent tire tracks, evidence of rogue bikers still making use of the now-wilderness route.

The long-arcing route finally brings you to the junction with Hot Springs Canyon and the Sespe Hot Springs **spur trail (8.5 miles, 2,650', 316857E 3829326N)**. This junction is before you cross Hot Springs Creek; if you reach the creek you've passed the trail to the hot springs. It's 0.5 mile up-canyon to the source of the Sespe Hot Springs at the confluence of Hot Springs Canyon and Poplar Creek.

Sespe Hot Springs is often called the hottest springs in Southern California. A longtime pleasure destination, the springs were accessible by automobile for much of the 20th century until the Sespe Road was closed in the late 1970s. It continued to be accessible by motorcycle (via the Johnston Ridge Trail) and mountain bike (by both Johnston and Sespe Trails) until the Sespe Wilderness was formed in 1992. Since then, its amenities have remained largely the same, and while still very popular, its distance from the closest trailheads means it receives less traffic than in its heyday.

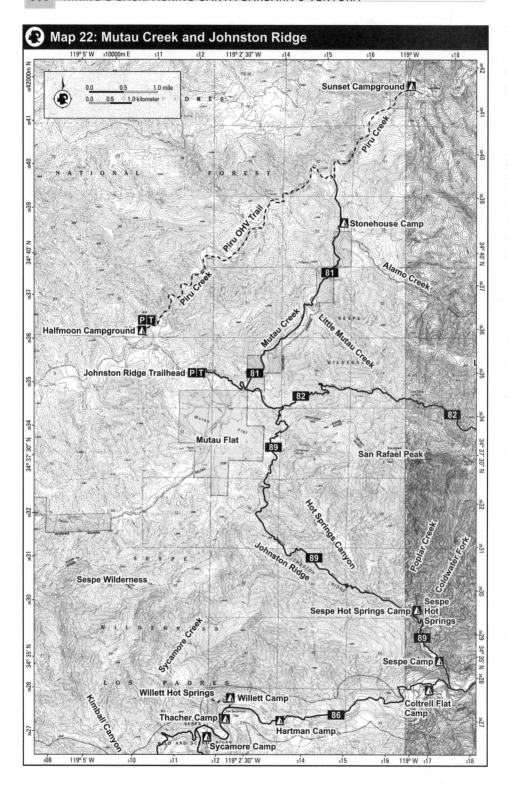

Map 22: Mutau Creek and Johnston Ridge

MAP 23 Alamo Mountain and Buck Creek 369

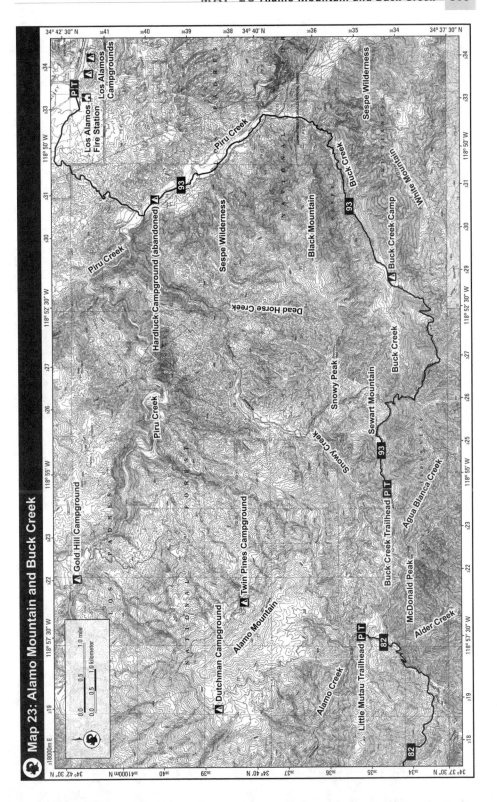

Map 23: Alamo Mountain and Buck Creek

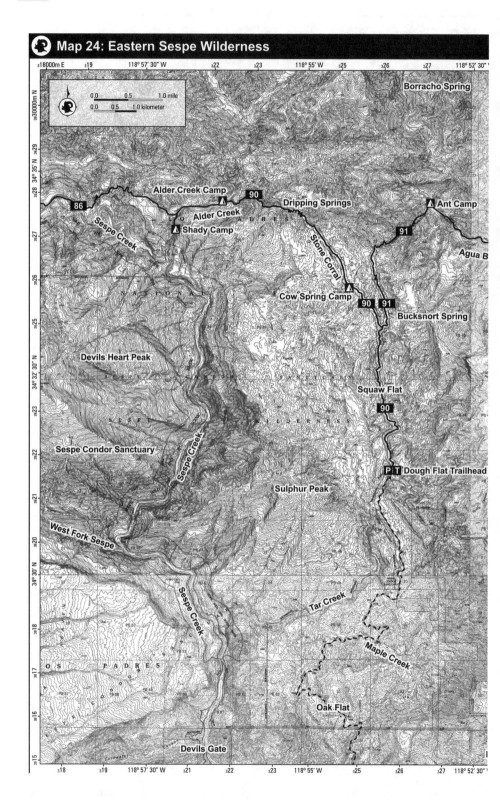

Map 24: Eastern Sespe Wilderness

MAP 24 Eastern Sespe Wilderness 371

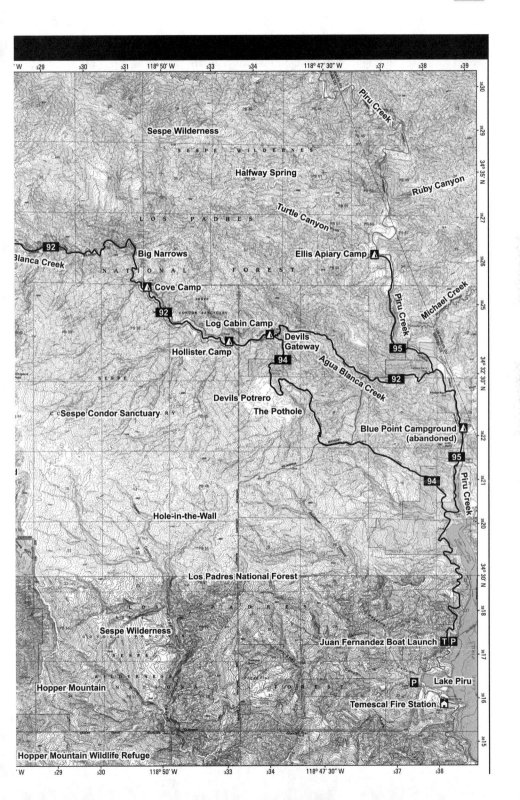

This stretch is dotted by a handful of introduced palms (you'll likely have noticed them while descending from the ridge); save for these shade-bearing trees (and an inordinate amount of cacti), there is little vegetation along this canyon floor, giving it something of an alien landscape appearance. The cascade where the hot water comes into the canyon is too hot for comfort; the numerous pools—which become cooler the farther downstream you are—vary in temperature. As it has often been said, camping near these springs is all about cold-water access.

The best spot to camp is usually near those palms, 0.25 mile downstream from the springs.

■　■　■　■　■　■　■　■　■　■　■　■　■　■　■　■　■

"HARMLESSLY PASSING YOUR TIME IN THE GRASSLAND AWAY..."

This stretch of the Sespe Wilderness—particularly along Johnston Ridge and the plateaus above Hot Springs Canyon—is home to the endangered desert bighorn sheep *(Ovis canadensis nelsoni)*. The present-day Los Padres was historically the far western extent of the desert bighorns' range. The creatures were hunted and had fallen to disease and other impacts that by 1914 they no longer inhabited the area. In 1985, however, a small population was transferred from the San Gabriel Mountains to the Sespe by the California Department of Fish and Game. Subsequent wilderness designation further ensured some protections, and though there have been challenges, the sheep have surmounted numerous obstacles and begun to thrive. You may be lucky enough to spot some of these creatures on your trek; Johnston Ridge is typically the best vantage point from which to spot them.

■　■　■　■　■　■　■　■　■　■　■　■　■　■　■　■　■

CAMP :: SESPE HOT SPRINGS

ELEVATION:	2,775'
MAPS:	USGS *Devils Heart Peak* (not shown); Harrison's *Sespe Wilderness*
UTM:	316913E 3829546N

More a series of unofficial sites that make use of camps built decades ago around the hot springs, Sespe Hot Springs Camp is not shown on the 1995 USGS *Devils Heart Peak* quad nor the 2008 LPNF visitor map. It is, however, shown on Harrison's *Sespe Wilderness*. A trio of palm trees, numerous cacti, and steaming, sulfuric runoff make this an almost-otherworldly stretch of the wilderness. The site beneath the palm trees—just right (east) of the trail—has a good kitchen with a well-built fire ring.

If continuing toward the Sespe from the junction with the Hot Springs spur, it's a quick 0.5 mile to the **old Sespe car campground (9.2 miles, 2,410', 317280E 3828544N)**.

CAMP :: SESPE

ELEVATION:	2,410'
MAP:	USGS *Devils Heart Peak* (not shown)
UTM:	317280E 3828544N

A drive-in campground when the Sespe Road led all the way to the hot springs, this site is a bit worse for wear but still features an old USFS table and cast concrete fire pit. A hitching post is also farther down along the flat here. Fire-scarred sycamores provide some shade. You'll even find the old concrete outhouse across the trail beneath (behind) a cluster of trees.

Note: This site is not shown on the 1995 USGS *Devils Heart Peak* quad nor the 2008 LPNF visitor map. It does however appear on Harrison's *Sespe Wilderness*.

From the old Sespe Camp, it's another 0.5 mile downstream to the junction with the **Sespe River Trail (9.6 miles, 2,400', 317531E 3827922N)**. See *Route 86* for your options here.

Route 90

DOUGH FLAT TO SHADY CAMP via Alder Creek (20W11)

LENGTH AND TYPE:	15-mile out-and-back
RATING:	Moderate
TRAIL CONDITION:	Clear to Alder Creek; passable to Shady Camp
MAP(S):	USGS *Devils Heart Peak*; Harrison's *Sespe Wilderness*
CAMP(S):	Cow Spring, Alder Creek, and Shady
HIGHLIGHTS:	Expansive views of the Topatopa and Santa Monica Mountains; unique geology of Stone Corral; riparian trekking along Alder Creek

TO REACH THE TRAILHEAD(S): Use the Dough Flat Trailhead to access this route.

TRIP SUMMARY: From the Dough Flat Trailhead, the Alder Creek Trail (20W11) ascends to Squaw Flat, climbing moderately to the fork with the Bucksnort Trail (19W18). Continuing via the left fork (northwest), the trail passes Cow Spring Camp and crosses through Stone Corral, eventually dropping steeply into the East Fork of Alder Creek and west to the confluence of Alder Creek to Alder Creek Camp and Shady Camp. Damage from the

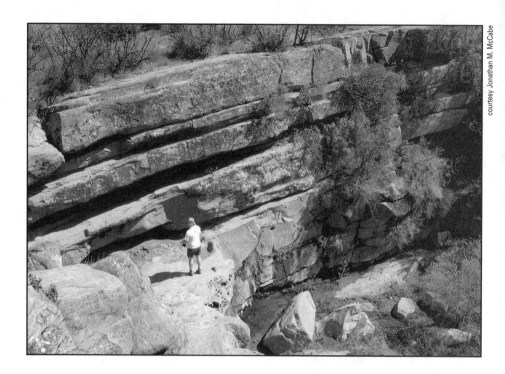

courtesy Jonathan M. McCabe

2006 Day Fire is glaring, but wildflowers are abundant and the scarred oaks and sycamores continue to recover.

This route also comprises a sizable portion of the old Horse Thief Trail, which in the 1870s was used by rustlers to feed a supply of easily nabbed horses to the Southern Pacific Railroad, which at the time was constructing the lines between Los Angeles and San Francisco. A stretch of the trail ran from Dough Flat past Cow Spring and Dripping Springs, and then along Alder and Sespe Creeks toward Sespe Hot Springs, using Mutau Flats as a stopover (with Old Man Mutah working literally as a middleman) before heading farther north.

Trip Description

From the **Dough Flat Trailhead (2,840', 326001E 3821693N)**, follow the trail along the course of the old Squaw Flat jeep trail; the route is wide for the first 3 miles of hiking, and since the fire, quite clear. Westward views are excellent for most of the hike.

After the first, short ascent you will follow and then cross a cobbled wash en route to Squaw Flat. Evidence of this region's geologic history is especially apparent along this stretch, with blocks of stone strewn along the trail and the creek bed inset with fossilized seashells. Wildflowers are abundant in spring; Lobb's poppies, chias, and Indian paintbrush are among the most commonly encountered.

Several well-defined tributaries cross the trail; these are usually dry except during or immediately after storms. After 1.25 miles you will enter the lower reaches of **Squaw Flat** (**1.3 miles, 3,150', 325751E 3823395N**), alongside Squaw Creek. A guerrilla picnic camp along the creek sits beneath a cluster of large oaks to the east of the trail. Beneath one of the oaks is a section of a 55-gallon oil drum used as a fire pit.

Equipment from early wildcatters is still scattered around the area, and the creek bank is heavy with poison oak here. Water is not always available, but there is a large spring that (in spring) bubbles out of the creek bank approximately 0.25 mile past Squaw Flat where you can often replenish.

From Squaw Flat, continue to (roughly) follow the creek's drainage, and a climb of nearly 700 feet in just over a mile out of the flat will lead you to an **open pass** (**2.4 miles, 3,690', 325694E 3824769N**), where southward and westward views are expansive. On an average day, the line of the Santa Monica Mountains is easily recognizable to the south. Just north of this viewpoint is the junction where trails 20W11 and 19W18 diverge; the junction is situated in a small bowl surrounded by red earthen hills. The old trail sign, long-abused by shooters and already rusting by the arrival of the 2006 fires, is now left to decay.

From the junction, continue northwest, following the Bucksnort Creek watershed and those of the creeks' various tributaries. You'll pass an incongruous Ventura County Watershed Protection District rain gauge, and after a mile will come upon the **Cow Spring Camp** (**3.4 miles, 3,510', 325008E 3825842N**) and the start of the Stone Corral section.

CAMP :: COW SPRING

ELEVATION:	3,510'
MAP:	USGS *Devils Heart Peak*
UTM:	325008E 3825842N

Cow Spring was once the literal end of the road for 4WD enthusiasts, as evidenced by the wide and level space and old concrete and cast-iron stove located beside the fire ring and grill at the southern end of the camp. A second fire ring with grill is positioned in the middle of the glade. Though it has room enough for a large group, the campground has only a trio of cottonwood trees, struggling to recover from the 2006 fires, and is very exposed (and quite hot in the summer).

The grazing permit for the namesake cattle was terminated in 1964, and in 1973 the site was closed to motor vehicles due to its proximity to the condor sanctuary and frequent vandalism.

If the creek next to camp and spring are both dry, standing pools of water can sometimes be found at the base of the falls (though seldom in summer).

Immediately north of Cow Spring Camp is a usually dry waterfall; this marks the beginning of the Stone Corral section of the trail. Here, the going is no longer along the former road, but easy nonetheless, as travel is on the whole quite level for the next 1.5 miles. This portion of the trail bisects a fascinating array of geologic formations and monoliths.

At the end of the formations, climb easily to another vista (3,670 feet), this time affording excellent views of McDonald Peak and the Alder Creek drainage along the ridge due north (the ridge in view is also the northern boundary of the Sespe Wilderness).

The northwesterly descent toward Alder Creek begins here, exchanging the arid and rocky terrain for the granite-cobbled streambeds and tree-lined washes of the riparian terrain below. The trail in parts can be quite steep. After a series of switchbacks is **Dripping Springs (5.25 miles, 3,100', 323614 3827566)**, a small grotto issuing from the mountainside.

After Dripping Springs you'll cross a number of additional washes, most of which are usually dry. After another 0.75 mile is the **junction (6 miles, 2,780', 322867E 3827970N)** of trails 20W11 and the old northern leg of the trail, no longer maintained by the Forest Service. The left (west) fork drops you into the East Fork of Alder Creek shortly thereafter, and in just under a mile the east fork converges with Alder Creek. The trail here makes some attempt to track along the banks and benches alongside the creek, but it is typically just as easy—if not easier—to trek along the streambed proper.

Alder Creek Camp (6.4 miles, 2,530', 322126E 3827858N) is just beyond the confluence, on the north bank, between the trail and creek.

CAMP :: ALDER CREEK

ELEVATION:	2,520'
MAP:	USGS *Devils Heart Peak*
UTM:	322126E 3827858N

Located on the north bank of Alder Creek just off the trail, Alder Creek Camp is a comfort-able site with easy access to the creek. Small oaks and sycamores surround the site. The creek can be dry during low rain years.

The kitchen currently possesses one fire ring with a grill; formerly there were two stoves here, but one was hauled over to a guerrilla site on the opposite bank and just downstream, beneath a stand of oaks.

From camp, continue nearly a mile along the creek bed to the **junction (7.2 miles, 2,410', 320961E 3827547N)** with the Sespe River Trail (see *Route 86*). These trails diverge just as Alder Creek begins its bend southward toward the narrows; the Sespe River Trail ascends

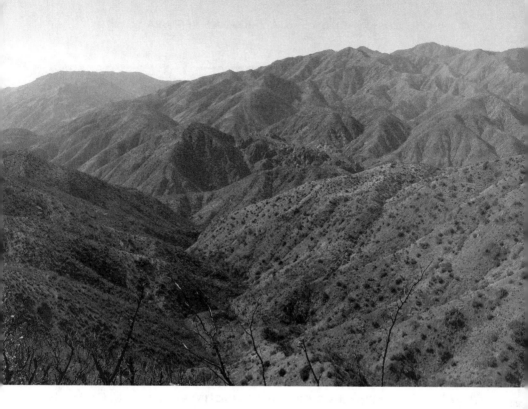

Dropping into Alder Creek

the drainage of a tributary to the northwest. Keep left (south) along the 20W11 from this junction; it's another 0.25 mile to **Shady Camp (7.4 miles, 2,400', 320958E 3827312N)**. The trail cuts across the brush here; you needn't follow the drainage.

Beyond Shady Camp, the trail ends almost immediately, but the old Devils Gate route (formerly USFS trail 20W14) can be navigated by the hearty for another 15 miles (one way) along the Sespe River.

CAMP :: SHADY

ELEVATION:	2,400'
MAP:	USGS *Devils Heart Peak*
UTM:	320958E 3827312N

Easily identified by the large, flat-topped boulder situated in the center of camp, Shady is the gateway to the Alder Creek narrows. The camp is set beneath two large oaks and has one fire ring with grill. Be advised that some older federal maps incorrectly show Shady Camp right at the junction of the trails to the north.

Route 91

BUCKSNORT TRAIL (19W18)

LENGTH AND TYPE:	11.2-mile out-and-back to Ant Camp
RATING:	Moderate
TRAIL CONDITION:	Clear (former service road) to passable (last mile sometimes overgrown)
MAP(S):	USGS *Devils Heart Peak*; Harrison's *Sespe Wilderness*
CAMP(S):	Ant
HIGHLIGHTS:	Fascinating geology; easy navigation along abandoned service roads

TO REACH THE TRAILHEAD(S): Use the Dough Flat Trailhead to access this route.

TRIP SUMMARY: This route follows the old service road to a saddle and then drops into the Agua Blanca drainage to an oak-dotted flat. This trip is a good overnighter.

Trip Description

From the **Dough Flat Trailhead (2,840', 326001E 3821693N)**, follow the trail as described in *Route 90* to the **split (2.4 miles, 3,750', 325779E 3824911N)** where the Alder Creek and Bucksnort Trails diverge.

From the junction, head right (northeast). After a very short climb, the trail splits from the old road atop a saddle and follows a short wash, meeting the road again below and leading to the **junction (2.6 miles, 3,600', 325902E 3825152N)** with the use trail leading toward Bucksnort Spring.

Pass through this flat and continue another mile over the old service road along a very easy grade to a second, more-defined **grassy flat (3.8 miles, 3,700', 325693E 3826441N)**. In the spring, the grasses can obscure the route a bit, but continue through the meadow toward the road cut to the northeast, climbing briefly to the **divide (3.9 miles, 3,750', 325644E 3826717N)** and a view of the Agua Blanca drainage below. Here the old roadbed finally ends, and you commit to the often brushed-in singletrack for the steady descent. Views of Cobblestone Mountain are impressive as you drop into the Agua Blanca drainage.

After several sets of switchbacks, you'll reach the **unnamed creek (5.2 miles, 2,875', 326590E 3827341N)** under the shade of big-leaf maples and sycamores. Follow the trail through the grasses along the banks of the creek and a second tributary to a faint **spur trail (5.5 miles, 2,760', 326883E 3827618N)** that leads eastward to **Ant Camp (5.6 miles, 2,750', 326997E 3827642N)**. The camp is set on the wide grassy flat beneath a cluster of mature live oaks; if you reach the fire-scarred 19W10 trail sign, you've overshot it and can simply triangulate eastward through the field to camp.

CAMP :: ANT

ELEVATION:	2,750'
MAP:	USGS *Devils Heart Peak*
UTM:	326997E 3827642N

A seldom-visited but still surprisingly serviceable site, Ant is situated just off the junction of the Bucksnort and Agua Blanca Trails. A table and large fire ring with grate stoves make up a functional kitchen; there is usually a second kitchen a bit farther off the table as well. There is room enough for a large group, as the field around camp is spacious and fairly clear. Accoutrements from campers of old (bed frames, pots, pans, and the like) can be found through the camp. Water can be had from Agua Blanca Creek; the tributary beside camp is intermittent.

Ant is usually the end of the hike for most folks; return the way you came for an easy overnighter. If continuing along the Agua Blanca Trail, see *Route 92* (and good luck!).

Route 92

AGUA BLANCA (19W10)

LENGTH AND TYPE:	11.4-mile one-way from Ant Camp to Blue Point Campground; shuttle
RATING:	Strenuous
TRAIL CONDITION:	Passable to difficult (unmaintained trail)
MAP(S):	USGS *Devils Heart Peak* and *Cobblestone Mountain*; Harrison's *Sespe Wilderness*
CAMP(S):	Ant, Cove, and Log Cabin
HIGHLIGHTS:	Narrows; fascinating geology; slot canyon

TO REACH THE TRAILHEAD(S): Use the Dough Flat and/or Juan Fernandez Boat Launch (Lake Piru) Trailheads for this shuttle.

TRIP SUMMARY: This trail follows Agua Blanca Creek from Ant Camp at the end of the Bucksnort Trail to the confluence of Agua Blanca and Piru Creeks above the old Blue Point Campground. The description is presented as a shuttle from Dough Flat to Blue Point, but you will first have to hike the Alder Creek and Bucksnort routes to Ant Camp (5.3 miles), and then afterward the old road from Blue Point to the Juan Fernandez Boat Launch (4.4 miles), in addition to the 11.4 miles described below for a total of more than 21 miles. This is a difficult multiday route.

Note: As of this writing, the Agua Blanca Trail—once a very popular route—receives virtually no traffic. I hope it will find a new life as part of the very eastern end of the proposed Condor Trail. Expect the going to be tough, with plenty of poison oak, scrambling over deadfall and blowdowns, and wet feet in all but the driest years (and if dry, then it will likely be hot and fairly miserable).

Trip Description

From **Ant Camp (2,750', 326958E 3827692N)** follow the fading singletrack eastward out of camp. Poison oak will dictate your route in many places, and you will be resigned to hiking along the creek bed for much of it, as the old stretches of trail are quite overgrown. After a mile along the creek, you'll reach a **small flat (1 mile, 2,550', 328144E 3826942N)**, where once stood Tin Can Cabin trail camp, so named for a cabin constructed of 5-gallon water tins. The site was abandoned during the 1974–1975 season. Virtually all evidence of it and the cabin has disappeared in the decades since, due to flooding, neglect, and fire.

Beyond the flat, continue along the creek, spending about as much time (likely more) rock-hopping as you will on any halfway decent piece of tread. Again, watch for poison oak here, as it seems to be especially thick along this stretch. You'll soon enter the upper mouth of the **Big Narrows (2.8 miles, 2,000', 330394E 3826766N)**, the simply but accurately named and very impressive formation cutting through Monterey formation sandstone and shale and winding downstream to the south. You may opt to follow the creek rather than bushwhack around the formation along the old route that stays south and west of the narrows; neither is easy (and mind the remnants of barbed-wire fences along the bypass), but at least in the creek you know you haven't lost the path.

Once finally clear of the Big Narrows, the canyon becomes considerably less claustrophobic and you'll reach **Cove Camp (4.3 miles, 1,900', 331344E 3825673N)** on the right (south) side of the creek.

CAMP :: COVE

ELEVATION:	1,900'
MAP:	USGS *Cobblestone Mountain*
UTM:	331344E 3825673N

This site—remote and seldom visited—features little but has room enough to pitch a tent or three, reliable water, and a fire ring set beneath a cluster of old live oaks.

From Cove, continue downstream another 2 miles to the old **Hollister Camp (6.1 miles, 1,620', 333350E 3824274N)**. Continue downstream, leaving the sanctuary corridor through which you've been traveling almost immediately to the east. The trail slowly improves along this stretch, thanks to the work of local volunteers. Next in the line of near-forgotten sites is the far more spacious **Log Cabin Camp (6.7 miles, 1,510', 334221E 3824593N)**.

CAMP :: LOG CABIN

ELEVATION:	1,510'
MAP:	USGS *Cobblestone Mountain*
UTM:	334221E 3824593N

Though another seldom-used site, Log Cabin still has potential. Numerous ice can stoves are clustered here, and the site also features a trio of barbecue stoves. Though brushy in spots, the camp nonetheless has plenty of space and is surrounded by pleasant oaks. There is room for several tents, and water can be retrieved from the creek.

Devils Gateway; courtesy Bardley Smith

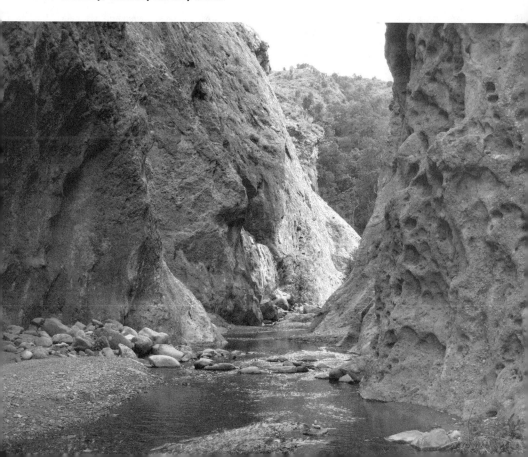

Only minutes downstream from Log Cabin Camp you'll reach the upper **junction (6.7 miles, 1,475', 334519E 3824472N)** with the Pothole Trail; see *Route 94*. Continue downstream through the Devils Gateway, another narrow slot (with a more menacing name than the Big Narrows, but it's actually less intimidating). The trail gains the south banks just past Devils Gateway, but then crosses several times en route to Kesters Camp and the old **service road (10.3 miles, 1,120', 337972E 3823642N)**. Follow this road south for a mile to the abandoned **Blue Point Campground (11.4 miles, 1,075', 338749E 3822238N)**; see *Route 95* for the description of the route south toward the Juan Fernandez Boat Launch.

Route 93

BUCK CREEK (20W01, 18W01, and 19W05)

LENGTH AND TYPE:	15.8-mile one-way (shuttle); 10.4-mile out-and-back to Buck Creek Camp from Buck Creek Trailhead; 21.2-mile out-and-back to Buck Creek Camp from Los Alamos gate (via Hard Luck Road)
RATING:	Moderately strenuous
TRAIL CONDITION:	Passable to difficult (unmaintained trail) and clear (paved and dirt roads along Piru Creek and through Hungry Valley OHV area)
MAP(S):	USGS *Alamo Mountain* and *Black Mountain*; Harrison's *Sespe Wilderness*
CAMP(S):	Buck Creek
HIGHLIGHTS:	Fantastic views from Sewart Mountain and ridge; fascinating geology along route and at Piru confluence

TO REACH THE TRAILHEAD(S): Use the Buck Creek and/or Los Alamos Trailheads for this route.

TRIP SUMMARY: This route navigates the length of Buck Creek from Sewart Mountain to the confluence with Piru Creek, and then hikes along Piru Creek and up and over a ridge to the east and down to the gate near the Los Alamos fire station. The route described below is west to east (downstream). This is a shuttle hike.

Note: Severely burned in the 2006 Day Fire, the Buck Creek Trail as of this writing has received virtually no maintenance in the years since. Several sections are nearly gone. Some volunteer clipping and flagging has been done, but be prepared for difficult, cross-country conditions even where your maps and GPS receivers may show trail. Further, the original lower Buck Creek Trailhead is no longer accessible since the closure of Hard Luck, resulting in an additional 3 miles along (paved) Hard Luck Road.

Trip Description

From the Buck Creek Trailhead, follow the old roadbed eastward through the charred remains of the pine forest that stood here pre–Day Fire. From the very outset you'll have excellent southward views of the Agua Blanca drainage, the Pothole, and the eastern end of the Topatopa Mountains (including the steel frame of the burned Topatopa Peak lookout tower) all the way out to the Pacific. Views to the east and north yield Antelope Valley, the Tehachapi Mountains, and—even when air quality isn't at its best—the snowcapped southern Sierra Nevada.

Make your way around tree fall as necessary to the **clearing** (**0.9 mile, 6,820', 325312E 3834810N**) atop Sewart Mountain (the summit, at 6,841 feet, is the rock outcrop just to the north). Here the old roadbed turns southeast, leading you another 0.5 mile to an easily missed **junction** (**1.4 miles, 6,220', 325858E 3834606N**). Head right (south) here and continue following the roadbed through the barren scrub- and yucca-dotted terrain until reaching a **seasonal pond** (**3.7 miles, 5,380', 327744E 3833401N**) and the junction with the Buck Creek Trail and abandoned White Mountain and Cobblestone Mountain Trails. (For those keeping track, the route you've been following is often plotted on maps as 18W01, which is the old Cobblestone Mountain trail's designation.) The old service road ends here— both routes reduce to singletrack from this point on.

Follow the lower, left (east) fork here past the pond and begin dropping sharply down into the Buck drainage along a series of long switchbacks. This stretch was spared major damage from the fire and is a pleasant and shady respite from the exposed and often hot terrain through which you have just hiked. Massive bigcone Douglas-firs provide a great deal of cover here.

After crossing a seasonal **tributary** (**4.6 miles, 4,690', 328237E 3833707N**) and turning one more switchback to follow said tributary, the trail leads you to the confluence with Buck Creek and Buck Creek Spring. Though somewhat difficult to find postfire, **Buck Creek Camp** (**5.2 miles, 4250', 328718E 3834431N**) is just downstream, on the right (south) side of the trail.

CAMP :: BUCK CREEK

ELEVATION:	4,250'
MAP:	USGS *Black Mountain*
UTM:	328718E 3834431N

A nearly forgotten camp, this site is shaded by mature bigcone Douglas-firs and some oaks. Little is left of this site other than a fire ring, and one can typically find a better spot to bivouac farther down the creek. Water is accessible in the creek.

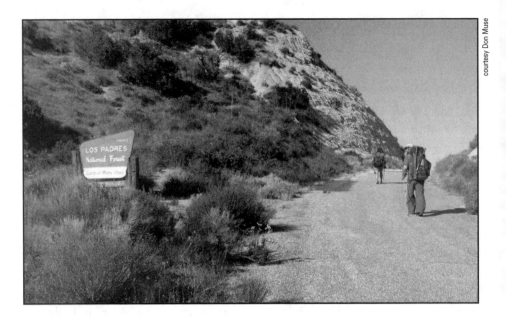

courtesy Don Muse

Forest's edge, Hard Luck Road

Note: Buck Creek Camp has been plotted at various points along the creek over the years; even Harrison's *Sespe Wilderness* map shows the site somewhat farther downstream (actually the site of one of the better unofficial camps).

From camp, the trail continues downstream. In years past this may have been a simple matter, but at present long portions of it are choked with downed alders, oaks, and firs and made further difficult by blackberry brambles, primroses, poison oak, and stinging nettles. Tread cautiously and navigate with care. Stretches of the old route, where they can be found, still provide a solid trail bed. The trail crosses the creek a few times, but look along the south side where a postfire flash flood has scoured a cobble-strewn plain along a minor **drainage (7.1 miles, 3,420', 331362E 3835573N)** and effectively cut a section of the trail off the canyon side. This is where the trail begins to climb out of the drainage and follow the southern banks along White Mountain's lowermost flanks, and the going is much smoother (if a bit overgrown). Views of the geology of both White Mountain (to the south) and Black Mountain (to the north) are quite impressive as you pass between these two granite ridges. Your terrain changes from the oak, alder, and conifer mix of the canyon to more exposed oak, scrub, and chaparral more typical of the Piru drainage.

After a fair amount of work and route-finding, you'll spy the incongruous conglomerate formations marking the Buck-Piru confluence. As you approach the confluence, the singletrack turns to an old roadbed and shortly meets the old **Buck Creek Road** (**8.8 miles, 2,740', 332701E 3837326N**). Follow the old road upstream (north) toward the southern end of the old **Hardluck Campground** (**10.9 miles, 2,870', 330862E 3839820N**), the former terminus for this route. There is very little shade along this stretch, but the occasional cottonwood can provide some respite on hot days.

A BIT OF HARD LUCK

Hardluck Campground was closed in 2009 due to its proximity to Piru Creek and its resident arroyo toads. For decades this 26-site car camp along the Ventura–Los Angeles county line—set along a quite barren river flat—served as the trailhead for those venturing down Piru and/or Buck Creeks. Those wishing to access this stretch of Piru Creek now must either hike or bike in.

Hike along the sealed road past the abandoned site, crossing **Piru Creek** (**11.4 miles, 2,900', 330459E 3840379N**)—and immediately thereafter pass the former site of the Buck Creek Guard Station—to start your ascent of the Buck Creek Road. You have two ways by which you can reach your vehicle parked at the Los Alamos gate. First, you can follow the sealed road 3 miles, climbing out of the drainage and dropping into the Hungry Valley Recreation Area back to the gate; or 0.7 mile from the Piru crossing, a **singletrack** (**12.6 miles, 3,050', 330983E 3841161N**) leaves the road to climb rather steeply through eroded badlands and scrub and then drops down the other side to meet the road. This route cuts about 0.5 mile from your total distance back to the **Los Alamos gate** (**15.8 miles, 2,980', 333256E 3841892N**).

Route 94

POTHOLE TRAIL (18W04)

LENGTH AND TYPE:	5.9-mile one-way from Pothole Trailhead to Agua Blanca junction; 10.2-mile out-and-back to Pothole Spring (Devils Potrero)
RATING:	Moderately strenuous
TRAIL CONDITION:	Passable
MAP(S):	USGS *Cobblestone Mountain*; Harrison's *Sespe Wilderness*
CAMP(S):	Pothole (unofficial)
HIGHLIGHTS:	Geologic sinkhole (Pothole); remote route with excellent views of Agua Blanca, Piru and surrounding watersheds, and Cobblestone Mountain

TO REACH THE TRAILHEAD(S): Use the Juan Fernandez Boat Launch (Lake Piru) Trailhead to access this route, and then hike 3 miles north along the road to the Pothole Trailhead.

TRIP SUMMARY: This route climbs rather steeply for about 5 miles before dropping into the Pothole and Devils Potrero. At its northern terminus, it connects with the Agua Blanca Trail (*Route 92*). While this route is described from south to north, it is just as enjoyable in reverse (perhaps even more so, as it makes for an ideal alternate exit for those following the Agua Blanca route).

Trip Description

From the **Pothole Trailhead (1,100', 338356E 3820479N)** beside Forest Road 4N13, follow the trail westward up the easy grade of a long-retired road, slowly curving northward to gain a small meadow and begin a series of switchbacks leading to the ridge of the drainage here. Some grazing does occur here, so in addition to the usual "land mines," after rains the tread can have some rough patches; mind your ankles accordingly. Further, since the Blue Point Campground closure in 1999 and the subsequent road closure, the Pothole route receives very little traffic. Save for a handful of dedicated local volunteers, the trail has been nearly forgotten. In decades past, a loop along this route and the lower 3 miles of Agua Blanca Creek—using the now-shuttered Blue Point Campground as the start and finish point—was a popular choice for hikers seeking a challenging two- or three-day route with varied terrain and relative solitude. While the terrain hasn't changed overly, in the years since, the solitude has only increased. It's rather uncommon to encounter other hikers on these trails, and rarer still to find backpackers camped at either the Pothole or Log Cabin Camps.

In the years since the 2003 Piru Fire, the decades-old firebreaks are better-defined than they have been in years, and you'll find yourself skirting the wide dozer line for much of this early portion. So once out of thick grasses that typically hinder progress along the lower stretch, navigation does become easier as you ascend. A steady 2-mile climb will grant you increasingly impressive views of not only Lake Piru but also the surrounding Sespe Wilderness, the massive Cobblestone Mountain formation, and stretches of the Dominguez, Canton, and other drainages.

Follow the **singletrack (2.7 miles, 3,240', 335471E 3822037N)** as it departs the dozer line and drops northward toward the Pothole and Devils Potrero. If you miss this sometime-obscured turnoff, there is an obvious sharp left in the firebreak about 200 yards later; head right (north) here and you can triangulate back to the singletrack shortly. The trail will lead you steadily down and around the chaparral-clad northern flank of Hill 2711 and then back southward toward the potrero. (Follow the thin use trail southward at the next bend to enter the actual potrero continuing down-trail.)

The **Pothole (4.4 miles, 2,300', 334450E 3823027N)**—and the Devils Potrero in which it is located—is the result of an ancient landslide, and is now dotted with grass and scrub and fringed by mature willows and cottonwoods.

From the Pothole, head back to that last bend and continue northward, crossing the creek twice before reaching the old Pothole cabin and (unofficial) **Pothole campsite (5.1 miles, 2,100', 334182E 3823721N)**.

CAMP :: POTHOLE

ELEVATION:	2,100'
MAP:	USGS *Cobblestone Mountain*
UTM:	334182E 3823721N

As this site is not a recognized system trail camp, it is neither maintained nor recognized by the US Forest Service. Set within the pleasant coppice of live oaks near the Pothole cabin, it typically boasts only a guerilla fire ring. Numerous farm implements from nearly a century ago are spread about the grounds near the cabin, and to the west is a swampy area. Water is best retrieved from Pothole Spring proper.

Do bear in mind that the property around the old cabin and Pothole Spring is privately held; treat the area as you would have others treat your property.

From camp, it's an easy and lush, fern-dotted (but often poison oak–choked) 0.75 mile in the company of the occasional bigcone Douglas-fir down to the **confluence (5.9 miles, 1,475', 334519E 3824472N)** with Agua Blanca Creek; just across the creek is the Agua Blanca Trail (see *Route 92*).

Route 95

LOWER COBBLESTONE TRAIL (18W03)

LENGTH AND TYPE:	3-mile one-way to Pothole Trailhead; 8.2-mile out-and-back from Juan Fernandez Boat Launch to Ellis Apiary
RATING:	Moderate (water levels and trail conditions)
TRAIL CONDITION:	Well maintained (sealed road) to challenging (wading and rock-hopping)
MAP(S):	USGS *Piru* and *Cobblestone Mountain*; Harrison's *Sespe Wilderness*
CAMP(S):	Ellis Apiary
HIGHLIGHTS:	Geology; some canyoneering opportunities (no ropes necessary)

TO REACH THE TRAILHEAD(S): Use the Juan Fernandez Boat Launch (Lake Piru) Trailhead to access this route.

LAKE PIRU ■ ■ ■ ■ ■ ■ ■ ■ ■ ■ ■ ■ ■ ■ ■ ■ ■

Formed in 1955 by the construction of Santa Felicia Dam on Piru Creek, Lake Piru (known as Santa Felicia Lake until 1956) is a popular boating and recreation area managed by United Water Conservation District. While the US Forest Service has been working with UWCD to obtain better access to the upper stretches of Piru Canyon for forest users, for now the first portion of all hikes up the canyon entails at least a 3-mile walk along a closed road. Because this road is in good shape and still receives maintenance, many hikers cycle this route in and then lock their bikes along the road, making the somewhat lengthy approach hike a bit more bearable. Whichever method you choose, this stretch is an easy endeavor of simply following the sealed road. I hope in the future a roadhead closer to the trails will be available, but as yet one is resigned to this somewhat limited (and limiting) access. You can check on the lake's road conditions (and get other general information) by phoning (805) 521-1500.

■ ■ ■ ■ ■ ■ ■ ■ ■ ■ ■ ■ ■ ■ ■ ■ ■ ■

TRIP SUMMARY: This route follows a sealed road to the abandoned Blue Point Campground, and then follows a dirt doubletrack to the Agua Blanca–Piru confluence. It then embarks along the abandoned Cobblestone Trail through a stretch of narrows along Piru Creek and then up the southwest flank of Cobblestone Mountain.

Trip Description

From the **Juan Fernandez Boat Launch** (1,100', 338307E 3817566N), follow the closed Forest Road 4N13 northward past the gate. You'll enjoy excellent views of the lake and surrounding hills and canyon along this walk.

Your first waypoint of note is the junction with a small **spur trail** (2.7 miles, 1,100', 338288E 3820077N) on your right (east) leading down the slope to a monument dedicated to Juan Fustero (see sidebar on the next page). Continuing farther up the road, you'll reach the **Pothole Trailhead** (3 miles, 1,100', 338356E 3820479N). See *Route 94* for this route.

As the northern end of the lake narrows and you continue along the road, you'll enjoy good views of Blue Point—named for the serpentine rock outcrop rising from the Sespe formation sandstone on the west side of the narrows—and beneath which you'll pass a gated service road leading to Canton Canyon on the east side of the lake.

On the north side of Blue Point, the geology changes abruptly from the trademark red claystone of the Sespe formation to the wind- and water-eroded mini-caves of the Matilija formation. It's a fascinating stretch and one worth investigating (though do be mindful of poison oak beside the road here).

■ ■ ■ ■ ■ ■ ■ ■ ■ ■ ■ ■ ■ ■ **JUAN FUSTERO**

Commonly referred to as the "last of the Piru Indians," Juan Fustero was the last full-blooded Tataviam male. (The Tataviams, distinct from the better-known Chumash, were a branch of Shoshone who migrated to the Santa Clarita Valley circa 400 AD.)

Fustero was born at the mouth of Holzer Canyon on the Temescal Ranch in 1841, and he was the great-grandson of the last chief of the Piru tribe. He was granted a US patent in 1885 and homesteaded on his ancestral land farther up Piru Canyon, where he earned a living farming, raising livestock, and making horsehair bridles and lariats. Fustero passed away in 1921: the marker set along the shores of Lake Piru—placed there in 1961—is in the area Fustero spent most of his life.

■ ■ ■ ■ ■ ■ ■ ■ ■ ■ ■ ■ ■ ■ ■ ■ ■ ■

Beyond, you'll reach the old **Blue Point Campground (4.4 miles, 1,075', 338749E 3822238N)**. The grounds, closed in 1999 to protect the habitat of the arroyo toad, were in decades past a very popular and heavily used campground, featuring 30 sites (most of which were well shaded) with tables and stoves (some on the road you now tread, but the bulk on the spur that crosses the creek just up a ways). All the camp facilities—including the five toilets—remain standing but are now closed to use.

From the old campground, you'll have two crossings of Piru Creek (usually a rock-hop or even a simple walk through a dry cobblestone creek bed, but other times a hip-deep wade) before reaching the privately held Whitaker Ranch. Please respect the owners' property and stay on the road. Leash any four-legged companions.

Just beyond Whitaker Ranch is an old **gate and turnstile (5.5 miles, 1,125', 338273E 3823662N)** set beneath the oaks shading this stretch. Beyond, the road curves to the west and drops you easily down to the **junction (5.7 miles, 1,150', 338090E 3823688)** with your route and the dirt road leading to Kesters Camp and the Agua Blanca Trail (19W10); head right (north) here. You'll quickly cross Agua Blanca Creek just before its confluence with Piru Creek, and then again make two more crossings of Piru Creek before the route disintegrates at the **confluence** of Michael and Piru Creeks **(6.4 miles, 1,170', 337487E 3824249N)**, where you'll find yourself entering the narrow walls of the Juncal formation, a fascinating geologic formation that includes large cobbles suspended in the sandstone matrix of the suddenly steep canyon walls. The Michael-Piru confluence also marks the Sespe Wilderness boundary along this stretch.

Even in the 1970s, the route from here up Piru Creek to Ellis Apiary and beyond was considered to be in poor shape. It has not improved since, and while a handful of volunteers make some efforts to clip a route and even on occasion flag that season's best option, you're

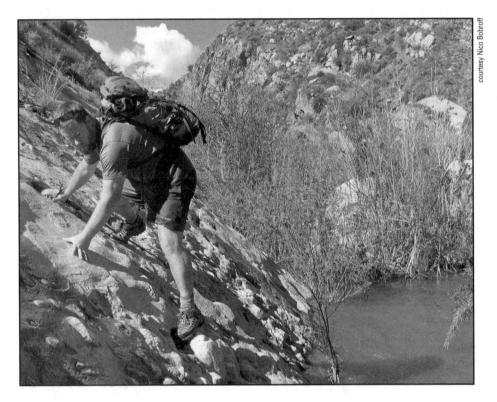

courtesy Nico Bobroff

Smear tactics, Piru Creek

pretty much resigned to slogging up the canyon here—depending on season and recent rain events, this nearly always entails wet feet. After passing through the initial narrows (keep to the right as you can, where you'll be able to pick up sections of the old trail), you'll pass through willow- and cottonwood-dotted flats along the remnants of the old system trail, now little more than a use/game trail. As your route bends to the north, you'll find yourself in a longer section of narrows, which again, depending on water levels, can be rock-hopped or waded across. The wide rock face on the left (west) side can also be used to stay out of the creek, but do mind your footing.

Follow the creek bed upstream for nearly 3 miles from where the road disappeared into the gorge to a flat, whereupon you'll keep to the left (west) side of the creek and follow the old roadbed (after slogging through the narrows, it's somewhat hard to believe a road was maintained through this area). Just beyond the remnants of an old hydraulic gold-mining operation, this much-improved stretch of trail will lead you to a flat of live oaks, under which you'll find **Ellis Apiary Camp (8.2 miles, 1,280', 336835E 3826379N)**.

CAMP :: ELLIS APIARY

ELEVATION:	1,280'
MAP:	USGS *Cobblestone Mountain*
UTM:	336835E 3826379N

The site of an early-1900s beekeeping operation, this site sees little use, and one might be surprised that it's even shown on current LPNF visitor maps—it receives no maintenance, and few amenities remain. Set beneath a cluster of oaks on a nice flat above Piru Creek, what was described as a dusty and overused site decades ago is now more often a quiet spot with a wide space of thick grass and miner's lettuce. Of particular interest to many visitors are the unique stoves here, pedestal-mounted affairs built of heavy-gauge steel with chimneys, stove plates, and a recessed grill. (Middle Matilija also features such a stove.)

From camp, the route up Turtle Canyon hasn't seen maintenance in half a century and isn't recommended.

Route 96

SLIDE MOUNTAIN (18W04)

LENGTH AND TYPE:	10.8-mile out-and-back
RATING:	Moderately strenuous (climb)
TRAIL CONDITION:	Well maintained to clear (heavily used singletrack partially along former service road)
MAP(S):	USGS *Whitaker Peak*, *Liebre Mountain*, and *Black Mountain*; Harrison's *Sespe Wilderness*
CAMP(S):	—
HIGHLIGHTS:	Fire lookout; 360-degree views of Los Padres and Angeles National Forests, Pyramid Lake, and Lake Piru; condor sightings possible

TO REACH THE TRAILHEAD(S): Use the Frenchman's Flat Trailhead to access this route.

TRIP SUMMARY: From the old US 99, this route follows the closed road a short way before heading up an abandoned dirt service road to Slide Mountain, a lookout peak straddling the Sespe Wilderness boundary. Though well within the boundary of the Los Padres National Forest, the area including Slide Mountain is managed by the Santa Clara–Mojave Rivers (formerly Saugus) Ranger District of the Angeles National Forest. Phone (661) 296-9710 for conditions and updates. There is no water along the route and very little shade.

Map 25: Slide Mountain

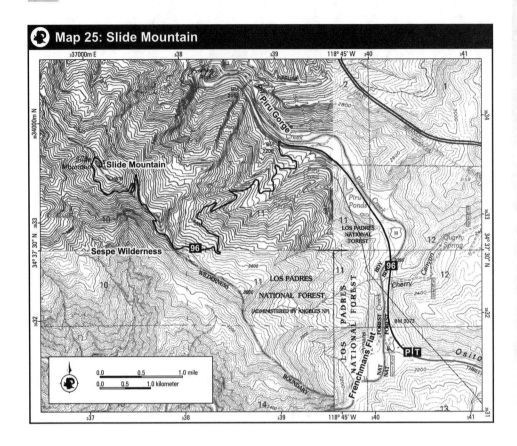

Trip Description

From **Frenchman's Flat** (**2,050', 340159E 3831869N**), follow the retired road 1.5 miles northward toward the dam. On your left (west) will be the gate marking the start of the **Slide Mountain Trail** (**1.7 miles, 2,200', 338953E 3833930N**), which follows the old road. Climb steadily along this road another mile to a small parking area known locally as **Kermit's Corner** (**2.6 miles, 2,910', 338395E 3833485N**). Here, even those vehicles with official access must park and their occupants continue on foot.

Turn left (south) at Kermit's Corner and continue the steady zigzagging climb—gaining views of the interstate and environs immediately to your east—until you reach an old dozer line at a **gap** (**3.8 miles, 3,800', 337825E 3832910N**) commanding fantastic views of the eastern Sespe Wilderness (into which you're now entering, as the ridgeline is roughly the wilderness boundary) and points west. From this vantage you'll gain an appreciation of the steep canyon walls of lower Piru Creek. On clear days, Lake Piru, the Santa Clara River Valley, and points to the southwest all the way out to the Pacific are visible from here.

Now atop a ridgeline, head to your right (north) and follow the singletrack through boulder and cobble formations—eased by the occasional group of switchbacks—to a second **gap (4.2 miles, 4,050', 337587E 3833267N)**, this one allowing your first clear view of Pyramid Lake to the northeast. Another series of switchbacks will then lead you along a less steep ascent of the western flanks of Slide Mountain in something of a 270-degree roundabout to the lookout and **peak (5.4 miles, 4,631', 337046E 3833770N)** atop Slide Mountain. Views of nearby Dome and White Mountains are fine here in all but the most inclement weather. This is also prime territory for condor sightings; the general remoteness of the Piru and Agua Blanca drainages to the immediate west, though not within the Sespe Condor Sanctuary, lend themselves to prime soaring territory for the massive birds.

There is also a portable toilet on the southwest edge of the tower here.

▨ ▨ ▨ ▨ ▨ ▨ ▨ ▨ ▨ SLIDE MOUNTAIN LOOKOUT

Built in 1969, the Slide Mountain lookout was delivered to the peak by helicopter in 1970. The 365-square-foot structure served but for a decade before its closure in 1980. On the whole, the Angeles National Forest's lookouts typically fared better than those in the Los Padres, which after World War II saw many of its lookouts fall into disrepair. In the Angeles, it wasn't until the 1970s and 1980s when budget cuts—compounded by increasingly poor air visibility—forced many of the Los Angeles–area lookouts out of use (a notable handful in the San Bernardino National Forest still remain). In October 2003, Angeles National Forest Fire Lookout Association (**anffla.org**) reopened the two-story metal-and-glass structure with the intent to man it solely with volunteers.

▨ ▨ ▨ ▨ ▨ ▨ ▨ ▨ ▨ ▨ ▨ ▨ ▨ ▨ ▨ ▨ ▨

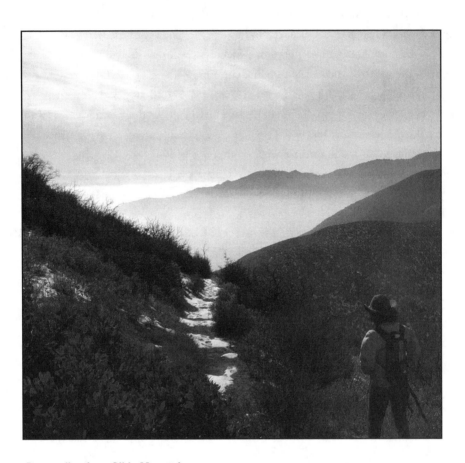

Descending from Slide Mountain

APPENDIX

■ ■ ■ ■ ■ ■ ■ ■ ■ ■ ■ ■ ■

Routes by Theme

Along the Condor Trail

Prime Condor Viewing Opportunities

Geologic Marvels

Geologic Marvels (continued)

14 Forbush-Mono

36 Montgomery Potrero and Rocky Ridge Trail

47 Bear, Deal, and Lower Rancho Nuevo Canyons

51 Upper North Fork Matilija Creek

62 Last Chance Trail, Santa Paula Canyon, and Topatopa Bluff

63 East Fork Santa Paula Canyon

68 Toad Springs

70 Mesa Spring

79 Fishbowls–Cedar Creek Loop

80 Thorn Point

85 Dry Lakes Ridge

86 Sespe River Trail

87 Lion Canyon

88 Red Reef Trail

90 Dough Flat to Shady Camp via Alder Creek

92 Agua Blanca

95 Lower Cobblestone Trail

Great Hikes for Little Explorers

3 Lizard's Mouth

4 The Playground

7 Upper Oso Canyon to Nineteen Oaks

18 La Cumbre Peak

23 Tangerine Falls

55 Wheeler Gorge Nature Trail

66 Rose Valley Falls

74 Raspberry Spring

77 Gene Marshall–Piedra Blanca National Recreation Trail

78 Potrero John

87 Lion Canyon

High Country

(Routes reaching 6000'+)

32 Mission Pine Trail

42 Madulce and Madulce Peak Trails

61 Hines Peak

69 Mount Pinos to Mount Abel (Vincent Tumamait Trail)

70 Mesa Spring

71 North Fork Lockwood Creek

72 McGill Trail

73 Boulder Canyon

74 Raspberry Spring

75 Chorro Grande

76 Reyes Peak Trail

77 Gene Marshall–Piedra Blanca National Recreation Trail

80 Thorn Point

82 Little Mutau

88 Red Reef Trail

93 Buck Creek

Hot Springs

1 Gaviota Peak via Gaviota Hot Springs

13 Agua Caliente Trail to Upper Caliente

86 Sespe River Trail

89 Johnston Ridge and Sespe Hot Springs

Peakbagging

1 Gaviota Peak via Gaviota Hot Springs

2 Broadcast Peak via Tequepis Trail

18 La Cumbre Peak

19 Cathedral Peak

32 Mission Pine Trail (San Rafael Mountain, West Big Pine Mountain)

33 Santa Cruz National Recreation Trail

35 McPherson Peak

Solitude

Swimming Holes and River Fun

Waterfalls

LIST OF MAPS

INDEX

CAMP INDEX

■　■　■　■　■　■　■　■　■　■　■　■　■　■

ABOUT THE AUTHOR

■ ■ ■ ■ ■ ■ ■ ■ ■ ■ ■ ■ ■ ■

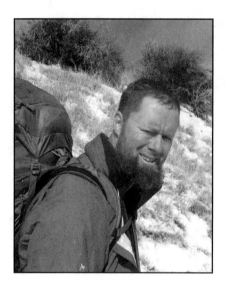

Currently based on California's Central Coast, Craig R. Carey grew up hiking and backpacking in the southern Los Padres. His work has appeared in *Wilderness, Islands, Hooked on the Outdoors, Rugby, The Green,* and *New Zealand Adventure.* Craig holds a BA in history from the University of California at Santa Barbara.